T0327584

Psychiatry of Intellectual Disability

Psychiatry of Intellectual Disability

A practical manual

Edited by

Julie P. Gentile, MD and Paulette M. Gillig, MD, PhD

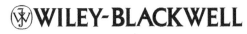

A John Wiley & Sons, Ltd., Publication

Library of Congress Cataloguing-in-Publication Data applied for.

A catalogue record for this book is available from the British Library.

Wiley also publishes its books in a variety of electronic formats. Some content that appears in print may not be available in electronic books.

Set in 10/12pt Times by Thomson Digital, Noida, India

Printed in Malaysia

First Impression 2012

Contents

Dedications   vii

Editor biographies   ix

List of contributors   xi

List of abbreviations   xiii

Foreword   xv

1 **Overview**   1
Allison E. Cowan, MD and Julie P. Gentile, MD

2 **Psychiatric Assessment**   14
Ann K. Morrison, MD and Paulette Marie Gillig, MD, PhD

3 **Medical Assessment**   26
Julie P. Gentile, MD and Michelle A. Monro, DO

4 **Neurologic Conditions**   51
Paulette Marie Gillig, MD, PhD and Richard Sanders, MD

5 **Traumatic Brain Injuries and Co-occurring Mental Illness**   75
Gretchen N. Foley, MD

6 **Interviewing Techniques**   90
Julie P. Gentile, MD and Paulette Marie Gillig, MD, PhD

7 **Mood Disorders**   125
Ann K. Morrison, MD and Christina Weston, MD

  8 **Anxiety Disorders**   146
     Kelly M. Blankenship, MD

  9 **Psychotic Disorders**   161
     Allison E. Cowan, MD

 10 **Personality Disorders**   191
     Julie P. Gentile, MD and Allison E. Cowan, MD

 11 **Aggression**   210
     Julie P. Gentile, MD and Paulette Marie Gillig,
     MD, PhD

 12 **Psychotropic Medications**   250
     Christopher T. Manetta, DO and Julie P. Gentile, MD

 13 **Psychotherapy**   278
     Carroll S. Jackson, LISW-S and Julie P. Gentile, MD

 14 **Behavioral Assessment and Interventions**   309
     Betsey A. Benson, PhD

 15 **Legal Issues for Treatment Providers and Evaluators**   325
     Jeannette Cox, JD

 16 **Syndromes of Intellectual Disability**   338
     Kelly M. Blankenship, MD and Christina Weston, MD

Index   366

Dedications

Dr. Gentile would like to dedicate this book to her husband John for his extraordinary love and support; to her daughters Sarah and Jess and her son-in-law Sayre for being sources of inspiration and pride every day; and to her parents Charlie (RIP) and Patricia, who always believed the sky was the limit. She would like to thank her patients with intellectual disability, and the people who stand with them, for being true survivors.

Dr. Gillig would like to dedicate this book to the memory of Uncle Al Petre, Peter Reilly and Patty Whibbs, childhood friends with intellectual disabilities. We had some good times.

Editor Biographies

Julie P. Gentile, M.D. (jen-TILL-ee) is Associate Professor of Psychiatry at the Boonshoft School of Medicine, Wright State University, Dayton, Ohio and the Project Director/ Primary Investigator for Ohio's Coordinating Center of Excellence in Mental Illness/ Intellectual Disability. She has been the Professor of Dual Diagnosis for the Ohio Department of Mental Health, the Ohio Department of Developmental Disability and the Ohio Developmental Disabilities Council since 2003, and the Medical Director for both the Montgomery County Board of Developmental Disabilities Mental Health Program and Consumer Advocacy Model (treating patients with traumatic brain injury, substance use, and mental illness). Dr. Gentile has evaluated more than 2,000 individuals with co-occurring mental illness and intellectual disability. She is the recipient of the American Psychiatric Association's Frank J. Menolascino Award for Excellence in Psychiatric Services for Developmental Disabilities, the Excellence in Contributions to Clinical Practice Award from the National Association for the Dually Diagnosed, and she is a member of Alpha Omega Alpha Medical Honor Society. She is a recipient of the Faculty Mentor Award, the Golden Apple Teaching Award, the Career Achievement Award, the Outstanding Achievement in Medical Education and Research Award of the Academy of Medicine, and the Nancy Roeske Award in Medical Education from the American Psychiatric Association. Dr. Gentile has been awarded more than $3,000,000 in grants and contracts to support her work in dual diagnosis since 2003. She is the Director of Medical Student Mental Health Services at Wright State University, is a member of the editorial board for the journal *Innovations in Clinical Neuroscience* and has published articles and book chapters on various topics in the area of co-occurring mental illness/intellectual disability.

Paulette Marie Gillig, M.D., Ph.D. is Professor of Psychiatry at the Boonshoft School of Medicine, Wright State University, Dayton, Ohio and on the Faculty of the Graduate School. She has been Ohio Department of Mental Health Professor of Rural and Underserved Populations since 1998, is listed in *Best Doctors in America*, *Who's Who in America*, *Who's Who in the World*, is Distinguished Fellow of the American Psychiatric Association and is a member of Alpha Omega Alpha Medical Honor Society. She also is a member of the Society of Neuroscience and the Russell DeJong Society. She is a recipient of the Faculty Mentor Award and the Golden Apple Teaching Award, the Outstanding Achievement in Medical Education and Research Award of the Academy of Medicine, and the Nancy Roeske Award in Medical Education from the American Psychiatric Association. Dr. Gillig has published three books and over 60 articles and book chapters in the several areas of Community

(Public) Psychiatry, Psychotherapy, and the Interface between Psychiatry and Neurology. She is the Section Editor for the journal *Innovations in Clinical Neuroscience*. She has completed residencies in both neurology and in psychiatry and she also holds a doctorate in Social Psychology in the area of cognitive processes. She is the past Area 4 representative to the American Association of Community Psychiatrists and Chair of the Training Committee. She was the Chair of the Committee on Minorities and Under-represented Groups for the Ohio Psychiatric Association, and a member of the Committee on Poverty and Homelessness of the American Psychiatric Association.

List of Contributors

Betsey A. Benson, PhD
Associate Professor, The Ohio State University, Columbus, Ohio, USA

Kelly M. Blankenship, MD
Assistant Professor, Indiana University, Indianapolis, Indiana, USA

Allison E. Cowan, MD
Assistant Professor, Wright State University, Dayton, Ohio, USA

Jeannette Cox, JD
Associate Professor, University of Dayton School of Law, Dayton, Ohio, USA

Gretchen N. Foley, MD
Assistant Professor, Wright State University, Dayton, Ohio, USA

Julie P. Gentile, MD
Associate Professor, Wright State University, Dayton, Ohio, USA

Paulette Marie Gillig, MD, PhD
Professor, Wright State University, Dayton, Ohio, USA

Carroll S. Jackson, LISW-S
Montgomery County Board of Developmental Disabilities, Dayton, Ohio, USA

Christopher T. Manetta, DO
Kirtland Air Force Base Medical Facility, Kirtland AFB, New Mexico, USA

Michelle A. Monro, DO
Edwards Air Force Base Medical Facility, Edwards AFB, California, USA

Ann K. Morrison, MD
Associate Professor, Wright State University, Dayton, Ohio, USA

Richard Sanders, MD
Associate Professor, Wright State University, Dayton, Ohio, USA

Christina G. Weston, MD
Associate Professor, Wright State University, Dayton, Ohio, USA

List of Abbreviations

AOC	altered consciousness
APD	antisocial personality disorder
ARND	alcohol related neurodevelopmental disorder
BD	bipolar disorder
BPD	borderline personality disorder
BPS	biopsychosocial
CBT	cognitive behavioral therapy
CDC	Center for Disease Control
CT	computerized tomography
DBT	dialectical behavior therapy
DC LD	Diagnostic Criteria – Learning Disorders
DM-ID	Diagnostic Manual – Intellectual Disability
DS	Down syndrome
DSM-IV-TR	Diagnostic and Statistical Manual, Fourth Edition Text Revision
DZ	dizygotic
ED	emergency department
EEG	electroencephalogram
EKG	electrocardiogram
EPS	extrapyramidal side effects
FAE	fetal alcohol effects
FAS	fetal alcohol syndrome
FASD	fetal alcohol syndrome disorders
FGA	first generation antipsychotic
FMR1	Fragile X Mental Retardation 1 gene
FXS	Fragile X syndrome
FXTAS	Fragile X tremor ataxia syndrome
GABA	gamma Aminobutyric acid
GAD	generalized anxiety disorder
GCS	Glasgow Coma Scale
GMC	general medication condition
HPD	histrionic personality disorder
ID	intellectual disability

IQ	intelligence quotient
LD	learning disorder
LOC	loss of consciousness
MDD	major depressive disorder
MI	motivational interviewing
MRI	magnetic resonance imaging
MZ	monozygotic
NADD	National Association for the Dually Diagnosed
NOS	not otherwise specified
OCD	obsessive compulsive disorder
ODD	oppositional defiant disorder
PD	personality disorder
PDD	pervasive developmental disorder
pFAS	partial fetal alcohol syndrome
PTA	post-traumatic amnesia
PTSD	post-traumatic stress disorder
PWS	Prader-Willi syndrome
SAP	Structured Assessment of Personality
SGA	second generation antipsychotic
SIB	self-injurious behavior
SP	supportive therapy
SSI	supplemental security income
SSDI	social security disability income
SSRI	selective serotonin reuptake inhibitor
TBI	traumatic brain injury
WS	Williams syndrome

Foreword

The field of Intellectual Disabilities (ID) is expanding along many fronts. Over the last 20 years, community-based placement has come to replace large residential facilities in many states. This transformation accompanied changes in treatment models, especially the legal and ideological shifts away from custodial to more active treatment programs. During this era, increased demands for community programs required a major restructuring of services to deal with many of our most complicated and difficult to treat patients. Adequate staffing and integration of complex services needs proved to be one of our greatest challenges- especially the gaps between availability and access to quality care and sociocultural-bound beliefs and values that might hinder utilization by the target population.

In part, availability and access to adequate care is often limited by maldistribution of qualified professionals, fragmentation of health care systems and persistent problems merging mental health and intellectual disability services. These are especially thorny issues since many of these individuals have either major problems with co-existing medical/neurological disorders, severe challenging behaviors or mental disorders. When specialized services are not available, any combination of these variables may overwhelm community programs and in many situations circumstances may jeopardize community placement. These challenging individuals seriously tax community resources and as a result finish up with multiple psychotropic medications or with an excessive reliance on acute hospitalization. In many cases these individuals end up in a pattern of revolving door admissions to mental health facilities. As a result, we are in the midst of a second psycho-pharmacological revolution; this one is generated by the increased overuse of polypharmacy that is due in part to limited clinical and behavioral management resources.

Over 25 years ago, the idea that individuals with ID might also be at risk for psychiatric disorders was clouded by many layers of diagnostic overshadowing. In addition, it became apparent that many individuals with ID did not fit either the standard psychiatric models of etiology or descriptive phenomenology, and therefore required modifications in the standard psychiatric evaluation and assessment. In the mid 1980s, the National Association for the Dually Diagnosed in the US attempted to remedy this confusing situation by providing direct training and educational programs designed for clinicians and direct care personnel in the field. In 2007, this Association published the Diagnostic Manual-Intellectual Disabilities. This two-volume edition modified and adapted the already existing DSM-IV-TR diagnostic criteria (American Psychiatric Association, 2000). These modifications, along with the ICD-based Diagnostic Criteria-Learning Disability already available, promoted a modified descriptive and categorical classification system for the field of dual diagnosis.

The DM-ID provided a starting place for improvements in clinical treatment using evidence and best practice-based diagnostic criteria.

This book edited by Drs. Gentile and Gillig is grounded in our growing understanding of the complex neurodevelopmental and biopsychosocial substrates for challenging behaviors and mental disorders. The authors provide abundant evidence for the value of criteria-based diagnosis and treatment planning founded on scientific evidence and our growing integration of genetics, behavioral neurosciences and neuropharmacology with psychosocial/behavioral therapies. Our biggest challenge is to keep our assessment and treatment approaches in step with the rapidly changing scientific evidence. One example of this problem is the difficulty we all face dealing with the rapid pace of change in our understanding of neurobiology of major psychiatric disorders. We now confront molecular genetics, intracellular mechanisms that are replacing our previous reliance on neurotransmitter models, behavioral neuropharmacology and genomics of drug metabolism and mechanisms of action, developmental changes that point to gene-environmental and epigenetic interactions rather than our older over-simplified models of nature versus nurture, neuro-endocrinological and neuro-immunological factors that influence brain function and psychopathology. If this isn't enough, we confront a second conundrum-dealing with the clinical heterogeneity and complex developmental neurobiology of ID.

The authors of this edition focus on integrating biopsychosocial models. In keeping with the medieval position taken by Bernard of Chartres and later borrowed by Isaac Newton: we make progress "by standing on the shoulders of giants" who came before us. This book is a testament to their vision and efforts. Their challenge to us is take the new knowledge gleaned from our marvelous technical and scientific research and integrate neurosciences into a person-centered, positive support program that provides humane care. This book reminds us how we might accomplish this.

Jarrett Barnhill MD DFAPA, FAACAP
University of North Carolina School of Medicine

1

Overview

Allison E. Cowan, MD, Assistant Professor, Wright State University, Dayton, Ohio
Julie P. Gentile, MD, Associate Professor, Wright State University, Dayton, Ohio

The history of intellectual disability and mental illness

The history of individuals with mental illness and intellectual disability (ID) is profoundly intertwined. Due to a lack of effective treatments, both groups have long occupied a status of *"otherness"* and have been relegated to the fringes of society. Individuals with ID and those with mental illness had to rely on support from the community if their families were unable or unwilling to care for them. Throughout history, such individuals have been diagnosed together as "mental defectives," have been treated or housed in asylums and have been singled out as somehow "less than human" or less deserving of the same rights and treatment as other individuals.

In more recent times, progress has been made in returning rights, choices and lives of their own making to individuals with ID and mental illness. There remains, however, a paucity of historical writings about people with a combination of both ID and mental illness. An overview of their separate histories and the subsequent development of the concept of dual diagnosis will serve as an appropriate starting point for *Psychiatry of Intellectual Disability*.

In prehistory, individuals with mental illness and ID were reliant on family and social structure. The earliest treatment of mental illness was likely through shamanism, spirituality and superstition, using herbs, rituals and amulets. From observations documented in the fossil record, other techniques were found, including psychosurgery.

Psychiatry of Intellectual Disability: A Practical Manual, First Edition.
Edited by Julie P. Gentile and Paulette M. Gillig.

For example, Neolithic humans used trepanation – the drilling of circular holes in the skull – to release evil spirits that were thought to cause mental illness. The practice of trepanation has been observed across varying cultures and geographical regions. For example, the Incans of Peru (Arnott *et al.*, 2002) and the Native Americans of North America (Stone *et al.*, 1990) performed trepanation, with most cases living long enough for the bones of the skull to heal. The great classical physicians Hippocrates and Galen used trepanation to treat phlegmatous lesions of the brain (Missios, 2007). There exists a painting by the Dutch Renaissance painter Hieronymus Bosch called *"Extracting the Stone of Madness"* that indicates that psychosurgery also was performed to alleviate mental illness.

The etiology of mental illness remains a mystery even now. The Judeo-Christian tradition teaches that disobedience to God will result in being cursed with madness, saying, "God will smite thee with madness" (The Holy Bible, King James Version, 1611). In the Hindu faith, a person suffering from schizophrenia would be treated by removing toxins presumed to be causing the illness in order to restore harmonious balance and mental health (Progler, 2008). Hippocrates also believed that mental illness resulted from an imbalance in the bodily humors, rather than a divine cause. He recommended that the body be allowed to restore itself, as opposed to using more invasive procedures and medicines.

Individuals with more severe intellectual or other disabilities historically did not survive into adulthood. In ancient times, infants who were considered "deformed" were often killed through what was called "exposure" (Bennett, 1923), in which the infant was abandoned outside, presumably to perish. Aristotle (Kraut, 1998) recommended, "Let there be a law against nourishing those [infants] that are deformed." Sparta, a culture infamous for rates of infanticide, had a process wherein the infant was brought for official inspection for "defects" and was abandoned if found to be "defective." Soranus of Ephesus, a 2nd Century C.E. physician, listed criteria that made an infant "worth rearing," which included having a healthy mother, being full-term, crying with vigor, being perfect in all its parts and having the right size and shape (Patterson, 1985). Soranus did, however, advocate for the humane treatment of persons with mental illness, recommending rest, sympathy and reading (Scheerenberger, 1983). He wrote:

> *"They [physicians] compare their patients to ferocious beasts whom they would subdue by the deprivation of food and by the torments of thirst. Misled without doubly by this error, they advise that patients be cruelly chained, forgetting that their limbs might be injured or broken and that it is more suitable and much easier to restrain the sick by the hands of men than by the weights of often harmful iron. They even advise bodily violence, like the use of the whip, as if such measures could force a return to reason."*

Slowly, the classical civilizations began outlawing infant exposure. The newly emerging major world religions promoted gentle treatment of people with intellectual and other disabilities. The Koran, the New Testament of the Bible, Confucius and Buddha argued for mercy and kindness for those with ID.

During the Middle Ages and through the Renaissance period, people with ID and mental illness continued to be treated as *other*. Some people with ID were employed as "fools," similar to court jesters, to provide a royal court or household with entertainment. The rights of individuals with ID and mental illness were restricted during these times by law. In England in the 1700s, Brydall recapitulated the earlier scholars Fitzherbert (who described "idiocy" as "not being able to count to twenty") and Swinbourne (who added that the definition should include not being able to do other activities like telling the days of the week or measuring fabric). A lunatick or "mad-man" was described by Brydall as "having sometime his Reason, and sometimes not" (Brydall, 1700).

When someone was pronounced an idiot, the individual's property would revert to the king; however, if someone was declared a "lunatick" – or mentally ill – their heirs would retain the rights to the family property. There is considerably more written about the distinction between mental illness and ID compared with their overlap. John Locke wrote that individuals with ID "[seem] to proceed from want of quickness, activity, and motion in the intellectual Faculties, whereby they are deprived of Reason: whereas *mad Men*, on the other side, seem to suffer by the other Extream. Or they do not appear to me to have lost the Faculty of Reasoning: but having joined together some *Ideas* very wrongly, they mistake them for Truths" (Locke, 1690).

While the rights of the individual were limited in the Middle Ages, there was also protection from prosecution; the insanity defense had been a viable defense in Roman and Greek times and made a return in the late 1500s. Richard Cosin wrote of the insane that "In which respects they are compared in lawe, to men absent, and utterly ignorant of any thing done by themselves, or in their presence" (Cosin, 1592).

The Middle Ages and the post-Reformation era were also times of great superstition. The *Malleus Maleficarum*, or "Hammer of Witches" (Kramer *et al.*, 1487, translated in Summers, 1948) was published to outline the correct prosecution of people (usually women) accused of witchcraft. There is no specific mention of individuals with ID, although descriptions of "witches" who drove men to insanity may have been about individuals suffering from mental illness. In writing about the Salem Witch Trials of 1692, Kai Erikson noted that some accused witches "were witless persons with scarcely a clue as to what happened to them" (Erikson, 1966). St. Vincent de Paul crusaded against the prosecution of people with mental illness and ID as witches.

The reformers

Treatment and attitudes toward people with ID and mental illness varied throughout history. Well-off families could afford to provide the additional support needed, but poorer families could not. When family or friends could not care for an individual with ID, mental illness or both, some communities as a group either actively or passively supported the individual.

In rural communities, a person with ID might be the "town idiot" and given food and shelter. However, circumstances were not always so benign. Scheerenberger quotes William Tuke, a Quaker philanthropist, who described: "Hardly a parish of any considerable extent in which there might not be found some unfortunate human creature, who, if his ill-treatment had made him 'frenetic,' was chained in the cellar or garret of a workhouse, fastened to the leg of a table, tied to a post in an outhouse, or perhaps shut up in an uninhabited ruin; or, if his lunacy were inoffensive, was left to ramble, half-naked and half-starved, throughout the streets and highways" (Scheerenberger, 1983).

In more urban communities, a person with ID would rely on begging or would be placed in an institution like an asylum. Asylums began as a way to house individuals with mental illness and ID. Treatment of people with mental illness and ID included cold baths, beatings and immobility, to calm what was thought to be demons or disturbed tempers. In some sections of the asylum, residents were not given clothes and were chained to walls without heat. During the time of the asylums, people with ID were still viewed as a form of entertainment, with the more famous asylums charging entrance fees to visitors.

Reformers like Tuke, who advocated for "moral treatment," sought to improve the living conditions for people with ID. Philippe Pinel, a French physician who also encouraged the humane treatment of people with ID and mental illness, wrote: "The managers of those institutions [the asylums], who are frequently men of little knowledge and less humanity, have been permitted to exercise towards their innocent prisoners a most arbitrary system of cruelty and violence; while experience affords ample and daily proofs of the happier effect of a mild, conciliating treatment, rendered effective by steady and dispassionate firmness."

Pinel is famous for removing the irons from the residents at Bicêtre upon taking charge at the facility. He and the superintendent of the hospital, Jean-Baptiste Pussin, worked closely in providing compassionate treatment to residents of the asylum (Gerard, 1997). Consistent with today's ethos concerning patient care, Pinel advocated "to allow every maniac all the latitude of personal liberty consistent with safety; to proportion the degree of coercion to the demands upon it from his extravagance of behavior, to use mildness of manners or firmness as occasion may require" (Pinel, 1806). A well-known American reformer and scholar in the field of mental health care, Dorothea Dix, addressed the Massachusetts legislature regarding recommendations to reform the state institutions; and Eduoard Séguin of France advocated that individuals with ID be educated for their own "improvement" (Scheerenberger, 1983).

Starting in the middle 20th century, attempts were made to deinstitutionalize individuals with ID or mental illness and integrate them back into the community. The discovery of the first effective antipsychotic, chlorpromazine (Thorazine), allowed for symptoms to be treated outside of the institutional setting, with varying results.

Current treatment recommendations

It is important to maintain the human rights and dignity of the individual with ID. This includes informed consent to treatment, accurate diagnosis, and formulation of a biopsychosocial treatment plan. Allow individual choice in small and large decisions. The rise of self-advocacy groups like Autism Speaks and People First have been influential in allowing individuals a voice where the forum did not previously exist.

Prevalence and classification

Approximately two percent of the population have co-occurring mental illness and ID and these individuals will be encountered in virtually every practice setting (Hardan & Sahl, 1997, Larson *et al.*, 2001, Silka & Hauser, 1997). There is a three to six times increased rate of psychiatric and behavior problems in individuals with ID compared to the general population. There are many etiologies currently known for ID, obviously a highly heterogeneous condition. Most causes of ID fall into the categories of chromosomal abnormalities, other genetic factors, prenatal and perinatal factors, acquired childhood disorders, environmental factors and socio-cultural factors.

ID is usually classified as profound, severe, moderate or mild, which can often be an indicator of the level of dependency or expressive language capabilities of the individual. The designation is frequently correlated with the level of risk for certain medical and neurological conditions.

- Generally, individuals with *mild* cognitive deficits live independently in the community in supported residential situations and participate in life-long supported employment. Special vocational and community socialization training is often required for success and to attain the highest quality of life.
- Persons in the *moderate* category will most often need varying levels of support from their families or community agencies. Because their expressive language skills are typically more limited, they are at higher risk of being unable to communicate subjective complaints about mental health and medical illnesses.
- Individuals with *severe* and *profound* ID are more likely to have very high levels of dependence on outside supports and to have associated medical conditions, with many requiring intensive support to be able to master activities of daily living. Significant medical complications, such as seizure disorders, swallowing difficulties, speech impairments, ambulation limitations, sensory deficits and reduced life expectancies are more common for persons in the profound impairment category. Multiple physical disabilities increase risk for medical complications irrespective of the level of ID, so the use of the biopsychosocial formulation is therefore vital in the mental health assessment.

Current and proposed diagnostic criteria for ID

It has been argued that the existing diagnostic manuals for mental disorders (i.e. The American Psychiatric Association Diagnostic and Statistical Manual for Mental Disorders, 4th Edition Text Revision 2000, and International Classification of Diseases 10th Revision, Criteria for Mental Retardation, 1996) are not a good fit for use in individuals with ID (see Tables 1 and 2). Publications such as the Diagnostic Manual – Intellectual Disabilities (DM-ID 2007) and Diagnostic Criteria – Learning Disabilities (DC-LD 2001)

Table 1 Diagnostic criteria for mental retardation.

Sub-average IQ	Decrease adaptive function in at least two areas	Onset before age 18
Mild MR	50/55 – ~70	85%
Moderate MR	35/40 – 50/55	10%
Severe MR	20/25 – 35/40	3–4%
Profound MR	<20/25	1–2%

Source: Reproduced with permission from the Diagnostic and Statistical Manual of Mental Disorders, Fourth Edition, Text Revision (DSM-IV TR), American Psychiatric Association, 2000, p. 41.

Table 2 International classification for diseases and other health-related conditions. Criteria for mental retardation.

F70 Mild mental retardation	**Clinical description**
	Mildly retarded people acquire language with some delay but most achieve the ability to use speech for everyday purposes, to hold conversations and to engage in the clinical interview. Most of them also achieve full independence in self-care (eating, washing, dressing, bowel and bladder control) and in practical and domestic skills, even if the rate of development is considerably slower than normal. The main difficulties are usually seen in academic school work, and many have particular problems in reading and writing. However, mildly retarded people can be greatly helped by education designed to develop their skills and compensate for their handicaps. Most of those in the higher ranges of mental retardation are potentially capable of work demanding practical rather than academic abilities, including unskilled or semiskilled manual labor. In a socio-cultural context requiring little academic achievement, some degree of mild retardation may not itself represent a problem. However, if there is also a noticeable emotional and social immaturity, the consequences of the handicap, e.g. inability to cope with the demands of marriage or child-rearing, or difficulty fitting in with cultural traditions and expectations, will be apparent. In general, the behavioral, emotional and social difficulties of the mildly mentally retarded, and the needs for treatment, are more closely akin to those found in people of normal intelligence than to the specific problems of the moderately and severely retarded. An organic etiology is being identified in increasing proportions of patients, although not yet in the majority.
	Diagnostic guidelines
	If the proper standardized IQ tests are used, the range 50 to 69 is indicative of mild mental retardation. Understanding and use of language tend to be delayed to a varying degree, and executive speech problems that interfere with the development of independence may persist into adult life. An organic etiology is identifiable in only a minority of subjects. Associated conditions such as autism, other developmental disorders, epilepsy, conduct disorders or physical disability are found in varying proportion. If such disorders are present, they should be coded independently.
	Includes: feeble-mindedness, mild mental subnormality.
F71 Moderate mental retardation	**Clinical description**
	Individuals in this category are slow in developing comprehension and use of language, and their eventual achievement in this area is limited. Achievement of self-care and motor skills is also retarded, and some need supervision throughout life. Progress in school work is limited, but a proportion of these individuals learn the basic skills needed for reading, writing and counting. Educational programs can provide opportunities for them to develop their limited potential and to acquire

some basic skills; such programs are appropriate for slow learners with a low ceiling of achievement. As adults, moderately retarded people are usually able to do simple practical work if the tasks are carefully structured and skilled supervision is provided. Completely independent living in adult life is rarely achieved. Generally, however, such people are fully mobile and physically active and the majority show evidence of social development in their ability to establish contact, to communicate with others, and, to engage in simple social activities.

Diagnostic guidelines

The IQ is usually in the range 35 to 49. Discrepant profiles of abilities are common in this group, with some individuals achieving higher levels in visuo-spatial skills than in tasks dependant on language, while others are markedly clumsy but enjoy social interaction and simple conversation. The level of development of language is variable; some of those affected can take part in simple conversations, while others have only enough language to communicate their basic needs. Some never learn language, though they may understand simple instructions and may learn to use manual signs to compensate to some extent for their speech disabilities. An organic etiology can be identified in the majority of moderately mentally retarded people. Childhood autism or other pervasive developmental disorders are present in a substantial minority and have a major effect upon the clinical picture and the type of management needed. Epilepsy and neurological and physical disabilities are also common, although most moderately retarded people are able to walk without assistance. It is sometimes possible to identify other psychiatric conditions, but the limited level of language development may make diagnosis difficult and dependent upon information obtained from others who are familiar with the individual. Any such associated disorders should be coded independently.

Includes: imbecility, moderate mental subnormality, moderate oligophrenia.

F72 Severe mental retardation

Clinical description

This category is broadly similar to that of moderate mental retardation in terms of the clinical picture, the presence of an organic etiology and the associated conditions. The lower levels of achievement mentioned under F71 are also the most common in this group. Most people in this category suffer from a marked degree of motor impairment or other associated deficits, indicating the presence of clinically significant damage to or maldevelopment of the central nervous system.

Diagnostic guidelines

The IQ is usually in the range 20 to 34.

Includes: severe mental subnormality, severe oligophrenia

F73 Profound mental retardation

Clinical description

The IQ in this category is estimated to be under 20, which means in practice that affected individuals are severely limited in their ability to understand or comply with requests or instructions. Most such

(*continued*)

individuals are immobile or severely restricted in mobility, incontinent and capable at most of only very rudimentary forms of nonverbal communication. They possess little or no ability to care for their own basic needs and they require constant help and supervision.

Diagnostic guidelines

The IQ is under 20. Comprehension and use of language is limited, at best, to understanding basic commands and making simple requests. The most basic and simple visuo-spatial skills of sorting and matching may be acquired and the affected person may be able, with appropriate supervision and guidance, to take a small part in domestic and practical tasks. An organic etiology can be identified in most cases. Severe neurological or other physical disabilities affecting mobility are common, as are epilepsy and visual and hearing impairments. Pervasive developmental disorders in their most severe form, especially atypical autism, are particularly frequent, especially in those who are mobile. **Includes**: idiocy, profound mental subnormality, profound oligophrenia.

Source: Reproduced with permission from the International Classification of Diseases Tenth Revision, Guide for Mental Retardation, World Health Organization, 1996. http://www.who.int/mental_health/media/en/69.pdf. Access date 06/27/11, pp. 9–13.

---

are adaptations of diagnostic manuals utilized for the general population, and they address the unique needs and presentations of individuals with ID (DM-ID 2007, DC-LD 2001 (see Tables 3 and 4). These classification systems are grounded in evidence-based methods and supported by the expert consensus principles. The manuals include review of scientific literature and research, etiology and descriptions of various mental disorders and, when appropriate and supported by literature, proposed alterations of criterion for use in individuals with ID.

The proposed criteria for the *Diagnostic and Statistical Manual*, 5th Edition, to be published in 2012 can be found in Table 5.

Current trends in nomenclature

For many years, the term 'mental retardation' has been used not only in diagnostic manuals, in writing and in reference to persons with ID, but has been used as a slang term and to ridicule persons with cognitive limitations. There has now been a shift to the use of either "intellectual" and/or "developmental" disabilities, with legislation in many regions to formally eliminate the term "mental retardation."

In September 2010, the United States Congress passed legislation eliminating the term "mental retardation" from all federal laws and utilizing the terminology "an individual with intellectual disability" in all health, education and labor law. This legislation made the language in federal law consistent with language used by the Center for Disease Control and Prevention, the United Nations and the United States federal government. It also determined that all references to individuals with ID would be referred to in the People First Language format, described below (United States 111th Congress Bill S2781, 2010).

Table 3 American Association on Intellectual and Developmental Disabilities.

AAIDD definition: "a disability characterized by significant limitations both in intellectual functioning and in adaptive behavior as expressed in conceptual, social, and practical adaptive skills. The disability originates before age 18" (American Association of Mental Retardation, 2005). To this they add "five assumptions essential to the application of the definition":

1. Limitations in present functioning must be considered within the context of community environments typical of the individual's age peers and culture.
2. Valid assessment considers cultural and linguistic diversity as well as differences in communication, sensory, motor, and behavioral factors.
3. Within an individual, limitations often coexist with strengths.
4. An important purpose of describing limitations is to develop a profile of needed supports.
5. With appropriate personalized supports over a sustained period, the life functioning of the person with mental retardation generally will improve.

(American Association on Mental Retardation, 2005)

Degrees of severity
Mild: 50–55 to 70
Moderate: 35–40 to 50–55
Severe: 20–25 to 34–40
Profound: below 20–25

AAIDD categories
Intermittent support
Limited support
Extensive support
Pervasive support

Source: Reproduced with permission from Fletcher, R., Loschen, E., Stavrakaki, C., & First, M. (eds., 2007). *Diagnostic Manual – Intellectual Disability (DM-ID): A Textbook of Diagnosis of Mental Disorders in Persons with Intellectual Disability*. NADD Press, Kingston, NY, pp. 64–66.

Table 4 Diagnostic criteria for learning disabilities for use with adults (DC-LD).

• Diagnostic criteria: used synonymously with the ICD-10 term Mental Retardation. The diagnosis of Mental Retardation is dependent upon the person having an intelligence quotient below 70, together with continued impairment in adaptive behavior/social functioning, and with onset during the developmental phase (i.e. before the age 18 years). The term *borderline learning disabilities* is not included in the ICD-10, nor is it included in DC-LD. Within most European and North American cultures, ICD-10 recommends the use of the Vineland Adaptive Behavior Scales as an assessment tool.
• Severity of learning disabilities:
   o Mild learning disabilities: IQ range = 50–69; mental age 9 to under 12 years
   o Moderate learning disabilities: IQ range = 35–49; mental age 6 to under 9 years
   o Severe learning disabilities: IQ range = 20–34; mental age 3 to under 6 years
   o Profound learning disabilities: IQ range = 20; mental age <3 years
   o Other learning disabilities
   o Unspecified learning disabilities.
• An example of a clinical summary sheet (this relates DC-LD descriptive classification to etiology, using the four dimensions of biological, psychological, social and development, and provides an example of other summary information relevant to clinical practice).
• Diagrammatic presentation of the hierarchical approach to diagnosis which is adopted throughout DC-LD.
• The text of DC-LD provides additional information on psychiatric assessment of adults with learning [intellectual] disabilities.

Source: Adapted from Royal College of Psychiatrists. DC-LD (Diagnostic Criteria for Psychiatric Disorders for Use with Adults with Learning Disabilities/Mental Retardation). London: Gaskell, 2001, p. 18.

Table 5   Proposed criteria for *Diagnostic and Statistical Manual* 5th Edition (Subject to change; to be published in 2013).

Intellectual Developmental Disorder is a disorder that includes both a current intellectual deficit and a deficit in adaptive functioning with onset during the developmental period. All three of the following criteria must be met.

A.   Intellectual Developmental Disorder is characterized by deficits in general mental abilities such as reasoning, problem-solving, planning, abstract thinking, judgment, academic learning and learning from experience. Intellectual Developmental Disorder requires a current intellectual deficit of approximately 2 or more standard deviations in Intelligence Quotient (IQ) below the population mean for a person's age and cultural group, which is typically an IQ score of approximately 70 or below, measured on an individualized, standardized, culturally appropriate, psychometrically sound test.

AND

B.   The deficits in general mental abilities impair functioning in comparison to a person's age and cultural group by limiting and restricting participation and performance in one or more aspects of daily life activities, such as communication, social participation, functioning at school or at work, or personal independence at home or in community settings. The limitations result in the need for ongoing support at school, work, or independent life. Thus, Intellectual Developmental Disorder also requires a significant impairment in adaptive functioning. Typically, adaptive behavior is measured using individualized, standardized, culturally appropriate, psychometrically sound tests.

AND

C. Onset during the developmental period.

Code no longer based on IQ level.

"People first" language

As Mark Twain once said, "The difference between the right word and the almost right word is the difference between lightning and the lightning bug." The Sapir-Whorf hypothesis of language (Chandler, 1994) proposes that language use significantly shapes perceptions of the world and forms ideological preconceptions.

"People First" language is a linguistic style that is becoming more widely recognized and considers the persons or individuals *first* and their associated disability or condition as a *secondary* attribute as opposed to being defined by their disability (Snow, 2009). It entails using the term "individual" or "person" first, followed by the condition or mental health issue. The purpose is to avoid perceived or subconscious dehumanization and is considered "disability etiquette."

For example, instead of "schizophrenic patient" or "intellectually disabled person," it is preferred by groups advocating "people first" to state "patient with schizophrenia" or "person with intellectual disability." In this sense, the person's identity is separated from their disorder or condition or disability. Along the same lines, instead of "a deaf person," People First Language recommends "person with a hearing impairment." Although critics of People First language may claim that is it awkward and repetitive. whether in written form or in oral presentation, it is significant that the aforementioned style is preferred by many individuals with disabilities and their advocates.

The interface between intellectual disability and mental illness

Patients with dual diagnosis often present to psychiatrists with behavioral problems. Because these patients often have communication difficulties, they may have medical conditions which are undiagnosed and that affect their behavior. Characteristics of ID may confound the usual procedures for psychiatric assessment and treatment. For example, it may be helpful to incorporate some child mental status examination techniques when assessing adult patients with ID. The psychiatric interview of patients with ID can be complicated by communication deficits or lack of verbal communication skills but, by utilizing certain question types and avoiding others and allowing sufficient time, one can yield a wealth of information as well as effectively develop rapport between mental health clinician and patient.

Most mental health (MH) care delivery systems have a different philosophy than most ID systems. For example, ID systems may meet the individual "where he is" without expecting significant change in functioning, and focus on habilitation. By contrast, MH systems typically focus on "cure" and are recovery-oriented, in that the expectation for mental illness is the achievement of clear short-term goals.

The ID professional relies on assessment of functioning, while the MH professional relies on diagnosis. When ID professionals refer individuals with ID to MH systems for assessment and care, they should request treatment for anxiety or mood instability or another appropriate MH diagnosis or symptom set, as opposed to services for "mild ID" or "Down syndrome," for example. ID assessments view the entire person (living environment, employment, medical), while MH assessments utilize the medical model and pursue diagnosis of disorders and underlying causes.

In many MH settings, evidence-based practices are preferred. ID settings sometimes use consensus and tradition, but most have been moving toward evidence-based practices in recent years. In the end, both systems must work in collaboration in order to treat individuals with ID and mental illness effectively. The ID system offers involvement over the lifespan, holistic consideration of the person in the environment, housing and employment services and detailed account of skills and behavior; the MH system offers crisis support, treatment of emotional distress, behavior as a form of communication and knowledge of mental illnesses which may affect all areas of functioning.

This book covers a curriculum of topics for the multidisciplinary treatment of individuals with co-occurring ID and mental illness. Patients with ID may present with emotional, behavioral, interpersonal or adjustment problems and may benefit from psychiatric input even when there is lack of a diagnosable psychiatric disorder, while the individual also works closely with a multidisciplinary team that receives input from caregivers, family, and interested others. Patients with ID can absolutely benefit from the full range of mental health treatment, but there are important alterations necessary to ensure that mental health assessment, diagnosis and treatment interventions are effective and relevant. Individuals with ID represent two to three percent of the general population, so it is reasonable to assume this specialized group will be integrated into virtually every practice setting.

Use of the biopsychosocial formulation is the key to determining the etiology and true meaning of the behavior in the person with ID. Patients with ID often function at higher levels when accurately diagnosed, when psychotropic medications are prescribed following best practices and evidence-based medicine principles, when polypharmacy is avoided, when medical conditions are appropriately treated, and when they have access to a full range of mental health treatments suitable to their developmental framework. Mental health care delivery systems can, and should, offer comprehensive treatment plans, including psychotherapy for patients with ID. Psychotherapy can be effective for patients with ID, and we discuss specific alterations and types of psychotherapy.

Patients with dual diagnoses are often medically fragile and often have co-occurring seizure disorders and other neurological conditions. These are described here, as are recommended modifications regarding the prescribing of psychotropic medications in this population. Best practices and evidence-based medicine principles formulated for the general population are recommended when there are no unique guidelines available for individuals with ID. Clinical vignettes created from composite cases are utilized to illustrate important practice points.

References

American Psychiatric Association (in preparation). *Diagnostic and Statistical Manual of Mental Disorders*, 5th Ed. Scheduled to be published May 2013. www.dsm5.org/ProposedRevision/Pages/proposedrevision.aspx?rid=384# (Access date 01/27/12).

American Psychiatric Association (2000). *Diagnostic and Statistical Manual of Mental Disorders*, 4th Edition, Text Revision (DSM-IV TR), Arlington, VA.

Arnott, R., Finger, S. & Smith, C.U.M. (2002). Trepanation: history, discovery, theory. Swets & Zeitlinger, Lisse, The Netherlands.

Bennett, J. (1923). The exposure of infants in ancient Rome. *The Classical Journal* **18**(6), 341–351. The Classical Association of the Middle West and South. URL: www.jstor.org/stable/3288906 (access Date 04/01/11).

Brydall, J. (1700). The Law Relating to Natural Fools, Mad-Folks, and Lunatick Persons. In Eghigian, G. (ed., 2010) *From madness to mental health: psychiatric disorder and its treatment in western civilization*. Rutgers University Press, NJ.

Chandler, D. (1994). Adapted from *The Act of Writing*. University of Wales, www.aber.ac.uk/media/Documents/short/whorf.html. Access date 05/18/11.

Cosin, R. (1592). Conspiracy for pretended reformation: viz. presbyteriall discipline. In Hunter, R.A. (ed., 1963) *Three hundred years of psychiatry 1535–1860*. Oxford, UK, pp. 73–6, 80–81.

Erikson K. (1966). *Wayward puritans: a study in the sociology of deviance*. Wiley, West Sussex UK.

Fletcher, R., Loschen, E., Stavrakaki, C. & First, M. (eds., 2007). *Diagnostic Manual – Intellectual Disability (DM-ID): A Textbook of Diagnosis of Mental Disorders in Persons with Intellectual Disability*. NADD Press, Kingston, NY.

Gerard, D. (1997). Chiarugi and Pinel considered: soul's brain/person's mind. *Journal of the History of the Behavioral Sciences* **33**(4), 381–403.

Hardan, A. & Sahl, R. (1997). Psychopathology in children and adolescents with developmental disorders. *Research in Developmental Disabilities* **18**, 369–82.

(The) Holy Bible, King James Version (1611). Deuteronomy 28:28.

Kraut, R. (1998). *Aristotle: Books VII and VIII*. Clarendon Aristotle Series, Oxford Press, USA.

Larson, S.A., Lakin, K.C., Anderson, L., Lee, N.K., Jeoung Hak Lee, J.H. & Anderson, D. (2001). Prevalence of mental retardation and developmental disabilities: estimates from the 1994/ 1995 National Health Interview Survey. *American Journal of Mental Retardation* **106**(3), 231–52.

Locke, J. (1690). An essay concerning humane understanding. In Hunter, R.A. (ed., 1963) *Three hundred years of psychiatry 1535–1860*. pages 37, 43, 68, 71. Oxford, UK.

Missios, S. (2007). Hippocrates, Galen, and the uses of trepanation in the ancient classical world. *Neurosurgery Focus* **23**(1), page E11.

Patterson, C. (1985). Not worth the rearing: the causes of infant exposure in ancient Greece *Transactions of the American Philological Association* **115**, 103–123.

Pinel, P. (1806). A treatise on insanity, translated from the French by D.D. Davis. In Eghigian, G. (ed., 2010) *From madness to mental health: psychiatric disorder and its treatment in western civilization*. Rutgers University Press, NJ.

Progler, Y. (2008). Ayurveda: the art of healing and being in an ancient Indian tradition. *Journal of Research in Medical Sciences* **13**(3), 156–157.

Royal College of Psychiatrists (2001). Diagnostic Criteria for Psychiatric Disorders for Use with Adults with Learning Disabilities/Mental Retardation. Occasional paper 48. Gaskell Press, London.

Scheerenberger, R.C. (1983). *A History of Mental Retardation*. Brookes, Baltimore.

Silka, V.R. & Hauser, M.J. (1997). Psychiatric assessment of the person with mental retardation. *Psychiatric Annals* **27**(3).

Snow, K. (2009). A Few Words About People First Language. www.nyla.org/content/user_1/ PeopleFirstLanguage-summary.pdf (access date 05/18/11).

Stone, J.L. & Miles, M.L. (1990). Skull trepanation among the early Indians of Canada and the United States. *Neurosurgery* **26**(6), 1015–1019.

Summers, M. (1948, repr. 1971). *The Malleus Maleficarum of Kramer and Sprenger (1487)*, ed. and trans. by Summers. Dover.

United States of America 111th Congress First Session (2010). S 2781 "Rosa's Law". www.gpo. gov/fdsys/pkg/BILLS-111s2781is/pdf/BILLS-111s2781is.pdf (access date 05/18/11).

WHO (World Health Organization) (1996). International Classification of Diseases Tenth Revision, Guide for Mental Retardation. www.who.int/mental_health/media/en/69.pdf (access date 06/27/11).

2

Psychiatric Assessment

Ann K. Morrison, MD, Associate Professor, Wright State University,Dayton, Ohio
Paulette Marie Gillig, MD, PhD, Professor, Wright State University,Dayton, Ohio

Overview

The psychiatric assessment of patients with intellectual disability (ID) presents both unique challenges and unique opportunities. The same elements that make for comprehensive assessment of all patients – which include a thorough history and mental status examination, a review of prior treatment records, obtaining collateral information, and ordering any additional diagnostic tests and consultations – are part of the psychiatric assessment of individuals with ID.

The patients themselves may be able to provide less direct access to historical information and subjective symptoms, so it is essential that the psychiatrist attempts to access the standard data which support any diagnoses. While individuals with ID may be accompanied by family, professional caregivers or care coordinators, it is still important to spend time directly observing and communicating with the patient. As an examiner gains experience working with individuals with ID, diagnostic acumen will improve, as will selection of effective treatments. People with ID have a high rate of comorbid medical conditions, often involving concurrent medications that might directly cause or contribute to psychiatric symptoms. A thorough and recent physical examination is essential, and coordination of care with the patient's primary care provider is a major task of assessment and management.

Psychiatry of Intellectual Disability: A Practical Manual, First Edition.
Edited by Julie P. Gentile and Paulette M. Gillig.
© 2012 John Wiley & Sons, Ltd. Published 2012 by John Wiley & Sons, Ltd.

Table 1 Challenges in the diagnostic assessment of psychiatric disorders in people with intellectual disabilities.

Cognitive disintegration	Vulnerability to decompensation under stress and subsequent overload of cognitive functioning may lead to bizarre, atypical and even psychotic-like presentations
Psychosocial masking	Limited life experiences and intellectual capacity can influence the content of psychiatric symptoms
Intellectual distortion	Diminished abstract thinking and communication skills limit the ability of the person to accurately and fully describe emotional and behavioral symptoms
Baseline exaggeration	Pre-existing maladaptive behavior not attributed to a mental illness may increase in frequency or intensity with the onset of a psychiatric disorder

Source: Sovner (1986).

Sovner (1986) described some of these challenges to the examiner when assessing individuals with ID (see Table 1).

Managing the interview

The first step in efficiently managing the interview is advance knowledge of who will be the collateral informants providing the information. It is also important to obtain records in advance, to facilitate a more efficient interview by having some data already available in order to prepare specific questions to fill in gaps or uncertainties in the history. In some cases, setting limits on the number of attendees in advance may be necessary.

Knowing the number and role of the informants and reviewing records prior to the appointment will also help in estimating the time needed for the initial interview. Usually, the initial psychiatric appointment will need to be longer than a standard diagnostic interview.

The great number of people involved in the life of an individual with ID, the distress that the patient and caregivers are experiencing due to the presenting problem, and the secondary distress from strains on relationships among all involved, can present additional challenges to obtaining an accurate history. There can also be complicating factors such as too much or too little information, as well as too many or too few reliable informants. Nevertheless, collateral data sources able to provide vital information should be present for the interview. If this is not accomplished, the clinician may be unable to determine the etiology of the presenting symptoms and may be also unable to formulate appropriate treatment interventions.

If the patient is non-verbal, has no usable language skills or has an extensive history of psychiatric and/or behavioral problems, the situation is even further complicated. If the only records brought to the interview are current medication records and notes from a recent visit to a primary care doctor, it may be necessary simply to politely reschedule for a time when records and informants will be available.

At the other end of the spectrum is the patient with mild ID, a cooperative demeanor and well-developed expressive language skills. Although this patient may have little difficulty providing information about history and symptoms privately, they may find doing so difficult in a roomful of concerned parents, supervisors and direct caregivers. It is important in such circumstances to allow the person private interview time, to direct a great deal of questions to the patient and to provide verbal support and encouragement for attempts to tell the story. This may involve setting limits with interested others who have accompanied the patient, who are anxious to discuss their points of view or who will tend to answer for the patient.

Most difficult to manage are those situations in which there has been a particularly challenging behavior, often involving aggression or property destruction, and where there are divergent beliefs about the origin of the behavior from the different informants. In some cases, if there are simply too many people to accommodate in the space or in the allotted time, one may request that someone from each sphere of the person's life is selected to be the spokesperson.

The examiner also needs to be alert for increased distress in the patient, particularly if informants relate material in a very critical or otherwise affectively charged manner. Having someone selected in advance to be able to provide a "time out" in either a less stimulating or, conversely, a distracting environment, may help to avoid causing unnecessary stress to the patient. The examiner should also consider removing, or keeping out of reach, objects that are in the person's repertoire of maladaptive behaviors.

Obtaining the history (adapted from Levitas & Silka, 2001)

Attempt to obtain the history directly from the patient, but be aware that modifications and corroborating information may be needed. The person's receptive language skills may be better than expressive skills, so patience is key. Use simple vocabulary and avoid complex sentences (particularly leading questions or those that involve more than one question at a time). The patient also may have limited ability to chronicle events, and one may need to use events such as birthdays, major holidays, seasons, time at a particular job, house or school to help establish a timeframe for symptoms and behaviors.

Be aware that some patients will respond affirmatively (or negatively) to any query, and some will respond with the answer they believe will please the examiner or others in the room. Parroting and perseverating habits may also interfere with the accuracy of responses. Encourage the patient to bring and use the communication assistance tools that are helpful and familiar to them (see Chapter 6 for a more detailed description of these techniques).

Limitations of attention and physical impairments in the individual may present challenges for the examiner and may also impact extensive history taking. Allowing time for breaks for the person and a flexible office space (such as having a larger space available suitable for walking or to simply get away from the often very stimulating environment of a large number of people talking about the person may be helpful. When possible, a variety of seating options such as single chairs (some of which are stationary, some with arms and some without, some hard and some soft), small couches, and sufficient space for wheelchairs and walkers, will provide for a more comfortable session.

Clinical Vignette #1

Mr. L. is a 20-year-old single white male who resides with his older brother and his brother's family. Mr. L. and his brother came for follow-up after a medical hospitalization. In the hospital there had been two episodes of acute agitation requiring emergency use of a benzodiazepine and an antipsychotic. The exact precipitants for these episodes were somewhat difficult to ascertain, but the patient's sister-in-law, who observed one of them, indicated that Mr. L. seemed to be "giving orders to the nursing staff as though he believed he knew what treatments other patients required."

Mr. L. was transported to the hospital when his family believed he was having a reaction to pain medication following a dental procedure, which they thought caused a dramatic increase in his level of energy and a complaint of feeling very anxious, irritable and unwilling or unable to focus and follow directions.

Mr. L was typically very introverted and quiet; indeed, the family was initially pleased when he appeared to be more social and talkative and more willing to spend more time with them. They had not noticed the initial decrease in his sleep, due to his tendency to spend time in his room alone most nights after dinner. About one week prior to hospitalization, the patient had insisted that he be allowed to play a video game despite having no prior interest in or skill at the game. Later, his brother discovered him endlessly looking at the graphics of the game, which featured voluptuous women, but not actually playing the game. Mr. L. now talked in an animated manner about wishing to get a car and driver's license; he was interested in becoming an emergency medical technician/firefighter and he began to make frequent requests for his allowance.

This vignette provides a brief example of how subtle changes in behavior may initially be overlooked due to the patient's usual functional limitations (**baseline exaggeration**), how the supported structure of the patient's environment and their own lack of experience may dampen the expression and detection of psychiatric symptoms (**psychosocial masking**) and how the patient's inability to articulate his thoughts and feelings more thoroughly also results in lack of recognition of psychiatric symptoms (**intellectual distortion**).

In this case, the patient had been experiencing symptoms of initial hypomania – and subsequently mania – that had been misinterpreted by his family. He began experiencing a decrease need for sleep, was more social, and developed increased sexual interest, a desire to spend more money, increased sense of self-esteem and confidence leading to grandiosity. At the hospital, the patient was diagnosed with Bipolar Disorder I-Most Recent Episode manic-provisional, and he was treated for his symptoms.

Although it could be argued that his presentation fell short of the full criteria (hospitalization was brief, harmful consequences were limited and the aspirations of driving and becoming an EMT were only grandiose in the context of his intellectual disability), this was primarily due to the supervision, support and urgent treatment he received, which limited the full expression of his emerging symptoms.

Observers may also overlook symptoms of psychiatric illness because the behaviors appear to be merely a worsening of previously noted maladaptive behaviors (baseline exaggeration). As in Clinical Vignette #1 above, a person with chronically poor sleep habits

Table 2 Selected assessment instruments.

General	Aberrant Behavior Checklist (ABC)
	Assessment of Dual Diagnosis (ADD)
	Developmental Behaviour Checklist (DPC-P)
	Developmental Behaviour Checklist for Adults (DBC-A)
	Psychiatric Assessment Schedule for Adults with Developmental Disabilities (PAS-ADD)
	Nisonger Child Behavioral Rating Form (NCBRF)
	Psychopathology Instrument for Mentally Retarded Adults (PIMRA), Self-report (PIMRA-SR), Informant (PIMRA-I)
	Diagnostic Assessment Schedule for Severely Handicapped-II (DASH-II)
	Reiss Screen for Maladaptive Behavior (RSMB)
Psychosis	Positive and Negative Syndrome Scale (PANSS)
	Psychotic Symptom Rating Scales (PSYRATS)
Depression	Children's Depression Inventory (CDI)
	Glasgow Depression Scale for people with a Learning Disability (GDS-LD), Glasgow Depression Scale for people with a Learning Disability Carer Supplement (GDS-CS)
	Mood, Interest, and Pleasure Questionnaire (MIPQ)
	Self-report Depression Questionnaire (SRDQ)
Behavior analysis	Motivational Assessment Scale (MAS)
	Motivation Analysis Rating Scale (MARS)
	Functional Analysis Interview Form (FAIF)
	Functional Analysis Checklist (FAC)

Source: Summarized and reproduced with permission from Hermans *et al.*, 2010; Hurley *et al.*, 2007; Hatton *et al.*, 2005; Silka & Hauser, 1997.

may not initially draw notice for insomnia caused by mania or depression, and someone who has a habit of talking to him/herself when frustrated or angry may not draw immediate attention when they begin to respond to auditory hallucinations.

Standardized assessment instruments

Standardized assessment instruments, whether developed for the general population or for use with people with ID, and completed by either the patient and/or caregiver, may be used to enhance the clinical exam (see Table 2) (Hermans & Evenhuis, 2010; Hatton *et al.*, 2005; Mohr *et al.*, 2005). However, experienced clinicians conducting traditional interviews with the patient and informants and performing examinations of patients, supplemented only with a Diagnostic and Statistical Manual (Fourth Edition) checklist for schizophrenia and depressive disorders, also showed a high level of inter-rater reliability (Einfield *et al.*, 2007).

Behavioral analysis is described in detail in Chapter 14 and also provides more objective information regarding current symptoms and behavioral changes.

Mental status examination: modifications and interpretation for persons with ID

(1) Observation

As the person's level of intellectual impairment increases, the formal mental status examination will rely more heavily on observation than on the individual's report of subjective states. General appearance gives one clues to the person's recent appetite, attention to grooming and self-care. This is true even for people who receive assistance with activities of daily living, because their cooperation can impact their appearance.

Note the presence of abnormal movements such as extrapyramidal side effects, tics and stereotypies. Speech abnormalities should be considered in the context of the patient's overall clinical condition, and they may have a medical etiology rather than being related to a psychiatric disorder alone. For example, loud speech may be due to hearing loss, or slurring of words may be caused by an underlying neurologic disorder or be related to over-medication or medication side effects.

(2) Orientation

Level of arousal should be noted (alert, sedated etc.). Orientation should be ascertained in the context of level of arousal. Fund of knowledge should be evaluated in the context of intellectual limitations and social restriction. For example, a patient with ID may be alert and may know he or she is in a hospital but may not know the name of the hospital; or they may know the month, season or a recent holiday, but not the specific date. This patient would be considered to be "oriented."

(3) Mood and affect

Individuals with less severe cognitive deficits usually are able to report feelings and other internal experiences of mood. Inquiry into feeling states with simple vocabulary or visual displays is usually understood, except for the more severely impaired. Inference of mood state by observation of affect and psychomotor behavior may be helpful when the person is unable to provide subjective report. Giddiness or childlike affect may be a result of the person's maturational age rather than a mood disorder. Chapter 7 describes assessment of mood disorders in more detail.

(4) Thought disorder

There is some evidence that psychiatric syndromes are expressed differently in people with ID. Hatton *et al.* (2005) summarized the psychotic symptoms reported by individuals with ID and noted that delusions are less complex and often insufficient to constitute a diagnosis of schizophrenia using standard diagnostic criteria. Auditory hallucinations are more reliably detected, but negative symptoms are unlikely to be helpful in the differential diagnosis (see also Chapter 9).

(5) Cognition

Excessive detail, rambling and tangential thought processes might be due to the person's underlying cognitive impairment rather than a thought disorder. Alzheimer's dementia, seen especially in patients with Down syndrome, is more likely to present with personality and behavior changes rather than episodic memory decline (Ball *et al.*, 2006). Memory may be tested by brief cognitive assessment in the clinical interview, but more formal testing is indicated if a new cognitive impairment is suspected. Chapter 5 describes in detail the cognitive assessment of persons with traumatic brain injuries and co-occurring mental illness, and Chapter 4 describes the assessment of neurologic conditions.

(6) Risk of harm

The evaluation of suicidal threats and self-harm behaviors also is complicated, because the person's understanding of the potential lethality of the plan or action may be inaccurate. A medically insignificant event may reflect a serious wish to die, while a clinically severe attempt may not have been intended to do more than attract attention, and the supervised environment may have limited the consequences of a dangerous act. Similarly, evaluating the person's threats or acts of aggression and harm toward others must take into account intent and opportunity, not just the overt behavior. Chapter 15 describes legal issues in treatment.

(7) Insight and judgment

Despite limited intellectual capacity, individuals with ID often display a significant amount of insight into their distress and the need for assistance, even when psychotically ill. They may say, for example, "I'm not right," "I can't think" or "I don't want to do anything." Even when formal insight is lacking, they may be willing to accept the opinion and advice of trusted family members, housing staff, work supervisors and others.

Diagnostic studies

Laboratory studies may be ordered when conducting psychiatric assessment of people with ID, especially if these tests have not been performed in another setting during a physical evaluation. These studies should include an electrocardiogram, complete blood count, comprehensive metabolic panel, thyroid function tests, urinalysis, folate, B12 and syphilis serology (Silka & Hauser, 1997). Chapter 3 describes medical assessment in persons with ID.

Including a lipid panel may be reasonable, given the overall prevalence of hyperlipidemia, especially in some affected populations such as individuals with Down syndrome, in addition to the need to monitor glucose and lipid levels regularly if one continues or initiates an atypical (second generation) antipsychotic. Blood levels of medications, an electroencephalogram, computerized tomography (CT) or magnetic resonance imaging (MRI) of the head may also be appropriate on an individual basis (Silka & Hauser, 1997). Including a toxicology screen for alcohol and illicit drugs should also be considered, especially for those individuals in community settings. Current prevalence rates of substance use disorders may be underestimates, as routine toxicology is seldom performed on this population.

Differential diagnosis and diagnostic overshadowing

After completing the history, the physical and mental status examinations and diagnostic studies, one is then faced with developing a differential diagnosis of the presenting problems. Often, the initial question is whether the problems represent an underlying, well-defined psychiatric illness such as schizophrenia, depression or panic disorder, or represent limitations of behavioral repertoire from the underlying ID.

The differentiation between psychiatric disorders versus the limitations of the patient's behavioral repertoire can sometimes be difficult. The concept of "diagnostic over-shadowing" has been proposed to explain the tendency to not recognize the presence of mental illness in individuals with ID because of the symptoms of ID. This phenomenon was described initially by Reiss *et al.* (1982) and Reiss & Szyszko (1983), but Spengler *et al.* (1990) found that the phenomenon did not generalize for the upper range of intellectual impairment (IQ 70 and 80), which represents the majority of people with intellectual impairment. White *et al.* (1995), in a meta-analysis, noted that while the effect of over-shadowing is reliable across studies, the effect size is small to moderate and the clinical significance in "real life" situations is unclear.

Personality factors, personality disorders and substance use issues in persons with ID

Not identifying personality disorders in people with ID leads to the same problems as it does in the general population (see Chapter 10). Attempts to treat the affective instability, relationship problems, sense of entitlement, intolerance of being alone, disproportionate reactions to slights, lack of consideration of others, over-dependency or reliance on others and other characteristics of an underlying personality disturbance by pharmacology alone, rather than through psychotherapeutic and behavioral inter-ventions, are often unsuccessful (Heber, 1964; Ziegler & Burack, 1989; Alexander & Cooray, 2003; Lidher *et al.*, 2005).

Substance use disorders, as a source of problem behaviors or distressing symptoms, also may be overlooked in persons with ID. Even when substance abuse or dependency is recognized, treatment for the person with ID is often difficult to access or may not meet the needs of the person. Programs may not accept people with significant cognitive impair-ments, and the rehabilitative approaches used may require cognitive and social skills which are beyond the reach of many people with ID.

Persons with ID begin using substances at a later age than the general population, but that difference may be decreasing. Individuals with ID appear to be at greater risk of developing problems related to substance use (McGillicuddy, 2006). Those individuals in more restrictive and supervised housing are likely to have lower reported rates of substance use and misuse (Burgard *et al.*, 2000), but these rates may be underreported. When assessing the patient with ID, providing some opportunity for a private interview during history taking may facilitate obtaining more accurate information about substance abuse.

Stressful life events and exaggeration of baseline symptoms (based on Hurley, 2001)

People with ID are vulnerable to the same life events as the general population. Exposure to one or more life events in the previous 12 months is associated with increased risk for affective disorder in adults with ID (Hastings *et al.*, 2004). Excessive reassurance-seeking is associated with depressive symptoms in the person with ID, as are negative social interactions with staff and interpersonal rejection (Hartley *et al.*, 2008).

Clinical Vignette #2

Ms. A is a 55 year old single African-American female with ID who was brought to the clinic by her father. He reported that she had recently been more argumentative and irritable at home, and quite uncharacteristically had thrown a phone and a glass at him on two separate occasions. He was also concerned that she had been talking more about her mother, who died about nine months ago, she had been up at night for several hours and she had decreased appetite, even at her favorite restaurants for about the last four months. Over the past month, he found her at times yelling when no one was there, and at times she seemed to be have been talking to her mother.

He had had similar reports of behavioral problems from workshop staff. About two months ago, at the urging of these staff members, he took her to her family physician, who initiated treatment with risperidone 1 mg twice per day and mirtazapine at 30 mg at bedtime.

Following this, Ms. A's father reported she was sleeping and eating somewhat better, but still seemed uninterested in bowling and movies and continued to talk and sometimes yells when no one is present. She had also been talking about "retiring" from the workshop and, indeed, had some recent problems with walking away from her station and several of instances of verbal arguments with peers, as well as a couple of physical episodes in which she had pushed supervisors.

The patient endorsed feeling sad since her mother's death and said that she missed the things they did together, such as shopping and crafts. Her mother had also regularly taken her to church, an activity that her father had never attended. She said she did hear her mother's voice, but this was comforting to her; however, she also heard two other voices, which were scary and told her she was a bad person and "no one will like her now that her mother is gone". Additionally, her father noted that she was quite tremulous, especially when trying to perform an action such as eating. He was not sure whether this was completely new as she would sometimes be shaking before treatment, especially when she became upset and appeared anxious in the last year. Indeed, he speculated that he may have noticed some milder problems with her walking and tremulousness over the previous one to two years, noticed with bowling and crafts. He reported that when he took her back to the family physician one month ago, she had been started on Sinemet (carbidopa/levodopa).

A telephone conference with the family physician revealed that she believed Ms. A may have Parkinson's disease. Attempts to increase risperidone worsened tremor, despite treatment with additional anti-Parkinsonian agents, although psychotic symptoms seemed to improve. The patient was eventually treated with olanzapine; however, even with this agent, her tremor worsened. Her gait also became impaired, and further progression of underlying Parkinson's disease were in fact confirmed.

This case illustrates multiple issues in diagnosis using a bio-psychosocial formulation. Ms. A. had an immediate stressor – the loss of her mother – preceding a major depressive episode. The depressive episode seems to have been accompanied by psychotic symptoms, as her hallucinations were not limited to hearing her mother's voice in a comforting manner. She also had loss of other support, namely the loss of her church family, as this was an activity tied to her mother. In addition, she was in danger of losing her work supports. Ultimately, the patient was discovered to have had Parkinson's disease, and this may also have played a role in the development or exacerbation of her psychotic depression.

Conclusion

Psychiatric assessment of individuals with ID is both challenging and rewarding. All of the psychiatrist's skills and knowledge about general medicine are called upon: psychiatric interviewing; psychodynamic, social, cognitive and behavioral theories; biopsychosocial formulations (Engel, 1977); psychotherapeutic techniques; ability to work with multidisciplinary teams; and knowledge of the systems of general medical care, mental health care and ID services. Satisfaction comes both from the relatively straightforward treatment of an individual with major depression or schizophrenia, and from the more complex management of challenging behaviors that have no specifically identifiable psychiatric disorder at the root, but which require the development of long-term strategies to try to improve quality of life and to preserve interpersonal relationships.

References

Alexander, R. & Cooray, S. (2003). Diagnosis of personality disorders in learning disabilities. *The British Journal of Psychiatry* **182**(S44), 528–31.

Ball, S.L., Holland, A.J., Huppert, F.A., Treppner, P., Watson, P. & Hon, J. (2006). Personality and behaviour changes mark the early stages of Alzhemier's disease in adults with Down's syndrome: Findings from a prospective population-based study. *International Journal of Geriatric Psychiatry* **21**, 661–673.

Burgard, J.F., Donohue, B., Azrin, N.H. & Teichner G. (2000). Prevalence and treatment of substance abuse in the mentally retarded population: An empirical review. *Journal of Psychoactive Drugs* **32**(1), 293–298.

Einfeld, S., Tonge, B., Chapman, L., Mohr, C., Taffe, J. & Horstead S. (2007). Inter-rater reliability of the diagnosis of psychosis and depression in individuals with intellectual disabilities. *Journal of Applied Research in Intellectual Disabilities* **20**(5), 384–390.

Engel, G.L. (1977). The need for a new medical model: A challenge for biomedicine. *Science* **196** (4286), 129–136.

Hartley, S.L., Hayes Lickel, A. & MacLean, W.E. (2008). Reassurance seeking and depression in adults with mild intellectual disability. *Journal of Intellectual Disability Research* **52**(11), 917–929.

Hastings, RP, Hatton, C, Taylor, J. & Maddison, C. (2004). Life events and psychiatric symptoms in adults with intellectual disabilities. *Journal of Intellectual Disability Research* **48**(P1) 42–46.

Hatton, C., Haddock, G., Taylor, J.L., Coldwell, J., Crossley, R. & Peckham, N. (2005). The reliability and validity of general psychotic rating scales with people with mild and moderate intellectual disabilities: an empirical investigation. *Journal of Intellectual Disability Research* **49**(7), 490–500.

Heber, R. (1964). Research on personality disorders and characteristics of the mentally retarded. *Mental Retardation Abstracts* **40**(1), 304–25.

Hermans, H. & Evenhuis, H.M. (2010). Characteristics of instruments screening for depression in adults with intellectual disabilities: Systematic review. *Research in Developmental Disabilities* **31**, 1109–1120.

Hurley, A.D. (2001). Axis IV and Axis V: Assessment of persons with mental retardation and 1developmental disabilities. *Mental Health Aspects of Developmental Disabilities* **4**, 17–20.

Hurley, A.D., Levitas, A., Lecavalier, L. & Pary R.J. (2007). Assessment and diagnostic procedures. Special considerations for the mental health diagnostic interview for individuals with ID. In: Fletcher, R., Loschen, E., Stavrakaki, C. & First, M. (eds.) *Diagnostic Manual-Intellectual Disability: A Clinical Guide for Diagnosis of Mental Disorders in Persons with Intellectual Disability.* Chpt 2: 9-23. NADD Press/National Association for the Dually Diagnosed, Kingston, NY.

Levitas, A.S. & Silka, V.R. (2001). Mental health clinical assessment of persons with mental retardation and developmental disabilities: history. *Mental Health Aspects of Developmental Disabilities* **4**, 31–43.

Lidher, J., Martin, D.M., Jayaprakash, M.S. & Roy, A. (2005). Personality disorders in people with learning disabilities: follow-up of a community survey. *Journal of Intellectual Disability Research* **49**(11), 845–851.

McGillicuddy, N.B. (2006). A review of substance use research among those with mental retardation. *Mental Retardation and Developmental Disabilities Research Reviews* **12**, 41–47.

Mohr, C., Tonge, B.J. & Einfeld S.L. (2005). The development of a new measure for the assessment of psychopathology in adults with intellectual disability. *Journal of Intellectual Disability Research* **49**(7), 469–480.

Perez-Achiaga, N., Nelson, S. & Hasiotis A. (2009). Instruments for the detection of depressive symptoms in people with intellectual disabilities. *A systematic review. Journal of Intellectual Disabilities* **13**(1), 55–76.

Reiss, S. & Szyszko, J. (1983). Diagnostic overshadowing and professional experience with mentally retarded persons. *American Journal of Mental Deficiency* **87**(4), 396–402.

Reiss, S., Levitan, G.W. & Szyszko J. (1982). Emotional disturbance and mental retardation: diagnostic overshadowing. *American Journal of Mental Deficiency* **86**(6), 567–574.

Silka, V.R. & Hauser, M.J. (1997). Psychiatric assessment of the person with mental retardation. *Psychiatric Annals* **27**(3), 162–169.

Sovner, R. (1986). Limiting factors in the use of DSM-III criteria with mentally ill/mentally retarded persons. *Psychopharmacology Bulletin* **22**(4), 1055–9.

Spengler, P.M., Strohmer, D.C. & Prout, H.T. (1990). Testing the robustness of the diagnostic overshadowing bias. *American Journal on Mental Retardation* **95**(3), 204–214.

Sturmey, P. (1994). Assessing the functions of aberrant behaviors: A review of psychometric instruments. *Journal of Autism and Developmental Disorder* **24**(3), 293–304.

White, M.J., Nichols, C.N., Cook, R.S., Spengler, P.M., Walker, B.S. & Look, K.K. (1995). Diagnostic overshadowing and mental retardation: a meta-analysis. *American Journal on Mental Retardation* **100**(3), 293–298.

Zigler, E. & Burack, J.A. (1989). Personality development and the dually diagnosed person. *Research in Developmental Disabilities* **10**, 225–240.

3

Medical Assessment

Julie P. Gentile, MD, Associate Professor, Wright State
University, Dayton, Ohio
Michelle A. Monro, DO, Edwards Air Force Base, Palmdale, CA

> *"Persons with physical and mental impairments are often granted a permanent visa
> to the kingdom of the sick."*
>
> (Tighe, 2001)

Introduction

In recent years, as medical care for individuals with intellectual disabilities (ID) has
improved, "some disability-related mortality has been replaced by disability-related
morbidity" (McDermott *et al.*, 2006). Today, persons with ID are more likely to live to
adulthood, reside in the community and look forward to a longer life, although longevity
among adults with ID still falls short when compared to the general population (Sutherland
et al., 2002). More severe cognitive deficits and increased dependency on community
supports are associated with shortened lifespan (Chaney & Eyman, 2000). Other risk factors
associated with increased mortality include the inability to ambulate or to feed oneself, poor
motor or communication skills, self-help limitations (Hayden, 1998), some degree of
neurological or other physical impairment (Janicki & Breitenbach, 2000) and the presence
of Down syndrome (Sutherland *et al.*, 2002).

By contrast, individuals with mild ID with only minimal need for community support
appear to share comparable life expectancies with the general population (Patja *et al.*, 2000).
According to the American Diabetic Association (2010), life expectancy for individuals
with ID has increased to the degree that those in their twenties are expected to have

Psychiatry of Intellectual Disability: A Practical Manual, First Edition.
Edited by Julie P. Gentile and Paulette M. Gillig.
© 2012 John Wiley & Sons, Ltd. Published 2012 by John Wiley & Sons, Ltd.

analogous longevity when compared to other persons (American Diabetic Association [ADA] Guidelines, 2010). Given this information, it is important that individuals with ID receive appropriate medical care and that organic causes are considered when behavioral changes and mental health symptoms exist.

There are few specific guidelines in the literature to help medical practitioners who are caring for patients with ID, especially with regard to prevention and management of cardiovascular disease and cancer (ADA Guidelines, 2010). Unfortunately, people with ID are at increased risk for chronic diseases such as heart disease and obesity, and they often have decreased capacity and opportunity for conditioning and fitness. Patients with ID also have a higher incidence of seizures, hearing and vision problems, as well as low bone mineral density. The frequency of co-occurring medical conditions in the ID population who also receive mental health care is twice that of other mental health populations (Ryan, 2003), and common conditions may present in unusual ways.

Knowledge of commonly occurring and potentially undiagnosed medical conditions that arise in patients with ID is important for mental health clinicians, especially because medical conditions may present with behavioral changes in this population. Patients with ID usually have limited verbal skills, and therefore behavior should be viewed as a form of communication, a potential health-related problem or resulting from medication intolerance or some other side effect. The patient with significant behavioral changes should also be seen by a primary care physician who knows the patient's previous medical history, has performed a recent and thorough physical examination and has obtained laboratory testing as needed. An abbreviated history or physical examination without laboratory studies may be unrevealing (Ryan, 2003), and more than the usual number of tests may be needed to reach a diagnosis.

Syndrome-specific medical conditions

Down syndrome

Down syndrome (DS) is the most common genetic cause (trisomy 21) of ID, and occurs in 1 in 1,000 births. Individuals with DS are vulnerable to many medical conditions, involving virtually every organ system. Endocrine disorders such as hypothyroidism are more common, and symptoms include weight gain and fatigue. The Canadian consensus guidelines for primary health care of adults with developmental disabilities (Sullivan *et al.*, 2006) recommends a regular thyroid screen every 1–3 years for all individuals with ID and more often in high risk subgroups, such as those with DS.

About 70% of children with DS have visual impairment, and it is estimated that approximately 60% have some type of hearing loss (Goldstein & Reynolds, 1999, Van Dyke *et al.*, 1995). Autoimmune disorders (including alopecia areata) are more common. Patients with DS may not mount fevers (or at least not to the same extent as someone in the general population), so conditions such as neuroleptic malignant syndrome and infectious processes may be more difficult to diagnose. Unfortunately, hematologic abnormalities and chronic or recurrent infections of the upper and lower respiratory system (ears, nose, sinuses, throat and chest) are common. Pulmonary infections are especially prevalent in individuals with hypotonia who may have a weak cough. Premature aging, Alzheimer's disease and early menopause are more common, as is sleep apnea.

Joint and muscle disorders are highly prevalent, including atlantoaxial instability, which is increased mobility of the cervical spine at the level of the uppermost cervical vertebrae (the atlantoaxial joint). As many as 20% of individuals with DS experience this condition and it can present in a variety of ways, including incontinence of bowel or bladder, gait problems, odd sensations in hands or feet, proprioception problems (difficulty in judging where to step) or whipping the head forward (Goldstein & Reynolds, 1999, Van Dyke et al., 1995). If the condition is suspected, the patient should be referred to a primary care physician for further evaluation. If it is not diagnosed and treated, the patient can suffer spinal cord compression at the high cervical level, and therefore the condition can lead to total paralysis and is potentially fatal. Atlantoaxial instability is evaluated by x-ray measurement of the space between the posterior segment of the anterior arch of the first cervical vertebra and the anterior segment of the odontoid process of the second cervical vertebra. This is accomplished with a series of x-rays. The space should be < 5 mm. People with DS also experience other orthopedic conditions at a higher rate than that of the general population, including scoliosis, joint dislocation, hip and knee cap instability, weak ankles and flat feet.

Cardiac conditions are quite common in persons with DS. Approximately 30–45% have congenital heart conditions, the most common being atrioventricular septal defect, and this condition can present with abrupt squatting or "sit down strikes" (Van Dyke et al., 1995, Dykens, 2000).

Several gastro-intestinal disorders are more common in DS, including aganglionic megacolon, annular pancreas, duodenal atresia and stenosis, imperforate anus, trachea-esophageal fistula and pyloric stenosis, esophageal motility disorder and gastroesophageal reflux disease (Goldstein & Reynolds, 1999, Van Dyke et al., 1995).

Fragile X syndrome

Individuals with Fragile X syndrome (FXS) experience seizure disorders at a rate of approximately 20% and experience higher rates of joint laxity, flat feet, endocrine disorders and scoliosis (Dykens, 2000, Goldstein & Reynolds, 1999). Weak connective tissue can predispose individuals with FXS to medical conditions such as hernias and recurrent middle ear infections. The same connective tissue alterations may be the etiology of alterations in the valves and vessels of the heart, causing mitral valve prolapse, which occurs in about 50% of persons with FXS. Fifty percent of these patients also experience *vision problems*, with the most common presentation being myosis (nearsightedness) (Dykens, 2000, Goldstein & Reynolds, 1999).

In contrast to DS, there is no shortened lifespan and no increased incidence of dementia. In more recent years, cerebellar changes have been noted in males with the pre-mutation for FXS but who do not have the syndrome; this presents as a tremor-ataxia syndrome called FXTAS (Fragile X Tremor-Ataxia Syndrome).

FXS affects females in different ways. About 16–19% of females who have a pre-mutation gene experience premature ovarian failure (POF), where their ovarian function stops before normal menopause – sometimes well before the age of 40 years, and sometimes as early as in their mid-twenties (Dykens, 2000, Goldstein & Reynolds, 1999).

Prader-Willi syndrome

Prader-Willi syndrome (PWS) occurs in 1 in 10,000 births. It is one of the most frequent microdeletion syndromes and it is nearly always accompanied by ID (Rubin & Crocker, 2006). It is also the most common cause of genetic obesity. Seventy percent of cases are related to a deletion of the long arm of chromosome 15. The major criteria for the diagnosis of PWS are neonatal hypotonia, hyperphagia, cognitive impairments, hypogonadism, and behavioral problems including skin picking.

Individuals with PWS have an insatiable appetite, in combination with poor exercise tolerance (Ryan, 2003). They experience neuropsychiatric issues, including incomplete development of the hypothalamus, minimal or absent satiety cells, reduced muscle strength and mass, early muscle fatigue, sleep hypoxemia, slowed metabolism of stored nutrients, skin changes and paresthesias (Ryan, 2003, Dykens, 2000). The insatiable appetite can lead to obesity and related complications such as type II diabetes and cardiovascular disease.

Edema and right heart failure are all more prevalent in individuals with PWS (Goldstein & Reynolds, 1999), as are cerebro-vascular disease (stroke), arthritis, and sleep apnea. Obesity represents the greatest risk to good health. In addition, the proclivity to eat large amounts of food quickly increases the risk of stomach necrosis and rupture. These acute gastro-intestinal conditions can be life-threatening (Dykens, 2000, Goldstein & Reynolds, 1999).

Patients with PWS are also at risk for scoliosis, and this should be monitored regularly. Pulmonary problems are common and include central hypoventilation and apnea. Gastro-esophageal reflux and aspiration are of concern as well (Goldstein & Reynolds, 1999). Individuals with PWS have low levels or absent sex hormones, which places them at risk for osteoporosis. The additional weight due to over-eating, combined with weak and brittle bones, leads to a higher susceptibility to falls, fractures and other injuries (Dykens, 2000).

Williams syndrome

Most individuals with Williams syndrome (WS) have alterations in their blood vessels which can cause problems in various organ systems, i.e. cardiac (narrowing of the aorta, leading to supravalvular aortic stenosis), pulmonary, renal, etc. The narrowing of other blood vessels can lead to hypertension (Goldstein & Reynolds, 1999, Dykens, 2000). Hypothyroidism is often present, and elevated calcium levels are also common, but the cause is poorly understood. This calcium abnormality can cause "colic-like" symptoms during infant years and often resolves on its own. However, if this is not the case, both calcium and vitamin D should be monitored and treated as needed (Goldstein & Reynolds, 1999, Dykens, 2000). Failure to thrive is not uncommon, nor is slow weight gain. In adulthood, slightly smaller stature is common.

Hearing loss typically has an early onset and may be progressive. Individuals with WS who appear to have normal hearing, as defined by behavioral thresholds, should be screened for subclinical impairment or undetected cochlear pathology (Marler et al., 2010). The clinician should have an increased index of suspicion for outer hair cell dysfunction in otherwise normal hearing individuals. Paradoxically, some patients may experience hyperacusis, or increased sensitivity to noise.

Accelerated aging (early puberty, graying of the hair, early menopause) appears to be related to reduction in elastin protein due to an elastin gene deletion in individuals with WS (Goldstein & Reynolds, 1999, Dykens, 2000). Low muscle tone is over-represented in this syndrome, as is joint laxity; as the individual ages, physical therapy may be helpful for joint stiffness and contractures (Goldstein & Reynolds, 1999). Both inguinal and umbilical hernias also occur at a higher frequency than in the general population. Dental problems (especially widely spaced teeth) are also common.

Table 1   Behavioral presentations commonly associated with medical conditions in the patient with intellectual disabilities.

Fist jammed in mouth	Gastroesophageal reflux disease, eruption of teeth, asthma, rumination, nausea, anxiety, painful hands/paresthesia and gout.
Biting side of hand	Sinus problems, eustachian tubes, ear problems, eruption of wisdom teeth, dental problems, pain or paresthesia in hands.
Whipping head forward	Atlantoaxial subluxation, other syndromes with joint laxity, dental problems, headaches.
Intense rocking	Visceral pain, headache, depression, anxiety, medication side effects.
Head-banging	Depression, headache, dental problems, seizure, otitis, mastoiditis, sinus problems, tineacapitis.
All behavior problems (most common cause)	Pain, medication side effects, sleep disorders, psychiatric illness.
Waving head side to side	Attempts to supplement visual field, vertigo, hypervigilance, headache syndrome, vitreous humor.
Walking on toes	Arthritis and hips or ankles or knees, tight heel cords.
Won't sit	Akathisia, anxiety, depression, back pain, other pain, sleep deprivation.
Sudden sitting down	Heart problems, syncope, orthostasis, medication side effects, vertigo, otitis, atlantoaxial instability, seizures, panic.
Waving fingers in front of eyes	Migraine, corneal scarring, cataracts, seizures, glaucoma, diplopia, medication side effects.
Wears multiple layers of clothing	Rule out endocrine and medication problems, post-institutional behavior.
Covers eyes or ears	Consider psychosis, expression of hypersensitivity, preferences or fears, pain or depression.
Places unusual wrappings on ankles, wrists, or other openings	Post-institutional coping, temperature regulation, or sensory integration issues.
Glares with hostility at previously liked others or strangers	Rage or paranoia secondary to abuse or trauma history, psychosis.
Wears costumes	Psychosis, expressing a wish or a fact from past or present.
Brushes unseen material off body	Psychosis, dissociative, or neuropathy.
Biting thumb or object with front teeth (or thumb sucking or bruxism)	Sinus problems, eustachian tube, ear problems, finger pain, paresthesias, gout.

Refuses to sit evenly or at all	Hip pain, low back pain, genital or rectal discomfort, ongoing abuse, clue to past abuse.
Unpleasurable masturbation	Prostatitis, urinary tract or genital infection, rectal injury or infection, peer acidic infection, syphilis, repetition phenomenon, i.e. past abuse, never learned pleasurable masturbation.
Odd food refusals, (e.g. cravings or combinations, unusual aroma), family history of miscarriages or dysmorphic features of developmental disability	Serum and urine amino acids, organic acids, and mucopolysaccharides, very long chain fatty acids, ammonia, lactate, pyruvate, white cell enzymes.
Spells which are not generalized tonic clonic seizures	Most are related to anxiety disorders or tic disorders; however if the usual treatment is not successful consider testing for cardiac events or unusual metabolic conditions such as porphyria or G6PD deficiency.
Intermittent fatigue	Multiple sclerosis, chronic viral infections, serum protein electrophoresis, lactate, pyruvate, comprehensive metabolic panel, glucose tolerance test, calcium, carnitine, B vitamins, iron levels.
Ataxia	Atlantoaxial subluxation, heavy metals, fatigue list
Joint swelling	ANA, rheumatoid factor, ESR, TB, syphilis screening.
Partial seizures	B1, B2, B6, B12, folate, niacin, pantothenic acid, titanic acid.
Snoring, history of airway obstruction or history of brain injury	Sleep apnea, hypopnea, hypoxemia, or seizures.
Flushing, rash, or other autonomic instability	Pheochromocytoma, carcinoid syndrome, porphyria, G6PD deficiency, autoimmune disorders, lime, TB, syphilis, viral including HTV.

Source: Ryan (2003).

Primary care evaluation and preventive health planning

Atypical presentation of symptoms, combined with behavioral and communication difficulties, increase the potential for medical and mental health care to be compromised in the ID population. McDermott *et al.* (2006) reported that some medical conditions are more prevalent in adults with ID, when compared to their peers without disabilities. There is a greater likelihood of dementia, seizure disorders, chronic obstructive pulmonary disease, congestive heart failure, diabetes and transient ischemic attacks in patients with ID; in addition, patients diagnosed with psychiatric disorders (without and with ID) are at increased risk for many medical conditions (McDermott *et al.*, 2006).

The evaluation of a patient with ID has similarities to that of an individual with memory loss, or one with acute mental status changes, such as delirium (Silka & Hauser, 1997). For example, the presentation involves detective work, emphasis on observation in the light of less subjective data and interpretation of behavioral presentations. See Table 1 for some behavioral presentations of medical conditions in the ID population. Reliable collateral information is essential.

Appropriate preliminary laboratory studies usually consist of an electrocardiogram (EKG), electrolyte levels, a complete blood count, screening blood chemistry, urinalysis, folate/B12 levels, syphilis serology, and thyroid function tests (Silka & Hauser, 1997). Depending on the differential diagnosis, other tests may include an electroencephalogram (EEG), a brain imaging scan, serum drug level measurements and other pertinent tests, as indicated (Silka & Hauser, 1997, Rueve & Welton, 2008).

Making decisions about additional laboratory testing

The United States Preventive Services Task Force published guidelines for preventive medical care which are now considered evidence based practices. These guidelines are accepted as standard of care in the United States (Wilkinson *et al.*, 2007). To be appropriate for screening, a disease must:

1 be serious and have important consequences;

2 be progressive, with early treatment more effective than later treatment;

3 possess a preclinical phase that is easily identified by screening tests; and

4 have a preclinical phase with a relatively long duration that is prevalent in the screen population (Wilkinson *et al.*, 2007, US Preventive Services Task Force, 2007).

See Table 2 for screening recommendations for adults with ID based on current evidence. Wilkinson *et al.* (2007) reviewed the available literature pertaining to screening tests in those with ID and generated a new SORT rating specific for patients with ID.

Table 2 Screening recommendations for adults with ID based on current evidence.

Screening	USPTF guideline for adults in the US	Evidence-based recommendations for adults with ID
Obesity/body mass index	B	B
Cholesterol/lipid	A	C
Diabetes	B	I
Hypertension	A	C
Tobacco/smoking cessation	A	I
Colon cancer	A	B
Breast cancer (women)	B	C
Cervical cancer (women)	A	B
Prostate cancer	I	I
Skin cancer	I	I
Osteoporosis	B	B
Vision and hearing	B	B
Mental health	B	C

A rating of A is for screens with patient oriented, consistent and good quality of evidence, B for inconsistent or lesser quality evidence, C for consensus or disease oriented practices, and I for inconsistent data.
Source: Adapted with permission from Wilkinson, J.E., Culpepper, L. & Cerreto, M. (2007). Screening Tests for Adults with Intellectual Disabilities. *Journal of the American Board of Family Medicine* **20**, 402.

Medication side effects

With the increased incidence of polypharmacy practices, drug interactions and medication, side effects should always be considered in the differential diagnosis (Silka & Hauser, 1997). For example, individuals with autism are especially prone to ataxia when prescribed benzodiazepines.

Many psychotropic medications are known to cause sedation in some individuals, including several mood stabilizers and antipsychotics. Antipsychotic drugs can cause serious side effects, including extrapyramidal side effects (EPS), which are documented to be more common and potentially more serious in patients with ID. The various forms of EPS are described in chapter 12.

Akathisia is one example of EPS which is more likely to go undiagnosed. The symptoms may resemble agitation or residual psychosis, leading the prescriber to increase the dose of the antipsychotic medication, resulting in exacerbation of the problem. Other categories of medications should be monitored closely in patients with ID, including (but not limited to) antihypertensive drugs, gastrointestinal medications, beta blockers and allergy medications, almost all of which are anti-cholinergic or antihistaminic (Silka & Hauser, 1997).

More common and less common conditions in the general ID population

Obesity, osteoporosis and smoking were found to be more prevalent in adults with ID, and therefore enhanced screening for these conditions has been recommended (Wilkinson *et al.*, 2007). Abnormal results for Papanicolaou tests (cervical screening for cancer) were less common in adults with ID; due to the influence of lifestyle and sexual activity of the patient on the need for preventive care, the recommendation is to individualize gynecologic screening schedules based on these variables.

When compared to the general population, patients with ID in an Australian study had increased frequency of thyroid disease, non-ischemic heart disorders and visual impairment (Beange *et al.*, 1995). Other researchers have found a high prevalence of cardiac conditions such as hypertension, as well as hearing impairment, epilepsy, endocrine problems (especially thyroid disease), skin anomalies and higher rates of oral and dental issues (Sutherland *et al.*, 2002). Sutherland *et al.* (2002) also report that adults with cerebral palsy are especially vulnerable to musculoskeletal deformities, bowel and bladder problems and gastro-esophageal reflux disease (GERD).

Organ system review

Metabolic changes and the cardiovascular system

The ID population is at increased risk of having metabolic and cardiovascular conditions when compared to their average-intelligence cohorts, whether or not psychiatric illness coexists. Several studies have noted higher rates of diabetes, obesity, high blood pressure, hyperlipidemia and sedentary lifestyles (Stanish *et al.*, 2006). Additionally, Stanish found that a review of the literature indicates that treating clinicians are less likely to recommend preventive or maintenance medical care for individuals with ID. Subsequently, undiagnosed and under-treated medical conditions lead to increased morbidity and mortality associated with cardiovascular and metabolic disorders. It has been suggested that this disparity explains the estimation that persons with moderate to severe ID have 20% less "expected life" versus the general population (Bittles *et al.*, 2002).

It is well known that there are identified risks for both medical and psychiatric conditions. If an individual has risk factors for both, the vulnerability is even greater. McDermott *et al.* (2006) found that patients in the general population with psychiatric illness were at an increased risk of all medical conditions seen in a primary care setting (including other psychiatric illnesses, cancer, coronary artery disease, congestive heart failure, emphysema, dementia, diabetes, hypertension and obesity), when compared to those without psychiatric diagnoses. It has been well documented that the use of antipsychotics in patients is associated with metabolic syndromes, hyperlipidemia and weight gain, and that diagnoses of hypertension, hyperlipidemia, obesity and/or diabetes are associated with higher incidences of cerebrovascular and cardiac injuries (Tasman *et al.*, 2003).

Both first and second generation antipsychotics, alternatively known respectively as typical and atypical antipsychotics, have long been associated with adverse metabolic effects in the general population (Tasman *et al.*, 2003). Weight gain after ten weeks of treatment with a second generation antipsychotic can range from nearly no discernible weight change for ziprasidone and quetiapine, to 9–10 pounds for olanzapine and clozapine. The most commonly accepted etiology for this weight gain is an increase in appetite, resulting in an increase in body fat. Accompanying the weight gain is a higher incidence of hyperlipidemia, hyperglycemia and new onset type 2 diabetes associated with the use of clozapine and olanzapine (and to a lesser extent with risperidone and quetiapine).

Clinical Vignette #1

Sam is a 37 year old individual with Fragile X Syndrome who presents for follow-up treatment of schizophrenia, paranoid type. Since he was started on quetiapine for treatment of his paranoid delusions and auditory hallucinations, his symptoms have improved significantly, but he has gained 32 pounds and his most recent laboratory results showed elevated total cholesterol and fasting glucose. He has family history for hypertension (mother) and coronary artery disease (father) and, during the appointment, the lab values are discussed with the patient and his parents.

Prior to initiation of the quetiapine, a complete informed consent was accomplished, describing both extrapyramidal side effects as well as metabolic syndrome. Because of the combination of significant family history, weight gain and abnormal lab values, a decision was made to cross-taper Sam to an alternate atypical or second generation antipsychotic medication. Aripiprazole was chosen, and the new medication was started and increased prior to the taper process of the quetiapine, so as to avoid decompensation and recurrence of the psychotic symptoms.

The cross-taper was ultimately accomplished without incident, but the physician also recommended consultation with a dietician and the family practice physician, as well as regular exercise, to be incorporated into Sam's daily programming schedule. At the sheltered workshop, Sam was placed in a program which included walking around the campus twice daily; he was also signed up at a local swimming club for water aerobics twice weekly. He was provided with healthy meals and snacks following the dietician's recommendations.

After eight months on the aripiprazole and the institution of the aforementioned nutritional/exercise program, Sam not only remained psychiatrically stable but he also lost 24 pounds and his laboratory values returned to normal limits without any additional medication prescribed by the family practice physician.

Reiss & Aman (1998) postulate that individuals with ID are as likely to develop adverse effects from use of an antipsychotic as the general population, although there is little research comparing the ID population with other groups. However, special consideration to those with ID should be made, as the recognition and explanation of the possibility of side effects may be more difficult, given the lack of subjective data from the patient.

Common side effects of antipsychotic medications include not only metabolic conditions but also extrapyramidal side effects (EPS), and the latter can indirectly potentiate the former. For instance, it is well documented that antipsychotics are capable of producing both acute and chronic extrapyramidal side effects, including akathisia, dystonias, parkinsonism, and tardive dyskinesia (described in chapter 12). If a patient experiences EPS, it may become an impediment to physical activity as it can decrease opportunities for ambulation and mobility. There is cumulative risk in individuals with ID, given the increased prevalence of functional limitations; these side effects may further complicate risk of cardiac pathology.

Initiatives such as *Healthy People 2010* (2000) and *Closing the Gap* (2003) noted unique risk factors and imbalances in funds of knowledge particular to those with ID, in contrast to the general population. Specifically, obesity and physical inactivity were identified as problems that persons with ID were more likely to face, and more research and preventative health measures were needed in order to address these risks. Research conducted in the aftermath of these initiatives has bolstered the findings noted in *Healthy People 2010* and added to the slowly growing collection of data pertaining to individuals with ID.

Stanish *et al.* (2006) performed a literature review on the physical activity of adults with intellectual disabilities. Standard guidelines per the Health and Human Services regarding physical activity are 30 minutes of moderate physical activity on most, but preferably all, days of the week, and/or 10,000 steps per day. Additionally, research has shown that less than eight minutes of continuous activity is not sufficient (Le Masurier, 2004). Stanish *et al.* (2006) reviewed all literature to date that applied these guidelines to those with ID. The outcome revealed that only 17.5–33% of persons with ID meet these criteria. However, these estimates drop significantly when the continuity of activity is considered, as those with ID are much less likely to engage in more than five minutes of physical activity at a time.

Also of note is that the types of activity patients with ID engage in (such as walking, chores, and work) may not be sufficient to meet the guidelines of "moderate" intensity. The barriers to meeting recommendations were both congruent with the general population (time, money, and weather) and particular to those with ID (more restrictive environments that decreased independence and choices), which may account for the lower percentage of this population meeting standard guidelines.

Screening for serious diseases such as heart disease can prevent associated morbidity and mortality provided those screens meet certain standards (Wilkinson *et al.*, 2007). See Table 2 for recommendations specific to cardiac disease and metabolic side effects of medications. Cardiovascular screens in the general population were obesity/body mass index measures, lipid panels, annual glucose tests, annual blood pressure measurements and smoking cessation counseling. The original and revised SORT ratings can be found in Table 2.

These results demonstrate significant variance between the quality and applicability of routine screening measures in those with ID and those with typical intelligence. Again, it is logical to conclude that this disparity places the ID population at a disadvantage in the identification and/or prediction of heart disease, and subsequently for greater risk of morbidity and mortality.

Fleming *et al.* (2008) conducted a literature review on the prevalence of and potential treatment options for obesity in the ID population. As noted by their colleagues, Fleming *et al.* found that those with ID had higher rates of obesity than the general population. However, these increases were predominantly isolated to persons with ID with the following risk factors: female gender; elderly; residential placement with family or in non-residential/supervised facilities; and Down syndrome. Furthermore, among those with ID, persons diagnosed with mild ID were more likely to be obese than those with more severe cognitive deficits.

Individuals with mild ID are more likely to live in supported residential settings in the community or with their families, which are settings known to be associated with overweight and obesity. Sedentary lifestyle, as well as less access to preventative medical care in persons with ID, was also noted. Fleming *et al.* (2008) outlined conceivable explanations for the elevated rates of obesity, including:

- limited or no ability to understand typical methods for information dissemination (books, pamphlets, structured lectures);

- limited or absent opportunities to participate in social physical activities (team sports or organized exercise lessons);

- lack of trained staff or caregivers;

- inadequate facilities (not handicap-accessible or unstaffed);

- overprotective caregivers and parents.

In an attempt to determine what treatments might prove more effective for those with Down syndrome, Fleming *et al.* (2008) constructed a randomized control trial comparing nutrition and activity education alone (NAE) versus NAE plus behavioral intervention training for caregivers. When caregivers were taught behavioral intervention strategies, Down syndrome patients lost more weight.

Both Down syndrome (DS) and Prader-Willi syndrome (PWS) have been linked with increased prevalence of heart and metabolic disease. Approximately 1% of persons with DS have insulin-dependent diabetes and, by the age of three years, 30% of children with DS meet criteria for obesity. 40–60% of children with DS are born with congenital heart disease, such as atrio-ventricular canal defects, that in some cases will result in pulmonary hypertension.

PWS is the most common cause of genetic obesity, which is a direct consequence of the associated hyperphagia (Rubin & Crocker, 2006). Individuals with PWS suffer from impaired insulin production impairment and insulin resistance (secondary to obesity), and are therefore at increased risk for insulin-dependent diabetes mellitus.

Smoking is a risk factor for both cardiovascular disease and lung cancer, but limited data exist on smoking in adults with ID. Lower smoking rates have been noted among adults with severe/profound ID (more likely to reside in more restrictive settings), and equivalent or higher rates were found among adults with mild ID (more likely to live in less restrictive settings). Individuals with ID were more likely to quit if encouraged to do so by their doctor. Smoking cessation counseling should be provided by treating prescribers, as this is known to be effective; the interventions must be tailored to meet the needs of the individual's level of cognitive functioning (Wilkinson et al., 2007).

In a study of factors associated with obesity and coronary heart disease in people with ID, 78.8% of the patients had an elevated body mass index (BMI), 43% of persons were found to be obese, 19.9% had hypertension, 26.5% had hypercholesterolemia and 4.5% had diabetes mellitus (Sohler et al., 2009). Coronary heart disease is becoming more prevalent in the ID population, and one explanation is increasing life expectancy. There is evidence that secondary conditions related to coronary heart disease such as hypertension, hypercholesterolemia and diabetes are also becoming more prevalent in the ID population, and that these conditions may begin to affect people with ID at younger ages than in the general population.

Several factors may contribute to the high rate of obesity in the ID population (Melville et al., 2007). These include living in the community rather than in institutional settings, adopting poor diets, lack of physical activity, and the prevalence of prescription of certain psychotropic medications. Existing weight-loss programs may be difficult to access and utilize for individuals with ID given their limited cognitive abilities and skills. Most individuals with ID rely on their caregivers to access and institute such interventions. Obesity is significantly associated with age and negatively correlated with the presence of a seizure disorder (Sohler et al., 2009).

Fleming et al. (2008) found obesity rates in patients with ID similar to those in the general population, but with higher prevalence among women, the elderly and persons with Down syndrome. Higher rates of obesity were found in adults with ID who live with their families, versus those living in more structured and supervised community or institutional settings.

Gender comparisons from the medical records showed that women with ID are at greater risk of overweight and obesity when compared with men. Pertaining to age, Wilkinson et al. (2007) report that adults with ID are at risk of developing obesity at an earlier age; in fact, it appears that this is likely to occur approximately twenty years earlier when compared to the general population. When taking into account the severity of cognitive deficits, obesity is higher among adults with mild to moderate ID (27–53%) compared with adults with severe to profound ID (11–29%) (Wilkinson et al., 2007). Individuals with ID who live in more restrictive environments such as institutions or in supported group homes have a lower mean BMI than do persons who live with their families or independently. Thirty to fifty percent of adults with ID received psychotropic medication, and antipsychotic medication is associated with weight gain of adults with ID. Wilkinson et al. (2007) recommended weight measurement at least yearly and a discussion of diet and exercise with all adult patients with ID and their caregivers.

Diabetes mellitus

With the side effect profile of the second generation (or atypical) antipsychotic medications, there has recently been more attention paid to metabolic changes, especially insulin resistance and "metabolic syndrome" in adults with ID. There is little research about diabetes specific to the ID population (Wilkinson *et al.*, 2007).

Adults with ID were significantly more likely to have diabetes than their counterparts in the general population, according to Havercamp *et al.* (2004). Sohler *et al.* (2009) reported that the history of seizures and use of mood stabilizers were both associated with increased prevalence of diabetes mellitus. A complicating factor is the association between prescription of mood stabilizer/anticonvulsant medications and weight gain; however, Sohler *et al.* (2009) found an association between diabetes even after adjustment for body mass index.

According to the American Diabetic Association (ADA, 2010), people with ID and others with specialized health care needs frequently have nutrition concerns. These may include, but are not limited to, growth alterations (i.e. failure to thrive, obesity or growth retardation), metabolic disorders and poor feeding skills. Poor health habits, limited access to services and long-term use of multiple medications are considered health risk factors, and these are frequently present in individuals with ID. Individuals with special needs are more likely to develop comorbid conditions such as obesity, putting them at risk to develop diabetes.

There are recommendations for the general population to monitor for diabetes; Wilkinson *et al.* (2007) proposes that patients with ID may have risk factors that indicate earlier and/or more frequent screening is essential for glucose monitoring.

The pulmonary system

Children with severe neurologic impairments will have a higher incidence of respiratory problems, and treating these conditions is inherently more complicated due to multiple contributing factors (Seddon & Khan, 2003). Common respiratory problems tend to be over-represented in the ID population; for example, Toder (2000) reported that individuals with ID and co-occurring cerebral palsy and/or traumatic brain injury have the highest prevalence of pulmonary pathology. These conditions typically do not directly affect pulmonary structure or function but may lead secondarily to lung damage due to aspiration and ineffective cough, for example, related to neurologic dysfunction. These patients are at increased risk of morbidity and mortality of respiratory infections, due to decreased airway clearance caused by muscular weakness and inadequate lung capacity. It is vital that these individuals maintain dental hygiene and engage in physical activity fitting to their capabilities.

Conditions that adversely affect the lungs include drooling, feeding problems, gastro-esophageal reflux, aspiration, spasticity and scoliosis, and these conditions should be managed medically to the best extent possible.

Poor airway clearance may result in pneumonia and sleep apnea. Children and adolescents with cerebral palsy, other muscular disorders and traumatic brain injuries commonly experience consequences such as ineffective cough, difficulty swallowing, and lung restriction from chest wall abnormalities (Marks, 2008). If underlying respiratory conditions exist, evaluation and compliance with treatment recommendations are even more complicated. There is increased risk of jaw instability, neurologic abnormalities and recurrent aspiration. These patients are at risk for chronic airway damage, recurrent lower respiratory infections, and death.

Gastroesophageal reflux and drooling (sialorrhea) increase the prevalence of these consequences. These pulmonary conditions are associated with significant morbidity, and appropriate medical care and compliance have the potential to greatly improve quality of life for individuals with pulmonary conditions and co-occurring ID (Marks, 2008). Regarding the pulmonary system, the Canadian consensus guidelines for primary health care of adults with developmental disabilities (Sullivan *et al.*, 2006) state that it is vital to ensure vaccinations such as *Haemophilus influenzae* and *Streptococcus pneumoniae* are current.

The gastrointestinal system

Children with neuro-developmental disabilities such as cerebral palsy, spina bifida or inborn errors of metabolism, commonly experience gastrointestinal problems. Feeding difficulties, aspiration and malnutrition are all potential consequences (Sullivan, 2008).

Gastro-esophageal reflux disease (GERD) is common in children with ID (Marks, 2008). The frequent and long-term use of medications (such as antibiotics for recurrent urinary tract and/or respiratory infections) may produce or exacerbate existing gastrointestinal symptoms. Constipation is a side effect of many medications (i.e. psychotropics, anticonvulsants, etc.), which may result in fecal impactions (Marks, 2008).

The prevalence of GERD in institutionalized adults with ID with IQ < 50 is high; in Bohmer *et al.* (2000), it was reported that 50% of subjects had GERD. Identified risk factors for GERD in patients with ID include cerebral palsy, IQ < 35, scoliosis, prescription anticonvulsants or benzodiazepines, and being non-ambulatory (Bohmer *et al.*, 2000). It is imperative that individuals presenting with hematemesis (vomiting blood), dental erosions or rumination be evaluated for GERD or other gastrointestinal pathology. If GERD is suspected in a patient with ID, a 24-hour pH measurement should be ordered. Researchers recommend a low threshold for the use of proton pump inhibitors. Both GERD and constipation are very common in the ID population and may not respond to classic management interventions (Sullivan, 2008).

Clinical Vignette #2

Angelo was a 45 year old non-verbal male with history of severe ID and no previously diagnosed psychiatric disorder. He was referred for mental health evaluation for problem behavior and specifically physical aggression, which had begun approximately four years prior but had escalated in frequency and severity in recent weeks. He lived with his mother, who had raised him as a single parent since birth.

His mother explained at the first appointment that not only was the aggression directed toward her, but she had developed several medical issues herself and had concerns about who would provide care for her son if she were no longer able to do so. Angelo was taking diazepam (valium) and Percocet, both on an "as needed" or "PRN" basis since the aggression began four years prior. Angelo's mother was instructed to administer one or both medications when Angelo's problem behavior reappeared, and the medications typically sedated him.

The mother's initial comment was, "I think he's in pain but no one seems to be able to figure out the cause." Despite visits to the primary care physician every six months to get the medication refills, Angelo had not received any objective testing, nor had he been provided any preventive care typically advised for a 45 year old man. No dental care had been provided for over ten years. Angelo's mother reported that the pain seemed to be worse when he was lying in bed, and at times when he was offered food or drink, although this was episodic in nature.

Angelo was scheduled for general anesthesia at a local hospital; during a period of several hours, he underwent a thorough dental exam and teeth cleaning, computerized tomography of his abdomen and genito-urinary examination. An esophagogastroduodenoscopy (EGD) was performed to evaluate his upper gastrointestinal tract. He was found to have severe esophageal reflux disease (GERD) and an acid blocker was recommended. All other tests were normal, as was his laboratory work-up.

After a week on the appropriate medication, the aggression ceased completely. He no longer required the diazepam or the Percocet, having been on both of these for several years. He was discharged from the mental health clinic as he did not suffer from any mental disorder.

Continued untreated GERD puts patients at higher risk for developing gastrointestinal (esophageal) cancer.

Helicobacter pylori (*H. pylori*) bacterium is an identified type I carcinogen which is correlated with peptic ulcers, gastric ulcers, gastric carcinoma and primary B-cell lymphoma (Kitchens *et al.*, 2007). The prevalence of *H. pylori* infection in patients with ID is twice the rate of the general population, and even more alarming is that they experience recurrence after triple drug treatment at a rate nearly seven times that of the general population (Kitchens *et al.*, 2007). The Canadian consensus guidelines for primary health care of adults with developmental disabilities (Sullivan *et al.*, 2006) recommend that the physician check for *H. pylori* infection if there are persistent signs of dyspepsia or unexplained behavioral changes, and to retest for *H. pylori* in three to five years after eradication of the bacteria. Untreated GERD and other gastrointestinal (GI) pathology place the individual at risk for malignancies; in fact, GI malignancy accounts for almost 50% of all cancer deaths in the ID population.

Khalid & Al-Salamah (2006) reported that the general surgical problems related to the gastrointestinal system necessitating admission in adult patients with ID included history of pica in 33% of cases. Volvulus of the colon (22.2%) and pseudo-obstruction (18.5%) were the most common causes of acute abdomen in this study. In cases of upper GI bleeding, the most common cause (57.7%) was reflux esophagitis. This is replicated in other studies (Khalid *et al.*, 2008, Orchard *et al.*, 1995). Khalid & Al-Salamah (2006) speculated that patients with ID not only experience these conditions at a higher prevalence, but also may have a higher threshold to pain when compared to the general population. To complicate matters, they do not communicate symptoms or display signs early in the course of the illness.

Identified risk factors for acute abdominal disorders in this study were male gender and history of pica. Orchard *et al.* (1995) reported that identified risk factors for erosive esophagitis in the ID population included hiatal hernia, sedentary lifestyle, incontinence, hypoalbuminemia, kyphoscoliosis and spastic quadriplegia. The clinician should have a high index of suspicion for acute abdomen pathology if a patient with ID presents with vomiting, abdominal distension, fever or acute increase in irritability.

Clinical Vignette #3

Suzanne, a 52 year old non-verbal female with history of profound intellectual disability, osteoarthritis and cerebral palsy, was referred to the mental health clinic by direct care staff, who had requested the referral for "behavioral problems."

Suzanne had no previous history of mental health problems and, in fact, had never been evaluated by a mental health professional. However, her caregivers reported a four-month history of anger outbursts, paranoia, physical aggression toward staff, weight loss of 13 pounds and attempts to ingest non-food items such as towels, pieces of clothing and blankets, and also unused incontinence pads. Her appetite was described as "decreased" and, in the previous four weeks, she had begun to gag herself, with no identified pattern, antecedents or precipitants to this behavior. Interventions up to that point included attempts to introduce a behavior support plan, wherein she was rewarded when not aggressive, but this had evoked no improvement. The aggression was notably more prevalent when Suzanne was offered food and drink.

Significant psychosocial factors include the death of Suzanne's sister, almost exactly one year prior to the date of the psychiatric assessment. She had been very close to her sister and she had spent every weekend with her until the sister found herself with terminal illness. Following her sister's death, Suzanne's uncle had taken over guardianship of her person and also had begun spending more time with Suzanne until approximately four months prior, when the uncle moved from the area. Since that time, the uncle had been unable to interface with Suzanne nearly as frequently as before, due to his own medical treatment and deteriorating medical condition.

The direct care staff also reported that the patient had been in the same supported residential placement for over ten years with consistent direct care staff but, with her recent history of aggression, they had initiated an assessment to have her moved to a Developmental Center, the only remaining institutional setting in the state for individuals with intellectual disabilities. They no longer felt they could support her in the community setting and felt that a more restricted environment was necessary.

Suzanne was referred to a gastrointestinal specialist, due to the ingestion of non-food items and her weight loss and loss of appetite. After objective testing, she was found to have a sigmoid volvulus and it appeared as though the sigmoid was twisted, which resulted in inadequate blood flow and bowel obstruction. This resulted in a sigmoid resection with colostomy. Since her behavior had changed dramatically over the previous four months until the surgery was performed, it was thought that perhaps her bowel had been twisting and untwisting during that time.

Following recovery from her surgery, the management of the supported living setting had Suzanne re-evaluated, with a new comprehensive psychological evaluation, and it was determined that she could successfully remain at the same residential placement where she had resided for over ten years.

At follow-up three months after intake, Suzanne presented appearing calm and relaxed with her direct care staff. She was able to continue to live in her supported living situation in the community. The transfer to the Developmental Center had been cancelled, and no further psychiatric follow-up was necessary.

Menstrual-related issues

One of most significant inequalities in medical care reported in the ID population is breast and cervical cancer screening. In a study by Havercamp *et al.* (2004), 11.5% of women with

ID reported never having visited a gynecologist, and as a group they were significantly less likely to have ever undergone mammography. Despite the recommendation in the United States for women to have mammograms every 1–2 years beginning at age 40 years, 26.8% of the women with ID aged 40 and older in Havercamp's study had no previously documented mammogram.

The start of menstruation involves layers of complication, because of privacy issues and the need for additional assistance in managing personal care and hygiene in the ID population which likely had pre-existing dependency needs. Dizon *et al.* (2005) studied menstrual and contraceptive issues among young women (ages 8 through 17 years) with ID. Caregivers often approach physicians (~90% of the time in this study) for menstrual suppression prior to menarche (in 40% of cases), with the primary concern being personal hygiene or "problems coping" with impending onset of menstruation. With current pharmacologic interventions, menstrual periods can be regulated and/or suppressed. Depo-Provera was the most commonly prescribed and accepted method of menstrual suppression in Dizon's study population.

Currently there is no identified standard or consensus on how to best meet the gynecologic needs of the ID population. Dizon *et al.* (2005) found that 49% of the subjects complained of spotting or breakthrough bleeding. Monitoring must be done for adverse effects of Depo-Provera including, but not limited to, decreased bone density, osteopenia, weight gain and abdominal pain.

Of post-menarchal women with ID, only 40% had irregular menstrual bleeding, so the request for suppression of menses was frequently made for non-medical reasons. Many caregivers feared that patients with baseline bowel or bladder incontinence would not be able to navigate the addition of menstrual hygiene care. The mean age of menarche in this study population was 12.13 years, which is not significantly different from the mean age in general for North American females (Dizon *et al.*, 2005).

Prior to the study, the hypothesis was that the majority of caregivers would be concerned with fertility issues, but this was not the case. Regarding the use of alternate forms of birth control, intrauterine devices should be utilized with great caution, due to the apparent increased pain threshold and therefore decreased ability of patients to report discomfort. Weekly transdermal patches may be promising in this population.

Burke *et al.* (2010) studied the gynecologic issues of adolescents with ID. Adolescent girls with diagnoses of Down syndrome, autism and cerebral palsy presented for gyneco-logic treatment most frequently for menstruation problems (menorrhagia, dysmenorrhea, irregular bleeding and hygiene issues) and mood/behavior changes. Medications frequently prescribed to patients with ID, such as anticonvulsants and antipsychotics, can affect cycling and nutritional issues. Bleeding abnormalities were the most prevalent complaint, and oral hormonal medications were the most commonly prescribed intervention. Burke *et al.* (2010) found that menarche may occur later on average in patients with cerebral palsy, compared to the general population.

Female patients with autism were much more likely to present with mood disturbances related to their menses (Burke *et al.*, 2010). There is inconclusive data regarding the efficacy of hormonal treatment for mood disorders; in fact, some patients report worsening symptoms. Oral contraceptives have been shown to improve physical symptoms related to menses, and suppression of the menstrual cycle is an option in these cases. Because other patients may benefit from anti-inflammatory drugs, Burke's study recommends this medication class be considered a good first line option, using caution in patients who may be at risk for GI upset with NSAIDs.

As with other medical conditions, patients with ID may have limited capacity to report pain, and the result may be externalization of their discomfort, with behavioral and/or mood changes. Selective serotonin reuptake inhibitors (SSRIs) have been shown effective for severe mood and physical symptoms in premenstrual syndrome, as well as pre-menstrual dysphoric disorder in placebo-controlled studies.

Quint *et al.* (1999) studied behavior problems in females with ID, including self-mutilation, aggression and other behavior problems, and found that 65% showed improvement with the use of non-steroidal anti-inflammatory drugs (NSAIDs). Oral contraceptives were effective in decreasing behavior issues in 40%. Depo-Provera injections were successful in treating 66% of the women in this study. The study posited that, with respect to the cyclical behavior seen in females with ID, approximately 18% appeared to be related to pain secondary to menstruation, based on 65% of the patients who responded to NSAIDS.

Various presentations of aggression are fairly common among people with ID. It can be caused by any chronic painful condition or it may be a form of communication. Because NSAIDs were helpful in 65% of patients, there should be a high index of suspicion for painful dysmenorrhea to be high with behavioral presentations. It was proposed by Quint *et al.* (1999) that NSAIDs be considered as an initial intervention, with birth control pills and depo-medroxyprogesterone tried subsequently. These hormonal options improved behavior in 40–66% of patients.

Premenstrual symptoms are common in women in the general population, and it is estimated that 80% of women of reproductive age in the general population experience

Clinical Vignette #4

Joanie is a 27 year old female with moderate ID who presented to a local mental health clinic for assessment of aggressive behavior toward others, with more severe and frequent episodes in her habilitation setting.

Upon interview, it was discovered that Joanie wore incontinence undergarments due to a urinary tract condition, and she was embarrassed by this. She started wearing the undergarments approximately three months prior to the assessment because her direct care staff discussed the "accidents" with her primary care physician. At that time, she underwent urinalysis to check for urinary tract infection and this was ruled out. To further investigate possible urinary tract pathology, the PCP ordered a bladder ultrasound. The direct care staff did not communicate this to the group home manager, so the test was never scheduled or performed.

Approximately one month later, the staff became frustrated with the frequency of changing sheets due to bed wetting and the amount of laundry Joanie required, and they asked that her aunt (an infrequent visitor, but her guardian, who made herself available for additional expenses that Joanie's disability income would not cover) supply the undergarments. Joanie was angry about this decision, but she was required to wear them both during daytime hours and overnight.

At work, her staff would ensure she was provided a new undergarment each time she used the restroom. Her co-workers become aware of this and teased her about it. There was a temporal relationship between the onset of aggression toward others and the introduction of the undergarments. During the assessment, the psychiatrist reviewed the medical records and found that the bladder ultrasound had been ordered but not scheduled or performed. Joanie verbalized her embarrassment regarding the undergarments, but denied anxiety, depression or other mental health symptoms.

Arrangements were made to schedule the ultrasound, which showed several small cysts. These were subsequently biopsied and found to be benign, but they were causing interruption in the control and flow of urine from the bladder to the urethra. Joanie underwent surgical removal of the cysts and the urinary incontinence was resolved. She no longer needed to use the incontinence undergarments, and the aggression resolved shortly afterward.

premenstrual syndrome or menstrual-related mood disorders (Quint *et al.*, 1999). Of these, 20–40% of women report "some difficulty" and 5% report a "significant impact on work and lifestyle."

Cancer

Certain cancer types appear to be slightly more prevalent in adults with ID, although rates of adenomatous polyps in institutionalized adults with ID approximated that of the general population in one small study. Constipation is a common problem for adults with ID living in group homes, making early detection of colon cancer symptoms difficult, and this is complicated by the prevalence of psychotropic medications prescribed in this population. Wilkinson *et al.* (2007) recommended that the United States Task Force Guidelines for colon cancer screening should be followed without alteration for adults with ID.

Breast cancer in women with ID was only slightly lower than that of the general population. It is it well documented that parity and history of breast-feeding have an impact on the prevalence rates of certain cancer types. Women with ID are less likely to have children and thus to breast-feed. Unfortunately, they are also less likely to undergo mammography. It appears that providers do not recommend standard preventive care to individuals with ID, so this is not an issue with compliance or patient cooperation. Since women with ID are living longer, primary care providers should make every effort to obtain mammograms at regular intervals, as recommended for individuals in the general population.

Cervical cancer screening for women is a topic of controversy. Cervical cancer is related to the number of sexual partners and frequency of sexual activity. Fewer women with ID are sexually active, putting them at a much lower risk group for cervical cancer. Two studies of institutionalized women with ID showed that the incidence of abnormal cervical cytology was extremely low (Wilkinson *et al.*, 2007).

Women with ID living in the community are more likely to be sexually active, however, but were not included in these studies. Therefore, no generalizable conclusions can be made for cervical screening. There exist other indications to do periodic gynecologic examinations, i.e. to evaluate for fibroids, ovarian masses, or dysmenorrhea. The available data argues against routine annual Pap tests in women with ID, but Wilkinson *et al.* (2007) ultimately recommends the decision be based on the woman's sexual and family history, as opposed to her cognitive ability. The physician should individualize the interval for cervical screening, based on the individual patient's risks.

Prostate cancer screening was shown in two large studies to document lower rates in men with ID, compared to the general population (Wilkinson *et al.*, 2007). Symptom detection and reporting are important for early detection and evaluation of these types of cancer. Wilkinson *et al.* (2007) recommended that physicians should screen their adult patients with ID as they would other adults, until more data is available.

Osteoporosis

Adults with ID have a documented increased prevalence of osteoporosis. This even applies to premenopausal women and men and is not limited to postmenopausal women (Wilkinson *et al.*, 2007). Risk factors for osteoporosis were identified in a 2006 review of the literature and included inactivity, long-term anticonvulsant use and possibly Down syndrome (Wilkinson *et al.*, 2007). Multiple previous studies documented the high rates of osteopenia and osteoporosis in adults with ID and cited the same risk factors, in addition to low serum vitamin D levels.

Zylstra *et al.* (2008) reported that significant risk factors for osteoporosis included subject age, race and level of ambulation. Other studies confirm these results. Center *et al.* (in Sutherland *et al.*, 2002, p. 8) also reported that individuals who were unable adequately to bear weight, such as people with mobility problems, are likely candidates for osteoporosis. The total rate of osteoporosis for the ID study population, as measured by dual-energy x-ray absorptiometry (DXA) scans of the femur, was 17.1%; the total rate of osteopenia for the same subjects was 51.0%. Neither gender, nor the severity of ID, affected prevalence.

Interestingly, individuals with diagnosis of metabolic errors had a significantly lower rate of osteoporosis. Zylstra *et al.* (2008) found the rate of osteoporosis to be higher in men with ID, when compared to males in the general population. The researchers proposed that asymptomatic males in the general population may be under-represented. They concluded that prevention and treatment of osteoporosis will be of increasing importance for the ID population as life expectancy increases.

The literature identifies a significant relationship in the rate of osteoporosis with both age and race; medical conditions associated include Celiac disease, Crohn's disease, amenorrhea and disabilities that limit weight bearing, among many others (Zylstra *et al.*, 2008). While there is limited data on osteoporosis in the ID population, it is documented that fractures are more common, and this may signify a causal relationship. Caucasians are at higher risk than African Americans in both community and institutionalized populations. Studies suggest that bone density improves with physical activity.

The rates of 19.2% for men and 14.5% of women are similar to those reported by others in the ID population, but they are distinctly different from those in the general population, as reported by the Centers for Disease Control and Prevention (CDC) (2% for men and 16% for women) and the National Osteoporosis Foundation (7% for men and 20% for women) (Zylstra *et al.*, 2005, Table 5). The recommendation from the Wilkinson study is that, given the high rates of osteoporosis documented among adults with ID, earlier screening should be implemented, beginning at younger ages (40 years if living in an institution, 45 if community dwelling) (Wilkinson *et al.*, 2007).

Sensory deficits

Visual problems are more common in adults with ID in all literature reviewed by Wilkinson, including both domestic and international studies (Wilkinson, 2007). The patients with ID, however, may be less likely to report visual symptoms or to have regular ophthalmic care. The method of screening must be individualized for patients with communication and perceptual limitations. Both vision and hearing problems can have a disproportionate influence on adults with ID; sensory input is one compensatory mechanism to assuage the cognitive deficits. The Canadian consensus guidelines for primary health care of adults with developmental disabilities (Sullivan *et al.*, 2006) recommend referral of patients with ID for vision and glaucoma assessments at least once before age 40 (age 30 for patients with DS), then every two years after age 40.

Hearing problems also have been found to be more prevalent in adults with ID. Studies conducted in the Netherlands (Zarchi *et al.*, 2011) show higher rates of hearing loss in older patients with ID, and emphasize the role of cerumen impaction, which is easily treatable. High rates of hearing loss are reported in Turner syndrome, Down syndrome, Williams syndrome and velocardiofacial syndrome (also known as 22q11 deletion syndrome). The high rates suggest a relationship between the auditory system and variety of genetic defects (Zarchi *et al.*, 2011).

Mild hearing loss can have devastating costs, even for typically developing children, particularly with vocabulary comprehension and syntax skills, receptive language skills and development of attention and concentration patterns (Marler *et al.*, 2010). Vision and hearing screening should be performed regularly for adults with ID, because the consequences of not screening are potentially substantial (Wilkinson *et al.*, 2007). The Canadian consensus guidelines for primary health care of adults with developmental disabilities (Sullivan *et al.*, 2006) recommend referral of patients with ID for hearing assessment every five years after age 45 (every three years throughout life for patients with DS). The guidelines also recommend consideration of screening of both vision and hearing at times when unexplained behavioral changes are noted.

Conclusion

Individuals with ID are a substantial and important part of the general population. Research and data gathering pertaining to those with ID has increased, but it is still quite deficient when compared to that for their non-ID peers. The limited available data suggest that there is an essential need to understand, and therefore appropriately treat, these individuals' unique needs. See Table 3 for clinical pearls.

Individuals with ID are at a significantly higher risk of having comorbid medical, genetic and psychiatric conditions that, in turn, place them at greater risk for medical conditions involving every organ system. The over-prescribing of antipsychotic medications and general polypharmacy issues further complicate this situation. The use of older, or first generation, antipsychotics can cause extrapyramidal side effects, and the use of newer, or second generation, neuroleptics increases the risk of cardiac and metabolic problems, including diabetes, obesity and hyperlipidemia. Developmental syndromes are each associated with specific medical conditions, and the knowledgeable clinician will be cognizant of conditions which occur with higher prevalence. This ensures that the patient's biological needs, as well as psychological needs, are met.

Patients with ID are less likely to participate in, or be exposed to, traditional preventative and treatment methods. There are sometimes logistical considerations when attempting to screen patients with ID, but the barriers to treatment must be overcome at all costs. It is well

Table 3 Clinical Pearls.

- When being weighed or measured, some patients with moderate to severe ID can be anxious or frightened because they may feel somewhat unsteady. These patients can be weighed at home on a bathroom scale in a more familiar environment. For patients who are unstable when standing, or who have comorbid physical disabilities, the scale may need to be larger and with more supports.
- Blood pressure could be assessed in a similar manner. "White coat hypertension" might be more prevalent in people with ID. Portable electronic blood pressure monitors are relatively inexpensive and can be used at any time. Home monitors can measure the blood pressure in a relaxed, familiar environment.
- Blood draws can be done at home under certain circumstances, and this technique may be preferable to a laboratory environment, where the patient is very fearful. For cholesterol and glucose testing, it is sometimes acceptable to use finger stick measurements if this is easier. Studies have shown that finger stick measurement is acceptable for screening purposes, especially in low to moderate risk patients younger than 65 years. However, finger stick values can overestimate HDL and underestimate LDL, so treatment decisions should ideally be based on venous samples.
- Vision screening often requires adaptive methods in patients with moderate to severe ID, and it should be done by specialists if it cannot be done reliably by the primary care provider.
- Clinicians must always look for cerumen as the first step in hearing screening. Patients can then have a basic hearing test, either in a primary care office or with an audiologist if needed.
- For some adults with ID, sedation is required for routine procedures like dental work, endoscopic procedures or minor surgery.
- With menstrual-related psychopathology, consult OBGYN to discuss regulation of menstrual periods (i.e. q 3 months)
- If a patient has any chronic pain condition, rule out exacerbation at the onset of any problem behavior, as well as PCP exam and lab work up.

Source: adapted from McDermott *et al.* (2006) and Wilkinson *et al.* (2007).

documented that individuals with severe and chronic psychiatric illnesses have greatly reduced life expectancy. It is also clear from the literature that preventive medical care and treatment of existing medical conditions is lacking in patients with ID. The result is a higher prevalence of morbidity and mortality when compared to individuals in the general population.

Since many patients with communication deficits exhibit behavioral changes or acute psychiatric symptoms when experiencing medical conditions, the mental health clinician often plays a vital role in facilitating access to appropriate care.

References

American Diabetic Association (2010). Providing Nutrition Services for People with Developmental Disabilities and Special Health Care Needs. *Journal of the American Dietetic Association* **110**, 296–307.

Beange, H., McElduff, A. & Baker, W. (1995). Medical disorders of adults with mental retardation: a population study, *American Journal on Mental Retardation* **99**, 595–604.

Bittles, A.H., Petterson, B.A., Sullivan, S.G., Hussain, R., Glasson, E.J. & Montgomery P.D. (2002). The influence of intellectual disability on life expectancy. *Journals of Gerontology Series A: Biological Sciences and Medical Sciences* **57**, M470–M472.

Bohmer, C.J., Klinkenberg-Knol, E.C., Niezen-de Boer, M.C. & Meuwissen, S.G. (2000). Gastroesophageal reflux disease in intellectually disabled individuals: how often, how serious, how manageable? *American Journal of Gastroenterology* **95**(8), 1868–1872.

Burke, L.M., Kalpakjian, C.Z., Smith, Y.R. & Quint, E.H. (2010). Gynecologic Issues of Adolescents with Down Syndrome, Autism and Cerebral Palsy. *Journal of Pediatric and Adolescent Gynecology* **23**, 11–15.

Chaney, R.H. & Eyman, R.K. (2000). Patterns of mortality over 60 years among persons with mental retardation in a residential facility. *Mental Retardation* **38**, 289–293.

Dizon, C.D., Allen, L.M. & Ornstein, M.P. (2005). Menstrual and Contraceptive Issues among Young Women with Developmental Delay: A Retrospective Review of Cases at the Hospital for Sick Children, Toronto. *Journal of Pediatric and Adolescent Gynecology* **18**, 157–162.

Dykens, E.M., Hodapp, R.M. & Finucane, B.M. (2000) *Genetics and mental retardation syndromes: A new look at behavior and interventions.* Paul H Brookes Publishing, Baltimore, MD.

Fleming, R.K., Stokes, E.A., Curtin, C., Bandini, L.G., Gleason, J., Scampini, R., Maslin, M.C.T. & Hamad, C. (2008). Behavioral Health in Developmental Disabilities: A Comprehensive Program of Nutrition, Exercise, and Weight Reduction. *International Journal of Behavioral Consultation and Therapy* **4**(3), 287–296.

Goldstein, S. & Reynolds, C.R. (1999). *Handbook of neurodevelopmental and genetic disorders in children.* Guilford Press, New York.

Havercamp, S.M., Scandlin, D. & Roth, M. (2004). Health Disparities Among Adults with Developmental Disabilities, Adults with Other Disabilities, and Adults Not Reporting Disability in North Carolina. *Public Health Reports* **119**, 418–426.

Hayden, M.F. (1998). Mortality among people with mental retardation living in the United States: Research review and policy application. *Mental Retardation* **36**, 345–359.

Janicki, M.P. & Breitenbach, N. (2000). Aging and intellectual disabilities – improving longevity and promoting healthy aging: Summative report. Geneva, World Health Organization.

Khalid, K. & Al-Salamah, S.M. (2006). Spectrum of general surgical problems in the developmentally disabled adults. *Saudi Medical Journal* **27**(1), 70–75.

Khalid, K., Al-Salamah, S.M., Al-Teimi, I. & Al-Dossary, N.F. (2008). Gastrointestinal tract bleeding in intellectually disabled adults. *Southern Medical Journal* **101**(1), 29–34.

Kitchens, D.H., Binkley, C.J., Wallace, D.L. & Darling, D. (2007). *Helicobacter pylori* infection in people who are intellectually and developmentally disabled: a review. *Special Care in Dentistry* **27**(4), 127–33.

Le Masurier, K. (2004). Pedometer sensitivity and specificity. *Medicine & Science in Sports & Exercise* **36**(2), 346.

Marks, J.H. (2008). Pulmonary Care of Children and Adolescents with Developmental Disabilities. *Pediatric Clinics of North America* **55**(6), 1299–1314.

Marler, J.A., Sitcovsky, J.L., Mervis, C.B., Kistler, D.J. & Wightman, F.L. (2010). Auditory Function and Hearing Loss in Children and Adults with Williams Syndrome: Cochlear Impairment in Individuals with Otherwise Normal Hearing. *American Journal of Medical Genetics Part C* (Seminars in Medical Genetics) **154C**, 249–265.

McDermott, S., Moran, R., Platt, T. & Dasari, S. (2006). Variation in Health Conditions Among Groups of Adults with Disabilities in Primary Care. *Journal of Community Health* **31**(3), 147–159.

Melville, C.A., Hamilton, S., Hankey, C.R., Miller, S. & Boyle, S. (2007). The prevalence and determinants of obesity in adults with intellectual disabilities. *Obesity Reviews* **8**, 223–230.

Orchard, J.L., Stramat, J., Wolfgang, M. & Trimpey, A. (1995). Upper gastrointestinal tract bleeding in institutionalized mentally retarded adults. Primary role of esophagitis. *Archives of Family Medicine* **4**(1), 30–33.

Patja, M., Iivanainen, H., Vesla, H., Oksanen, H. & Ruopplia, I. (2000). Life expectancy of people with intellectual disability: A 35 year follow up study. *Journal of Intellectual Disability Research* **44**, 591–599.

Quint, E.H., Elkins, T.E., Sorg, C.A. & Kope, S. (1999). The Treatment of Cyclical Behavioral Changes in Women with Mental Disabilities. *Journal of Pediatric and Adolescent Gynecology* **12**, 139–142.

Reiss, S. & Aman, M.G. (1998). *Psychotropic medications and developmental disabilities: The international consensus handbook* (Chapter 4: Guidelines for the Use of Psychotropic Medication). The Nisonger Center UAP, Columbus, OH.

Rimmer, J.H., Braddock, D. & Fujiura, G. (1994). Cardiovascular Risk Factor Levels in Adults with Mental Retardation. *American Journal on Mental Retardation* **98**(4), 510–518.

Rubin, I.L. & Crocker, A.C. (eds, 2006). *Developmental Disabilities: Delivery of Medical Care for Children and Adults* (2nd ed.). Paul H, Brookes Publishing Co., Baltimore, MD.

Rueve, M. & Welton, R. (2008). Violence in Mental Illness. *Psychiatry* (Edgemont), **5**(5), 35–48.

Ryan, R. (2003). *Intensive Conference on Dual Diagnosis*. The Community Circle, Denver, CO. CME Event.

Seddon, P.C. & Khan, Y. (2003). Respiratory problems in children with neurological impairment. *Archives of Disease in Childhood* **88**(1), 75–8.

Silka, V.R. & Hauser, M.J. (1997). Psychiatric Assessment of the Person with Mental Retardation. *Psychiatric Annals* **27**(3), 162–169.

Smith, G.A. (1999). *Closing the Gap: Addressing the Needs of People with Developmental Disabilities Waiting for Supports*, National Association of State Directors of Developmental Disability Services (NASDDDS), "A Special Studies Initiative" Report, May 1999.

Sohler, N., Lubetkin, E., Levy, J., Soghomonian, C. & Rimmerman, A. (2009). Factors Associated with Obesity and Coronary Heart Disease in People with Intellectual Disabilities. *Social Work in Health Care*, **48**, 76–89.

Stanish, H.I., Temple, V.A. & Frey G.C. (2006). Health-Promoting Physical Activity of Adults with Mental Retardation. *Mental Retardation and Developmental Disabilities Research Reviews* **12**, 13–21.

Sullivan, P.B. (2008). Gastrointestinal disorders in children with neurodevelopmental disabilities. *Developmental Disabilities Research Reviews* **14**(2), 128–36.

Sullivan, W.F., Heng, J., Cameron, D., Lunsky, Y., Cheetham, T., Hennen, B., Bradley, E.A., Berg, J.M., Korossy, M., Forster-Gibson, C., Gitta, M., Stavrakaki, C., McCreary, B. & Swift, I. (2006). Consensus guidelines for primary health care of adults with developmental disabilities. *Canadian Family Physician* **52**, 1410–1418.

Sutherland, G., Murray, S. & Iacono, T. (2002). Health issues for adults with developmental disability. *Research in Developmental Disabilities* **23**(6), 422–445.

Tasman, A., Kay, J. & Lieberman, J.A. (Eds., 2003) *Psychiatry* 2nd ed. Wiley, Chichester, UK.

Tighe, C.A. (2001). "Working at disability": A qualitative study of the meaning of health and disability for women with physical impairments. *Disability and Society* **16**, 511–529.

Toder, D.S. (2000). Respiratory problems in the adolescent with developmental delay. *Adolescent Medicine* **11**(3), 617–31.

United States Dept. of Health and Human Services (2000). *Healthy People 2010* (2nd ed.). US Government Printing Office, Washington, DC.

United States Dept. of Health and Human Services, Agency for Healthcare Research and
Quality. US Preventive Services Task Force (cited 2007, February 27). Available from www.
ahrq.gov/clinic/uspsfix.htm

Van Dyke, D.C., Mattheis, P.J., Schoon, E. & Williams, J. (1995). *Medical and Surgical Care for
Children with Down Syndrome*. Woodbine House, Bethesda, MD.

Wilkinson, J.E., Culpepper, L. & Cerreto, M. (2007). Screening Tests for Adults with Intellectual
Disabilities. *Journal of the American Board of Family Medicine* **20**, 399–407.

Zarchi, O., Attias, J., Raveh, E., Basel-Vanagaite, L., Saporta, L. & Gothelf, D.A. (2011).
Comparative Study of Hearing Loss in Two Microdeletion Syndromes: Velocardiofacial
(22q11.2 Deletion) and Williams (7q11.23 Deletion) Syndromes. *Journal of Pediatrics* **158**
(2), 301–6.

Zylstra, R.G., Porter, L.L., Shapiro, J.L. & Prater, C.D. (2008). Prevalence of Osteoporosis in
Community-Dwelling Individuals with Intellectual and/or Developmental Disabilities.
Journal of the American Medical Directors Association **9**(2), 109–113.

4

Neurologic Conditions

Paulette Marie Gillig, MD, PhD, Professor, Wright State University, Dayton, Ohio
Richard Sanders, MD, Associate Professor, Wright State University, Dayton, Ohio

Introduction

A large number of persons with intellectual disabilities (ID) have other neuropsychiatric impairments (Kaufman, 2007; Gaultieri, 2002; Corbett, 1979). In many of these persons, the neurological impairments also are associated with psychiatric morbidity (Reiss *et al.*, 1982).

The most common presenting signs of ID are behavior disturbances, language delay, fine motor/adaptive delay, gross motor delay, and neurological and physical abnormalities. From a neurological perspective, the most common findings are the presence of frontal release signs such as a suck or snout reflex, a muscle tone decrease, strength and coordination problems, deep tendon reflexes being increased or decreased, ataxia or other gait disturbances, stereotypies (repetitive simple movements or behaviors) and electroencephalogram (EEG) abnormalities (often in absence of clinical seizures).

Dysmorphic features

The development of the brain, the rest of the nervous system, and its related vasculature, are very closely linked with the development of the structures of the face (Jones, 1988). As a result, a number of neurological syndromes that cause ID are accompanied by "dysmorphic features." Dysmorphic features are various atypical constructions of face and sometimes other parts of the body.

Psychiatry of Intellectual Disability: A Practical Manual, First Edition.
Edited by Julie P. Gentile and Paulette M. Gillig.
© 2012 John Wiley & Sons, Ltd. Published 2012 by John Wiley & Sons, Ltd.

Fragile X syndrome (see also Chapter 16)

Boys with Fragile X syndrome (FXS) develop macrocephaly and testicular enlargement in early childhood and prognathism after puberty, and often have large ears. FXS is probably the most common cause of inherited ID (Fatemi & Folsom, 2010). It is related to excessive repetitions of the CGG trinucleide on the X chromosome, so is said to be "X-linked." About 70% of boys who inherit the abnormal gene have moderate to severe ID. They may have a mild-to-profound learning disability, and 60% have features of autism and repetitive speech and other stereotypies (Finestack *et al.*, 2009; Hier *et al.*, 1980; Gerald, 1976). Most girls do not have major symptoms, although up to one third have subtle cognitive impairment (Rodriguez-Ravenga *et al.*, 2010). Patients may present to the psychiatrist because of emotional lability (Freund *et al.*, 1993).

Cornelia de lange syndrome (Bachman-de Lange syndrome)

Cornelia de Lange syndrome is a disorder that can occur sporadically or can be transmitted as an autosomal dominant disorder. People with this disorder have the physical features of small stature, brachycephaly, bushy eyebrows with long eyelashes, and a low posterior hairline. Neuropsychiatric symptoms include moderate to severe learning difficulties, autism and self-destructive behavior. The disorder is notable for the person's rejection of physical contact and an apparent lack of emotional expression, except for the enjoyment of rapid movement.

Prader-Willi syndrome

Prader-Willi syndrome is a sporadically occurring form of ID. These patients are obese and have strabismus, small stature and small hands and feet; boys have small genitalia, with cryptorchidism. Neurological symptoms include hypotonia and extreme flexibility. They have moderate to severe learning difficulties and they may be brought to the psychiatrist's attention because they have episodes of stubbornness, rages, a tendency to verbally perseverance on favorite topics and a compulsion to eat. These patients also may develop anxiety that is accompanied by skin picking, and sometimes they have hallucinations. They may develop paranoia and depression. Behavioral problems are the most common cause of hospitalization (Clark *et al.*, 1995; Holm *et al.*, 1993).

Angelman syndrome

Angelman syndrome occurs sporadically. Patients' appearance is notable because of microcephaly, maxillary hypoplasia, deep-set eyes, a large mouth with tongue protrusion, prognathia and widely spaced teeth. The patients maintain elbows and wrists in a flexed position. This disorder usually caused by a deletion or inactivation of the genes on chromosome 15 that were inherited from the mother, with the normal paternal copy having been genetically "silenced" by the maternal copy. This "silencing" is most prominent in the hippocampus and cerebellum, and it is reflected in the type of neurological deficits that patients have – an ataxic gait and severe learning difficulties.

These patients develop little or no speech, and have paroxysms of inappropriate laughter. They apparently have little need for sleep (or perhaps it may be an inability to sleep), and usually have epilepsy and an abnormal electroencephalogram (Dan, 2009; Williams *et al.*, 2006; White *et al.*, 2006; Williams, 2005; Anderson *et al.*, 2001; Lann *et al.*, 1996; Buntinx *et al.*, 1995; Williams *et al.*, 1995).'

Williams syndrome (see also Chapter 16)

Williams syndrome (WS) is a disorder of chromosome 7 and is associated with mild to severe ID and delayed acquisition of motor milestones. People with WS have a short, broad forehead, prominent cheeks, a flat-bridged nose, nostrils that are full and turn slightly upward, and hypoplastic teeth that are widely spaced. They have, unfortunately, a very poor sense of visual-spatial relationships (Lenhoff *et al.*, 1997). Sometimes they may have symptoms of generalized anxiety disorder and attention deficit hyperactivity disorder. However, these patients sometimes possess extraordinary talents in music and in verbal fluency. People with WS also may come to the attention of a psychiatrist because their behavior is getting them into difficult situations from which they need to be extracted. For example, they are sometimes "too" loquacious and "over-friendly," and they have a great deal of empathy for other people but few boundaries.

Clinical Vignette #1

An eleven year old boy with Williams syndrome reportedly was visiting his aunt. They were walking through a hotel lobby and the boy was talking amiably and non-stop about his piano lesson, at which he excelled. The boy suddenly was distracted and took a detour into the middle of a banquet hall, where a wedding ceremony was taking place. He immediately walked down the aisle, but with some difficulty (due to visuospatial problems) and approached the bride's mother, whom he thought was the bride. He began to tell everyone about how beautiful Mom had looked on her wedding day.

The mother was amused (and flattered) to be thought of as the bride and the boy immediately noticed the mother's pleasure and persisted in the conversation, despite efforts at redirection from the minister, the groom and the organist, delaying the ceremony but delighting the guests. When the boy saw the organ, he sat down and began to play "Here Comes the Bride."

Velo-cardio-facial syndrome and DiGeorge syndrome

Velo-cardio-facial syndrome (and DiGeorge syndrome, where there is additionally a severe immune deficiency due to lack of the thymus gland) involves a chromosomal deletion in the region of 22qll.2. Both conditions involve heart defects, and there are characteristic facial features which can include small ears with squared upper ear; hooded eyelids; cleft lip and/ or palate; asymmetric facial appearance when crying; and small mouth, chin and side areas of the nose tip. These facial features may be associated with changes in brain morphology, as seen on MRI scan. These persons may develop behavioral problems, and there is mild developmental delay associated with learning disabilities. As adults, these patients may develop "schizophrenia" (one third of patients) or bipolar disorder (Feinstein *et al.*, 2002; Vantrappen *et al.*, 2001).

Clinical Vignette #2

This individual is a 40 year old man with velo-cardio-facial syndrome. He left school in the 8th grade, when he was 16 years old. His parents had been told that he had a learning disability, and he had also difficulty in conforming to classroom rules, resulting in some school suspensions. He was teased and excluded by many of the other children and felt quite isolated.

At the age of 17, he became convinced that his father was "the devil." He was hospitalized at the age of 21 due to a suicide attempt. In-patient evaluation included an MRI, which was remarkable for cysts adjacent to the frontal horns of the lateral ventricles, a small cerebellar vermis and a small posterior fossa.

His symptoms of depression and suicidal feelings improved with treatment but, despite management with antipsychotics, he continued to periodically experience auditory and olfactory hallucinations, thought blocking, bizarre delusions and paranoid ideas.

Neurocutaneous stigmata

Neurofibromatosis

There are two types of neurofibromatosis, but only Type 1 is related to behavioral and cognitive impairments. Neurofibromatosis Type 1 is autosomal dominant in 50% of cases, affecting chromosome 17. The other 50% of cases are sporadic. Neurocutaneous stigmata include café-au-lait spots that develop after one year of age. Café-au-lait spots are simply areas of uniformly light brown, oval and flat skin. Also, patients may develop freckles in the axillary or inguinal areas by three years, and cutaneous neurofibromas, which are soft, palpable, subcutaneous growths. Each cutaneous fibroma ranges from a few millimeters to several centimeters in size and runs along peripheral nerves. They can also grow from nerve roots within the spinal canal and, when they do, they can compress the spinal cord or the cauda equina.

Patients with Type 1 Neurofibromatosis can also develop Lisch nodules, which are multiple asymptomatic, macroscopic yellow-to-brown nodules that are situated on the iris of the eye. The presence of Lisch nodules is pathognomonic of the disorder, although they do not cause functional impairment. Neurofibromatosis Type 1 also is associated with the development of intracerebral tumors, which can induce astrocytomas and optic nerve gliomas.

Neurofibromatosis Type 1 has a high association with attention deficit hyperactivity disorder and with learning disabilities. The patient also can present with seizures and headaches (due to intracranial pressure of the neurofibromas on important structures), have speech and language deficits, mild to moderate learning difficulties, immature coordination and hyperactivity. They may seek care from a psychiatrist because of anxiety or depression and may feel isolated, but there is no increased incidence of psychosis or bipolar disorder (Hyman *et al.*, 2005; Creange *et al.*, 1999).

By comparison, Neurofibromatosis Type 2 is much less prevalent. It is sometimes referred to as familial acoustic neuroma; patients can present with bilateral acoustic neuromas and pale café-au-lait spots. Neurofibromatosis Type 2 is associated with the development of meningiomas but it does not cause behavioral, learning or cognitive impairments. Neurofibromatosis is autosomal dominant, involving chromosome 22.

Tuberous sclerosis

Tuberous sclerosis usually occurs spontaneously, but many cases can be attributed to mutations in one of two tumor suppressor genes which are on chromosome 9 or chromosome 16. During infancy and childhood, there develop hypopigmented splotches on the skin which are referred to as "neurocutaneous depigmented macules." These macules sometimes have a feather-like configuration (described as "ash-leaf" because that is their shape).

Patients also may have scaly areas on the trunk (referred to as "shagreen patches"); smooth and firm nodules on the malar surface of the face (but, in contrast to other forms of acne, not on the trunk) called "adenoma sebaceum" that usually develop in adolescence but sometimes are present as young as five years of age; periungual fibromas on the fingers; retinal phakomas (which are tumors); and calcified intracerebral "tubers," which are potato-like brain nodules 1–3 cm in diameter, identifiable on plain skull x-rays and computerized tomography (CT) scans. The latter are not identifiable on magnetic resonance imaging (MRI), because the tubers contain no water molecules and so cannot be detected unless they are large enough to be displacing normal structures. These tubers can irritate the surrounding cerebral cortex, causing seizures, and sometimes they can undergo malignant transformation.

Tuberous sclerosis patients have cognitive ability which ranges from normal to various degrees of ID, and some individuals can appear autistic (Asano *et al.*, 2001). They may be referred to a psychiatrist because of aggressive or destructive behavior, stereotypies, sleep disturbances and bouts of screaming.

Sturge-Weber syndrome (encephalotrigeminal angiomatosis)

Patients with Sturge-Weber syndrome have a vascular malformation of the face which is associated with an underlying cerebral hemisphere vascular anomaly. There is no known genetic basis for this syndrome. Patients with Sturge-Weber syndrome have neurocutaneous deep red ("port-wine") colored, non-elevated hemangiomas, which are commonly located in the facial area of one branch of the trigeminal nerve facial distribution. These hemangiomas are usually unilateral. Flame-like nevi may be present over the trunk. The cerebral cortex is remarkable for calcified layers of cortex, and this is accompanied by cortical atrophy in the area underlying the facial vascular malformation. These calcifications are best seen on a plain skull film or a CT scan.

People with Sturge-Weber syndrome sometimes but not always have ID, and they can develop seizures that can become refractory to treatment because of the structural central nervous system abnormality. Not surprisingly, patients with seizures are more likely to have significant developmental delay and ID. Patients with Sturge-Weber syndrome have learning difficulties which may be progressive (Sujansky & Conradi, 1995). This is in part due to sclerosis that gradually surrounds the cerebral lesion, causing physical and cognitive deficits to worsen. Over the course of time, patients can develop hemiplegia or hemianopia. Patients may be referred to psychiatry because of various behavioral disturbances.

Ataxia-telangiectasia

This neurocutaneous disorder is included here because, although the disease itself is not associated with a specific behavioral syndrome, the progression of the neurological disorder can result in cognitive impairment and the neurocutaneous findings and gait disturbance can tax the patient's coping skills. Ataxia-telangiectasia is a disorder characterized at first by aggregations of small, dilated vessels (telangiectasia) on the conjunctiva of the eye, the bridge of the nose and the cheeks. At the age of three to five years, the cerebellar vermis begins to degenerate, which causes a steadily progressive gait ataxia. Subsequently, cognitive impairment develops. Ataxia-telangiectasia is inherited in a recessive pattern on Chromosome 11 (the genetic damage interferes with DNA repair). The disorder is also associated with immunodeficiency, lymphomas and neoplasms.

Abnormal head circumference

Macrocephaly

(a) Sotos syndrome   Patients with Sotos syndrome are large at birth and macrocephalic, with an advanced bone age and accelerated growth (above the 97th percentile) in the first five years. Growth rate later falls to within the normal range. Patients with Sotos syndrome have delayed early motor and language milestones, and their neurological examination is remarkable for fine motor and coordination difficulties. They have variable cognitive impairments which, if present, tend to lead to problems in verbal processing and short-term memory. In addition, patients with Sotos syndrome may suffer from attention deficit hyperactivity disorder.

They, or their caregivers, may seek treatment from a psychiatrist because of aggressive behavior and tantrums. Their interpersonal behavior may be remarkable for apparent "social and emotional immaturity," which also can be a focus of treatment. Clearly, if they have attained an unusual height because of their early growth spurt, this can result in rejection or ridicule by peers, damaging their self-esteem and confidence and causing them to appear more socially immature to others.

(b) Mucopolysaccaridoses   Patients with the mucopolysaccharidoses (Hunter, Hurler, Hurley-Scheie and Sanfilippo syndromes) have a progressive macrocephaly, "coarse features" and corneal clouding. The Hunter and Sanfilippo syndromes are remarkable because of marked behavioral problems, including hyperactivity, restlessness, uncontrollable laughing and crying, and biting bedclothes.

Clinical Vignette #3

The patient writes anonymously on an internet site that he is a 19 year old young man with Sotos Syndrome. He has multiple medical problems, including a large head circumference, and he is also 7 feet 6 inches tall.

The patient states that he has been belittled his whole life and ". . . every time someone says something about the way I look, even though they don't mean it in a bad way, all of the torment and pain keeps flooding back."

The patient states that, although adults are sympathetic, there is "nothing they can do." Sometimes, he admits, he lashes out angrily at his family when he becomes very frustrated. He states, "No amount of ice cream, no number of tissue boxes that you cry through can stop the hurt. You have got to find something that inspires you."

The patient takes comfort from a contemporary song against racial prejudice, because he identifies with minority populations. He also enjoys being in touch via an internet chat room with other people who have Sotos syndrome, hoping that he can "help someone out" and that "maybe someone can relate to something I've written."

"We need to know that we're not alone. We are worth so much more than people think."

(c) Proteus syndrome   Proteus syndrome is characterized by macrocephaly and an unusual craniofacial appearance. Patients present with dolicocephaly, a long face, down-slanted palpebral fissures, low nasal bridge, wide anteverted eyes and mouth open at rest. They also have some protrusion of the abdomen. Intelligence may be normal, but some individuals have ID and there can be an associated seizure disorder.

Proteus syndrome apparently is caused by a mutation during embryogenesis. Patients have a normal size at birth, but there is overgrowth during the first year that can involve the whole body, or one limb or the digits. Skin and subcutaneous tissues thicken, and sometimes this is associated with large, primitively formed cerebral hemispheres and/or various other brain malformations. In these cases, there is usually ID and, often, seizures. The patient with Proteus syndrome also may develop hyperpigmented areas, lipomas and lymphangiomas. Patients may seek care from a psychiatrist because of depression. Supportive psychotherapy during the developmental period can be helpful.

Microcephaly

(a) Rett syndrome   This disorder occurs in girls and results in microcephaly. The girls have a normal development during the first 9–12 months, then there is loss of purposive hand movements, slowing of head growth and the development of autistic behavior (Mount *et al.*, 2001). The disorder is caused by a faulty gene on an X chromosome (presumably lethal in the male fetus). Patients show characteristic hand stereotypies and ataxia. Two-thirds of patients never walk and, in the rest, walking ability is lost in their 20s. Patients also suffer from loss of language (Hagberg, 2002).

(b) Fetal alcohol syndrome   This disorder also is characterized by microcephaly, small stature and poor growth, short palpebral fissures, maxillary hypoplasia, short smooth

philtrum and thin upper lip. Patients have mild to moderate learning difficulties, with poor fine motor coordination and tremulousness. They display irritability in infancy and hyperactivity during childhood.

Motor syndromes associated with ID

(a) Congenital hemiplegia   Congenital hemiplegia is associated with learning and behavioral problems, hyperactivity and problems with the peer group, especially when severe hyperactivity is present.

(b) Ataxia   When ataxia occurs in boys, it commonly is associated with adrenoleukodystrophy. Ataxia begins between the ages of 4–8 years, with gait disturbances and subtle cognitive decline, progressing to spasticity, dementia and death. Ataxia also is seen in metachromatic and Krabbe leukodystrophies, where it is associated with regressive behavior and various psychiatric disorders.

(c) Tics   Tics are seen in Tourette's syndrome, where there are both motor tics and vocal tics. Tourette's syndrome is comorbid with obsessive-compulsive disorder, attention-deficit hyperactivity disorder, self-injurious behavior and anxiety and depressive disorders.

(d) Stereotypies   Stereotypies are seen in Fragile X syndrome (alluded to above), where the patient displays hand flapping, knuckle biting and waving of objects. Stereotypies also can be present in autism, learning disabilities, and in Rett syndrome, where there is repetitive hand-wringing and clapping.

(e) Chorea, dystonia and rigidity

1. *Huntington's Disease*: Chorea and dystonia usually are present in Huntington's Disease (HD). HD usually presents in adulthood but childhood presentation occurs. Rigidity is the dominant extrapyramidal feature in children with HD, and seizures occur in 50% of childhood cases. Dysarthria can be an early neurological sign of HD, but the patient may present to psychiatry before any physical findings are evident, because psychosis can often be the presenting sign. Cognitive deterioration also can precede the onset of extrapyramidal features.

2. *Wilson's Disease*: Wilson's disease is autosomal recessive, affects basal ganglia, and is associated with cirrhosis of liver and with Kayser-Fleischer rings in the junction of the cornea and sclera. It is a potentially treatable illness. Thirty percent of children with the disease present with neurological symptoms starting after eight years of age, with dystonia, mask-like-facies, dysarthria and dysphagia, chorea and myoclonic movements. Psychiatric symptoms are prominent in Wilson's disease, with personality changes, irritability, decreased threshold to anger, deteriorating school performance and depression.

3. *Atonia/agenesis of the corpus callosum*: Atonia is present in hereditary motor and sensory neuropathies associated with agenesis of the corpus callosum and with Anderman syndrome (Dupré *et al.*, 2003; Howard *et al.*, 2002; Deleu *et al.*, 1997; Larbrisseau *et al.*, 1984). There likely is a genetic association between these disorders. The disorders involving agenesis of the corpus callosum usually are diagnosed by their clinical features, electrophysiologic testing, and genetic testing. These atonic disorders are characterized by severe progressive sensorimotor neuropathy with hypotonia, areflexia and amyotrophy. The MRI is notable for variable degrees of dysgenesis of the corpus callosum. ID may become more obvious as time goes on. During adolescence, when most children make progress in abstract reasoning, problem-solving and social skills, the person with agenesis of the corpus callosum may gradually fall further behind. This is apparently related to the lack of development in the corpus callosum, which limits information processing. In addition to mild to severe ID, some patients have "psychotic episodes" during adolescence. It has been argued (Filteau *et al.*, 1991) that psychosis occurs only in patients who have associated posterior fossa (cerebellar) atrophy, and that the psychosis is not related to corpus callosum abnormalities in and of themselves.

4. *Myoclonus*: In children, myoclonus may be due to primary epilepsy, or may indicate a progressive degenerative disorder with progressive loss of cognitive abilities such as SSPE (subacute sclerosing panencephalitis). SSPE is caused by the measles virus. It affects children who suffered wild measles infection in the first two years of life and who had not been immunized. SSPE symptoms occur years after the primary infection; they are associated with subtle personality changes and intellectual deterioration, followed within months by myoclonus, seizures, spasticity and dementia.

Neurological "soft signs"

Many syndromes involving ID are associated with neurological "soft signs" (Villamonte *et al.*, 2010; Tavano *et al.*, 2010; Fuentes *et al.*, 2010; Nijhuis-van der Sanden *et al.*, 2000; Holden *et al.*, 1982).

Cerebellar and basal ganglia-related disorders

Williams-Beuren syndrome is caused by a deletion of approximately 26 genes from chromosome 7. Patients have dysmorphic facial features and developmental delay, as well as motor "soft signs" suggesting cerebellar and basal ganglia dysfunction. These soft signs are especially present in patients who have severe linguistic deficits (Tavano *et al.*, 2010).

Autism

Patients with autism have handwriting impairments that are associated with problems in perceptual reasoning (Fuentes *et al.*, 2010).

Special features of the neurological examination in patients with ID

Initial observation

Observe the patient's general behavior, especially for any evidence of self-injury or aggression (Sovner & Hurley, 1991, 1990). Sometimes, patients use these behaviors to communicate discomfort or other needs, although they can become habitual, especially in patients with severe disabilities (Sandman, 1990/1991). At times, the person is communicating or attempting to self-sooth emotional discomfort (Gaultieri, 2002), such as in major depression or mania (Lowry & Sovner, 1992, 1991).

Observe the patient's use of language and "communicative intent" (i.e. is the patient trying to communicate to someone?). Observe the patient's social skills – for example, does the person make eye contact? Can they follow requests, and are they willing to do so? What is the patient's attention span? Are they impulsive? Do they have any obvious dysmorphic features (with special attention to the face and fingers) or neurocutaneous stigmata? What are the patient's head circumference, weight and height? In general, are motor functions of the cranial nerves intact – especially eye movements? Are there any unusual motor movements such as muscle tics or vocalizations, choreiform movements, dystonia or repetitive behaviors ("stereotypies") such as hand flapping or knuckle-biting (Sovner & Hurley, 1991).

If the examiner learns that any self-injurious behavior is of acute onset, it usually is an expression of pain and discomfort, and often there is an underlying medical cause. Some common medical causes of this behavior are reflux esophagitis or peripheral neuropathy, the uncontrolled epilepsy, or a side effect from sedating anticonvulsants, stimulants, neuroleptics causing akathesia or dysphoria, or selective serotonin reuptake inhibitors (SSRIs), which can induce compulsive self-injurious behavior (Gaultieri, 2002).

When examining for dysmorphic features in a child or adult (if possible), it is important to observe both parents because, if the disorder is autosomally dominant, it may have been transmitted from *either* parent.

Look for neurocutaneous abnormalities in persons with ID who have psychiatric disturbances. Neurofibromatosis type 1 and tuberous sclerosis both are associated with significant neuropsychiatric problems. It is important to remember that neurocutaneous features may be found on examination of the parents' skin, even if a child does not show this finding.

Also, examine the head circumference of both parents as well as the child (you can pretend to be measuring for a hat). Familial macrocephaly affects more boys than girls; therefore, in assessing a child, the head circumference from both mother and father may be important. Over 40% of persons of neurofibromatosis type I have macrocephaly.

Short stature is seen in a number of syndromes, such as Noonan's syndrome and Cornelia de Lange syndrome. On the other hand, there is a tendency to early excessive growth in both Fragile X and Sotos syndromes (Schafer & Bodensteiner, 1992).

Cranial nerves

cranial nerve II: vision   Deterioration in vision, especially if it is accompanied by personality change, intellectual deterioration or motor difficulties, requires urgent evaluation (Kaufman, 2007; Campbell *et al.*, 2006). See Table 1 for ID associated with cranial nerve II.

Table 1 Intellectual disabilities associated with Cranial Nerve II (vision) findings and conjunctival abnormalities.

Myopia	Persons with Bardet-Biedl syndrome and Rubenstein-Taybe syndrome may have myopia.
Lisch nodules	Persons with neurofibromatosis have "Lisch nodules."
Cataracts	Persons with Lowe's syndrome have cataracts.
Telangiectasia	Persons with homocystinuria or Marfan's syndrome have lens dislocation; telangetasia is present in ataxia-telangectasia after age 3.
Kayser-Fleischer rings	Persons with Wilson's disease have Kayser-Fleischer rings after age 4.
Optic atrophy	Optic atrophy is found in leukodystrophy and gangliosidoses.
Papilledema	Papilledema is found in evolving hydrocephalus in persons who have neurofibromatosis or tuberous sclerosis.
Phakomas	Phakomas are found in tuberous sclerosis.
Cherry red spots	Cherry-red spots are found in gangliosidoses and sialidosis.
Pigmentary changes	Pigmentary changes are found in mitochondrial disease, juvenile neuronal ceroid lipofuscinosis (Batten disease) and Usher syndrome.
Conjunctiva	Observe for dilated conjunctival vessels in the angles of the eyes. In ataxia-telangiectasia, which is an autosomal recessive developmental disease, these are present after age 3. Other findings in ataxia-telangiectasia are progressive cerebellar ataxia and, sometimes, choreoathetosis, immunodeficiency and malignancy and intellectual decline.

Summarized from Kaufman (2007), Gualtieri (2002) and others.

- *Examining visual fields*: Have the patient look at you, and hold two fingers out to either side within lateral view. Call the patient's name so that the patient looks at you, then move your fingers on one side and see if the patient looks or points at them.

- *Examining fundi*: Have the caregiver stand in front of the patient and ask the patient if the caregiver is "making faces" to fixate their gaze; or hold a picture or an object (e.g. a toy) and wiggle it so that the patient fixes their gaze on it.

cranial Nerves III, IV, VI: eye movement problems

- *Observing eye movement*: Notice whether side-to-side eye movements are slow, requiring the patient to move the head or blink to relocate the target. Problems with eye movements and the presence of nystagmus are seen in juvenile Gaucher disease, ataxia telangiectasia, Niemann-Pick disease type C, spinocerebellar degeneration, Huntington's disease and Pelizaeus-Merzbacher disease.

- *Nystagmus* is also an important eye movement finding. Nystagmus is an involuntary, rhythmical oscillatory movement of both eyes in any plane. It is not found in cerebral palsy so, if nystagmus is present, other conditions should be considered. For example, boys may develop ataxia, nystagmus and progressive weakness in the X-linked leukodystrophy of Pelizaeus-Merzbacher disease, and this eye finding is present in the first three months of life.

- Difficulties with voluntary conjugate gaze (called "supranuclear opthalmoplegia") are present in juvenile Gaucher disease (horizontal opthalmoplegia), the adult form of GM2 gangliosidosis, and type C Niemann-Pick disease (vertical opthalmoplegia).

other cranial nerves   Observe for facial symmetry, the external formation of the ears, the presence of motor weakness (upper and lower face), the movements of the mouth, and look for the presence of dribbling. Worster-Draught syndrome, for example, is associated with upper motor neuron bulbar palsy with mild pyramidal tetraplegia, and is usually associated with learning difficulties and other neuropsychiatric disorders.

Motor disorders

examining posture and movement   Observe gait, power and coordination (Gillig & Sanders, 2010) by asking a person to catch something (for example, ask the child to catch a ball). See if the patient is able to walk on toes and heels, as this helps to check for weakness and spasticity of the lower limbs (Sanders & Gillig, 2010). If the patient has difficulty hopping, standing from a squat or climbing stairs, this suggests a weakness of the pelvic girdle, as is seen in muscular disorders associated with learning impairment and behavioral disturbances (e.g. the Duchenne and Becker muscular dystrophies).

examining reflexes   With children, you might allow the child to sit on a caregiver's lap, resting the child's legs in the examiner's lap. A toy or other object for the person to hold may help with distraction. Remember to do the Babinski reflex (plantar reflex) last, because it may be unpleasant to the patient and limit their ability to cooperate further.

examining tone and strength and balance   Flex and extend the passive limb to look for increased tone, and measure for weakness, especially in extensor groups of the upper limbs and the flexors of lower limbs. Brisk reflexes and a positive Babinski are seen in congenital hemiplegia, for example, which is associated with learning and behavioral problems. Balance problems are seen in a number of syndromes of ID, including Down Syndrome (Villamonte *et al.*, 2010).

The management of spasticity

Spasticity is a common problem for persons with ID. Their increased muscle tone can seriously impair their daily activities and make management of their care more difficult (Charles *et al.*, 2010). On the other hand, tone reduction is not necessarily a goal when a person is using the increased tone for better function (e.g. walking using an otherwise weakened limb).

Spasticity often coexists with other motor findings including increased reflexes, clonus, a positive plantar reflex (Babinski) – all upper motor neuron findings – and muscle weakness and problems with coordination. Patients who have spasticity in an extremity will show resistance to externally imposed movement, usually with a "spastic catch." After resistance to movement, the examiner will feel a rapid decrease in resistance, referred to as the "clasped-knife" finding.

Guidelines recently have been published by the American Academy of Neurology (2010) regarding treatment of spasticity in children with cerebral palsy. These recommendations likely may provide guidance regarding treatment of spasticity in persons with ID in general.

Spasticity is a type of excessive muscle tone, caused by upper motor neuron lesion(s), and aggravated by stretch. In its extreme forms, it can be difficult to distinguish from dystonia, because the flexed position persists, but they are clinically distinguishable. With spasticity, resistance to passive stretch is distinctly variable through the range of the movement, with the speed or angle of the movement, etc. In dystonia, sustained or intermittent contractions cause abnormal sustained or repetitive movements (Sanger *et al.*, 2003).

Spasticity is quite common in the ID population. Patients with severe spasticity are unmistakable, and most will have been diagnosed quickly with cerebral palsy. These patients have grossly impaired motor function and often cannot ambulate or eat independently.

It is worth noting that the definition of cerebral palsy (a static motor disability present at birth and attributed to prenatal cerebral injury) does not rely on spasticity. Spasticity is the major problem in most individuals with cerebral palsy but, in some cases, the picture is dominated by involuntary movements (chorea, athetosis and/or dystonia), and in some cases ataxia is dominant. Sensory and cognitive deficits and seizures are also common (O'Shea, 2008). Spasticity is not always due to a congenital static brain condition (cerebral palsy). Unless the diagnosis is clear, other possible diagnoses should be excluded. The most common among these are post-natal acquired brain or spinal cord lesions, chronic (tardive) dystonia and multiple sclerosis.

When less severe, spasticity has often not been diagnosed but can be important in understanding the common problems of falling and aspiration. Minor spasticity is frequently manifested in posturing and gait variants. Toe walking (little or no contact between heels and ground) is very common and is less stable than a full-footed gait. Parts of the gait cycle often appear abrupt and exaggerated. An example is hip flexion, which gives an unusual kicking or high-stepping appearance. Spasticity of the upper extremities in such milder cases is most often manifest in posturing, while walking or while using the other arm.

Spastic movements of the upper extremities can be confused with stereotypy, chorea or athetosis. Spastic movements can interfere with, or replace, movements that would normally serve to help maintain balance or break falls. Spasticity can also affect many of the muscles involved in chewing and swallowing, detracting from the efficiency of the act, predisposing to aspiration (Rekand, 2010; Delgado *et al.*, 2010).

Treatment may involve actively treating spasticity, or it may involve choosing among treatment options according to their potential to aggravate the motor disability. The mainstay of direct treatment is botulinum toxin type A, but this is useful only for regional treatment (Delgado *et al.*, 2010). Some evidence supports diazepam, tizanidine and baclofen (Hoving *et al.*, 2009) in the systemic treatment of spasticity.

Tizanidine may be useful, but the evidence is mixed (Simpson *et al.*, 2009; Delgado *et al.*, 2010) and it may have antidepressant effects (Saper *et al.*, 2001). It is an alpha-2 agonist (as are clonidine and guanfacine), and it has seen use for autism and attention deficit hyperactivity disorder (Henney & Chez, 2009), although there have been no published trials of tizanidine for the treatment of any psychiatric condition. Tizanidine has a narrow therapeutic index and the optimal dose varies significantly among individuals. It is metabolized to inactive metabolites by the cP450 1A2 isoenzyme, and it can be quite vulnerable to inhibitors, so care is warranted in prescribing to patients taking tizanidine (Henney & Runyon, 2008).

Baclofen is the only clinically available GABA-B agonist. It can be administered orally or intrathecally (Hoving *et al.*, 2009). Baclofen has anxiolytic effects in at least some conditions (Breslow *et al.*, 1989; Drake *et al.*, 2003; Garbutt *et al.*, 2010), but no apparent general antidepressant effects; it may even aggravate some mood disorders (Post *et al.*, 1991). It is primarily eliminated by the kidneys (85%) (Shellenberger *et al.*, 1999).

Diazepam, as a benzodiazepine, has well-known motor and cognitive adverse effects (Kalachnik *et al.*, 2002). The motor effects include postural instability and ataxia – manifested, for example, in increased falls and automobile accidents in the elderly (Madhusoodanan & Bogunovic, 2004). It has a rapid onset and long half-life, and is metabolized by cP450 isoenzymes 3A4 and 2C19 (Fukasawa *et al.*, 2007).

Antipsychotic medications are frequently used to assist with aggression and other challenging behaviors in the ID population. Although spasticity *per se* is not affected by antipsychotic or dopamine blocking drugs, motor disability is certainly increased by the side effects common to most of these medications. Parkinsonian side effects can include reduced stride height and length, with an increased tendency to stumble and postural instability. Akathisia (manifested as increased walking) is also common with most "atypical" antipsychotics; in those with gait instability, akathisia alone increases the fall risk. Parkinsonian motor impairment can include impaired mastication and swallowing. By detracting from marginal baseline performance of a relatively complex act, this can significantly increase the risk of aspiration.

Any medication with cognitive side effects, including benzodiazepines, anticholinergic drugs, antihistaminic drugs, tricyclic antidepressants and many antipsychotic drugs, obviously detract from the execution of complex functions. In most of the population, walking and eating are not counted among complex functions. However, in the population under discussion, these tasks can be among their highest achievements, and even minor cognitive setbacks can have a devastating impact.

Assessment and treatment of neuroleptic-induced movement disorders

Individuals with ID have a fragile central nervous system and are especially sensitive to the development of acute, subacute and chronic extrapyramidal reactions to neuroleptic medications. Medication management and management of acute side effects, including acute extrapyramidal symptoms and neuroleptic malignant syndrome, are addressed in Chapter 12.

Tardive dyskinesia is a serious, potentially permanent movement disorder that is usually related to chronic administration of antipsychotic medication and some other medications. Tardive dyskinesia can present in several different ways. The most common manifestation (93%) involves choreoathetoid movements mainly in the tongue and masticatory musculature and the distal extremities (Gaultieri, 2002).

Tardive dystonia is characterized by sustained contractions of skeletal muscles, and it must be differentiated from spasticity in the examination of the motor system. There also is a form of dyskinesia in which patients develop motor and phonic tics ("*Tardive tourettes*"), and a malignant respiratory form of dyskinesia that involves the respiratory musculature and compromises breathing (Davis & Cummings, 1988).

Finally, there is *tardive akathisia*, in which akathisia symptoms first start after prolonged introduction of neuroleptic drugs. Tardive akathisia is probably related to damage to the basal ganglia, and it is characterized by a chronic subjective state of motor restlessness and hyperactivity that is experienced by the patient as extremely unpleasant and is associated with depression. Tardive akathisia has been known to result in aggressive acting-out, as well as self-injury that can even progress to suicide. Patients feel they have to pace constantly, cannot remain seated and feel like they are "crawling out of their skin" (Gaultieri, 2002). As with all tardive dyskinesias and dystonias, and in contrast to extrapyramidal symptoms, the symptoms of tardive akathisia increase when the neuroleptic dose is *decreased*. This can create difficulties with differential diagnosis, when trying to determine whether emerging behavioral symptoms are related to inadequate medication for symptom control or tardive akathisia.

Treatments of all tardive conditions include tapering and discontinuing neuroleptics, especially typical neuroleptics, substituting atypical neuroleptics if needed (Gaultieri, 1993) –and later, if possible, trying again to lower neuroleptic dose and improve behavioral outcomes by adding beta-blockers (Ratey *et al.*, 1985), benzodiazepines, clonidine (Zubenko *et al.*, 1984) or buspirone, for example.

The motor side effects of dopamine-blocking drugs generally resemble Parkinson's disease (drug-induced Parkinsonism) within the first few months of exposure. With chronic exposure, the motor side effects can also include a syndrome resembling Huntington's disease (tardive dyskinesia). Any of the abnormal movements described below are most commonly caused by drugs which directly reduce dopamine transmission, but they are sometimes caused by serotonin reuptake inhibitors and rarely by other drugs.

The Parkinsonian syndrome consists of diminished movement (slow, less gesturing, less arm swing while walking, etc.), resting tremor (which may be less common in drug-induced Parkinsonism than Parkinson's disease), rigidity (consistent resistance to passive movement throughout the range of motion or "lead pipe" rigidity) and postural instability. When encountered in a person taking dopamine-blocking drugs, Parkinsonian signs are probably drug-induced. Important related problems include akathisia and dystonia.

In the patient with ID, it is quite easy to over- and under-detect Parkinsonian side effects. Accuracy is improved by knowing the patient longitudinally, and/or by clear observations from daily caregivers.

As with the general psychiatric population, one must choose between an anti-Parkinsonian drug, switching to an antipsychotic likely to produce less of the side effect, reducing the dose of the offending drug or discontinuing the drug. Notwithstanding evidence and expert advice, many patients with ID and problem behaviors are still on high doses of antipsychotic drugs.

In many individuals and systems, dose reduction is fraught with difficulties. It should be remembered that anticholinergic medications have cognitive adverse effects, which are predictably severe in some groups (e.g. aging patients with Down syndrome develop Alzheimer pathology). Patients with ID often have problems with bowel motility, also aggravated by anticholinergic drugs. Unfortunately, dopamine agonist drugs often seem to have behavioral side effects in this population.

Akathisia must be considered whenever the patient is ambulating excessively. Often, the important subjective element of feeling an urge to be walking, feeling unable to sit still, etc. is inaccessible in this patient population, and one must infer. If akathisia is not considered, the "agitation" or other behavior problems related to increase in walking may prompt dose increases, aggravating the problem. After removing the offending agent, there are numerous remedies, but the first-line agent is propranolol.

Mild drug-induced dystonia can be easily overlooked. In particular, in patients with baseline axial spasticity, drug-induced axial dystonia is difficult to appreciate. Oculomotor dystonia may be less dramatic than "oculogyric crisis," in which case it can resemble the oculomotor component of self-stimulating behavior. Knowing the behavioral baseline and incorporating the rest of the motor examination is key to making these distinctions. Treatment of acute dystonia starts with intramuscular antihistaminic (such as diphenhydramine) or anticholinergic (such as benztropine). If refractory, it can be followed with further doses along these same lines, or a benzodiazepine (such as lorazepam). Chronic segmental dystonia (such as torticollis) is preferably treated with botulinum A toxin. Alternatives, and treatments for generalized dystonia, include anticholinergic drugs, baclofen and deep brain stimulation (Scott, 2000).

Tardive dyskinesia is a movement disorder characterized by chorea and athetosis, sometimes also including akathisia (tardive akathisia) and dystonia (tardive dystonia). It develops after at least three months of exposure to dopamine blocking drugs, and is usually persistent, although variable in intensity (van Harten & Kahn, 1999). It is common in the ID population (Bodfish et al., 1996), perhaps due to heavy antipsychotic exposure, increased vulnerability among those with severe disability (Wszola et al., 2001) and an increased prevalence of tardive-like movements (Bodfish et al., 1996).

Standard advice is to remove the offending agent on first detection, which can help if early in the course of illness. Because early detection is important, routine monitoring using a standardized scale is strongly advised, often dictated by policy and even legislation. Scales for this purpose are the venerable Abnormal Involuntary Movement Scales (AIMS; Guy, 1976; Munetz & Benjamin, 1988); the DISCUS (Kalachnik & Sprague, 1993; Matson et al., 2008), which was constructed particularly for patients less able to participate in assessment; and the Matson scale, which covers more side effects and is intended for individuals with ID (Matson et al., 2008).

Unfortunately, medication withdrawal can also precipitate at least temporary increases in the severity of dyskinesia and behavioral disturbance alike, raising the call for a substitute. All antipsychotic drugs can temporarily quell tardive dyskinesia but, beyond this, some may actually improve the condition, as evidenced by continued lower levels of dyskinesia after the drug is reduced or withdrawn. Clozapine is often said to be the drug treatment of choice for tardive dyskinesia (Simpson, 2000), and most experienced clinicians would concur. It should be noted, however, that clozapine has considerable side effects and it has little empirical basis as a treatment for tardive dyskinesia (Bassitt & Louza Neto, 1998). Somewhat less complicated options with at least some evidence for helping tardive dyskinesia are olanzapine (Chan et al., 2010, Kinon et al., 2004), quetiapine (Emsley et al., 2004) and risperidone (Chan et al., 2010).

When antipsychotic drugs are not necessary and the dyskinesia is not highly disabling, the group of vitamins and nutraceutical agents are attractive. Vitamin E, usually in high doses, showed promise in several smaller studies, but a well-conducted negative study (Adler et al., 1999) and new concerns about the safety of high-dose vitamin E (Miller et al., 2005) has removed it from the thinking of all but a few (Soares-Weiser et al., 2011). Other treatments of this ilk with at least some supporting evidence include vitamin B6 (Lerner et al., 2007), melatonin (Shamir et al., 2001) and a blend of amino acids (Richardson et al., 2003).

Other medications appear capable of improving tardive dyskinesia to some extent. These include levetiracetam (Woods *et al.*, 2008), amantadine (Pappa *et al.*, 2010) and naltrexone combined with clonazepam (Wonodi *et al.*, 2004). These options are best when there are additional target symptoms for the drug in question, as the impact is usually not dramatic. Somewhat more dramatic results were noted in a study of deep brain stimulation of the globus pallidus for severe, refractory tardive dyskinesia (Damier *et al.*, 2007). The condition is by no means hopeless, but prevention and early detection are much preferred to the alternatives.

Seizure disorders

Children with ID and developmental delay frequently have seizures, which tend to start after the onset of other neurological symptoms (Gaultieri, 2002; Steffenburg & Steffenburg, 1999; Deykin & Macmahan, 1979). The onset of seizures is usually in early childhood but one third of patients develop seizures in adolescence or early adult life (Boettger, 2003). Frontal lobe dysfunction is associated with seizure onset in 58% of cases, based on EEG findings (Kurokawa *et al.*, 2010).

Seizures are a common finding in patients with ID and they can be of any type. Although every type of seizure occurs in people with ID, infantile spasms and Lennox-Gastaut seizures occur only in persons with ID. Seizures can be associated with intellectual decline and they are often accompanied by behavioral problems. The likelihood of seizures increases where there is more severe ID, and about half of patients with severe disability have seizures.

Generalized convulsions are the most common diagnosed seizure type in the population of ID, but severe partial seizures, with or without secondary generalization, tend to be most frequent to occur, possibly because they are often more difficult to control medically. Autistic regression sometimes related to ictal or subictal events. Epilepsy or epileptiform EEG patterns occurs in a significant minority of autistic children with a history of regression (Gaultieri, 2002), and the neuropathology of autism likely involves areas of the brain that tend to be epileptogenic.

Behavioral problems and emotional instability in persons with ID with seizures can be preictal, ictal or postictal, and they can be related to the seizure itself (if inadequately treated) or, sometimes, to toxic effects of the anticonvulsant medications themselves (Kurokawa *et al.*, 2010).

The Landau-Kleffner syndrome (LKS) is associated with aphasia and autism as well as epilepsy. LKS is a condition in which temporal lobe seizures are associated with gradual loss of language ability, sometimes with the related development of autism (Gaultieri, 2002). The syndrome of LKS and other syndromes where there are continuous spike and wave complexes during slow wave sleep may be related conditions characterized by developmental regression, especially associated with the loss of the capacity for language. It is hypothesized that the continuous aberrant electrical activity can interfere with appropriate pruning process during development (Salin-Cantegrel *et al.*, 2007), disrupting language development by affecting the temperoparietal cortex, or the higher integrative functions by affecting the frontal cortex or by disruption of temporal input that initiates frontal development.

Personality changes and depression often occur in patients who have seizures that originate in the temporal lobes. Most children who have co-occurring ID and seizures have emotional or behavioral disturbances of some sort (Hauser, 1997; King *et al.*, 1994).

Aggression, self-injury, hyperactivity and intermittent agitation are the most common problems for which children with ID and seizures are referred to psychiatry, and the most common psychiatric diagnosis in children with ID with epilepsy is autism. The prevalence of seizures in children with autism is many times higher than the basal rate in the population (Gaultieri, 2002).

When a patient with ID is referred to psychiatry due to a behavioral disturbance, it is important first to be sure that anticonvulsants are in therapeutic range. Unfortunately, patients who have severe ID, especially if they have severe sensorimotor impairments, may have seizures that are only partially responsive to anticonvulsant medications. This can have a persistent effect on their behavior and emotional state.

Conclusion

The most common neurologic findings in persons with ID include frontal release signs, decrease in muscle tone, strength and coordination problems, increased or decreased deep tendon reflexes, gait disturbances, stereotypies and electroencephalogram abnormalities. Knowledge of various syndromes of ID increases awareness of commonly occurring associated medical and mental health issues, and this can facilitate accurate diagnoses and effective treatment.

A neurologic evaluation should be sought for any patient with changes in motor or sensory function, as knowledge of the components of the neurologic examination will facilitate appropriate referrals. When prescribing psychotropics, one should be cognizant of all medical and neurologic conditions, as certain conditions increase the risk of medication side effects in patients with ID. Since neurologic conditions and ID are intimately intertwined, it is essential that the mental health clinician be well informed in both areas.

References

Adler L.A., Rotrosen J., Edson R., Lavori, P., Lohr, J., Hitzemann, R., Raisch, D., Caligiuri, M., Tracy, K. (1999). Vitamin E treatment for tardive dyskinesia. *Archives of General Psychiatry* **56**(9), 836–841.

American Academy of Neurology (AAN) and the Child Neurology Society guidance on how to treat spasticity in children with cerebral palsy (CP) (2010). *Neurology* **74**, 336–343.

Andersen, W.H., Rasmussen, R.K., Strømme, P. (2001). Levels of cognitive and linguistic development in Angelman syndrome: a study of 20 children. *Logopedics, phoniatrics, vocology* **26**(1), 2–9.

Asano, E., Chugani, D.C., Muzik, O., Behen, M., Janisse, J., Rothermel, R., Mangner, T.J., Chakraborty, P.K. & Chugani, H.T. (2001). Autism in tuberous sclerosis complex is related to both cortical and subcortical dysfunction. *Neurology* **57**, 1269–1277.

Bassitt, D.P. & Louzã Neto M.R. (1998). Clozapine efficacy in tardive dyskinesia in schizophrenic patients. *European Archives of Psychiatry and Clinical Neuroscience* **248**, 209–11.

Bodfish, J.W., Newell, K.M., Sprague, R.L., Harper, V.N. & Lewis, M.H. (1996). Dyskinetic movement disorder among adults with mental retardation: phenomenology and co-occurrence with stereotypy. *American Journal on Mental Retardation* **101**, 118–29.

Boettger, T., Rust, M.B., Maier, H., Seidenbecher, T., Schweizer, M., Keating, D.J., Faulhaber, J., Ehmke, H., Pfeffer, C., Scheel, O., Lemcke, B., Horst, J., Leuwer, R., Pape, H.C., Völkl, H.,

Hübner, C.A. & Jentsch, T.J. (2003). Loss of K-Cl co-transporter KCC3 causes deafness, neurodegeneration and reduced seizure threshold. *The EMBO Journal* **22**, 5422–5434.

Breslow, M.F., Fankhauser, M.P., Potter, R.L., Meredith, K.E., Misiaszek, J. & Hope, D.G. Jr., (1989). Role of gamma-aminobutyric acid in antipanic drug efficacy. *American Journal of Psychiatry* **146**(3), 353–356.

Buntinx, I.M., Hennekam, R.C., Brouwer, O.F., Stroink, H., Beuten, J., Mangelschots, K. & Fryns, J.P. (1995). Clinical profile of Angelman syndrome at different ages. *American Journal of Medical Genetics* **56**(2), 176–183.

Campbell W.W., DeJong, R.N. & Haerer, A.F. (2006). *DeJong's The Neurological Examination*, Lippincott: Philadelphia, PA.

Chan, H-Y., Chiang, S-C., Chang, C-J., Gau, S.S-F., Chen, J-J., Chen, C-H., Hwu, H-G. & Lai, M-S. (2010). A randomized controlled trial of risperidone and olanzapine for schizophrenic patients with neuroleptic-induced tardive dyskinesia. *Journal of Clinical Psychiatry* **71**(9), 1226–1233.

Charles, P.D., Gill, C.E., Taylor, H.M., Putman, M.S., Blair, C.R., Roberts, A.G., Ayers, G.D. & Konrad, P.E. (2010). Spasticity treatment facilitates direct care delivery for adults with profound intellectual disability. *Movement Disorders* **25**(4), 446–473.

Clark, D.J., Boer, H., Webb, T. (1995). General and behavioural aspects of PWS: a review. *Mental Health Research* **8**(195), 38–49.

Corbett, J.A. (1979). Psychiatric morbidity and mental retardation. In: Games, F. E& Snaith, R.P. (eds.) *Psychiatric Illness and Mental Handicap*, pp. 11–25. Gaskill Press, London.

Creange, A., Zeller, J., Rostaing-Rigattieri, S., Brugieres, P., Degos, J.D., Revuz, J. & Wolkenstein, P. (1999). Neurological complications of neurofibromatosis type 1 in adulthood. *Brain* **122**, 473–481.

Curry, C.J., Stevenson, R.E., Aughton, D., Byrne, J., Carey, J.C., Cassidy, S., Cunniff, C., Graham, J.M. Jr., Jones, M.C., Kaback, M.M., Moeschler, J., Schaefer, G.B., Schwartz, S., Tarleton, J. & Opitz, J. (1997). Evaluation of mental retardation: recommendations of a consensus conference. *American Journal of Medical Genetics* **72**, 468–477.

Damier, P., Thobois, S., Witjas, T., Cuny, E., Derost, P., Raoul, S., Mertens, P., Peragut, J-C., Lemaire, J-J., Burbaud, P., Nguyen, J-M., Llorca, P-M. & Rascol, O. (2007). Bilateral deep brain stimulation of the globus pallidus to treat tardive dyskinesia. *Archives of General Psychiatry* **64**, 170–6.

Dan, B. (2009). Angelman syndrome: Current understanding and research prospects. *Epilepsia*, **50**(11), 2331–2339.

Davis, R.J. & Cummings, J.L. (1988). Clinical variants of tardive dyskinesia. *Neuropsychiatry, Neuropsychology and Behavioral Neurology* **1**, 31–38.

Deleu, D., Bamanikar, S.A., Muirhead, D. & Louon, A. (1997). Familial progressive sensorimotor neuropathy with agenesis of the corpus callosum (Andermann syndrome): a clinical, neuroradiological and histopathological study. *European Neurology* **37**, 104–109.

Delgado, M.R., Hirtz, D., Aisen, M., Ashwal, S., Fehlings, D.L., McLaughlin, J., Morrison, L.A., Shrader, M.W., Tilton, A. & Vargus-Adams, J. (2010). Practice parameter: pharmacologic treatment of spasticity in children and adolescents with cerebral palsy (an evidence-based review): report of the Quality Standards Subcommittee of the American Academy of Neurology and the Practice Committee of the Child Neurology Society. *Neurology* **74**, 336–343.

Deykin, E.Y. & Macmahon, B. (1979). The incidence of seizures among children with autistic symptoms. *American Journal of Psychiatry* **136**, 1310–1312.

Drake, R.G., Davis, L.L., Cates, M.E., Jewell, M.E., Ambrose, S.M. & Lowe, J.S. (2003). Baclofen treatment for chronic posttraumatic stress disorder. *Annals of Pharmacotherapy* **37**, 1177–1181.

Dupré, N., Howard, H.C., Mathieu, J., Karpati, G., Vanasse, M., Bouchard, J.P., Carpenter, S. & Rouleau, G.A. (2003). Hereditary motor and sensory neuropathy with agenesis of the corpus callosum. *Annals of Neurology* **54**, 9–18.

Emsley, R., Turner, H.J., Schronen, J., Botha, K., Smit, R. & Oosthuizen P.P. (2004). A single-blind, randomized trial comparing quetiapine and haloperidol in the treatment of tardive dyskinesia. *Journal of Clinical Psychiatry* **65**, 696–701.

Fatemi, S.H. & Folsom, T.D. (2010). The role of fragile X mental retardation protein in major mental disorders. *Neuropharmacology* **30**, 1–6.

Feinstein, C., Eliez, S., Blasey, C. & Reiss, A.L. (2002). Psychiatric disorders and behavioral problems in children with velocardiofacial syndrome: usefulness as phenotypic indicators of schizophrenia risk. *Biological Psychiatry* **51**, 312–318.

Filteau, M.J., Pourcher. E., Bouchard, R.H., Baruch, P., Mathieu, J., Bédard, F., Simard, N. & Vincent, P. (1991). Corpus callosum agenesis and psychosis in Andermann syndrome. *Archives of Neurology* **48**, 1275–1280.

Finestack, L.H., Richmond, E.K. & Abbeduto, L. (2009). Language development with Fragile X Syndrome. *Topics in Language Disorders* **29**, 133–148.

Freund, L.S., Reiss, A.L. & Abrams, M.T. (1993). Psychiatric disorders associated with fragile X in the young female. *Pediatrics* **91**, 321–329.

Fuentes, C.T., Mostofsky, S.H. & Bastian, A.J. (2010). Perceptual reasoning predicts handwriting impairments in adolescents with autism. *Neurology* **75**(20), 1825–1829.

Fukasawa, T., Suzuki, A. & Otani, K. (2007). Effects of genetic polymorphism of cytochrome P450 enzymes on the pharmacokinetics of benzodiazepines. *Journal of Clinical Pharmacy and Therapeutics* **32**, 333–41.

Garbutt, J.C., Kampov-Polevoy, A.B., Gallop, R., Kalka-Juhl, L. & Flannery, B.A. (2010). Efficacy and safety of baclofen for alcohol dependence: a randomized, double-blind, placebo-controlled trial. *Alcoholism: Clinical & Experimental Research* **34**, 1849–1857.

Gerald, P.S. (1976). Sex chromosome disorders. *New England Journal of Medicine* **294**, 706–708.

Gillig, P.M. & Sanders, R.D. (2010). Psychiatry, neurology and the role of the cerebellum. *Psychiatry* **7**, 38–43.

Gualtieri, C.T. (1993). The problem of tardive akathesia. *Brain Cognition* **23**, 102–109.

Gualtieri, C.T. (2002). *Brain injury and mental retardation: psychopharmacology and neuro-psychiatry.* Lippincott, Williams & Wilkins, Philadelphia, PA.

Guy, W. (1976). *Abnormal Involuntary Movement Scale (AIMS); ECDEU assessment manual for psychopharmacology.* pp. 534–537. U.S. Dept. of Health, Education and Welfare, Rockville, MD.

Hagberg, B. (2002). Clinical manifestations and stages of Rett syndrome. *Mental Retardation and Developmental Disabilities Research Review* **8**, 61–65.

Hauser, M.J. (1997). The role of the psychiatrist in mental retardation. *Psychiatric Annals* **27**, 170–174.

Henney, H.R. 3rd& Runyan, J.D. (2008). A clinically relevant review of tizanidine hydrochloride dose relationships to pharmacokinetics, drug safety and effectiveness in healthy subjects and patients. *International Journal of Clinical Practice* **62**, 314–324.

Hier, D., Atkins, L. & Perlo, V. (1980). Learning disorders and sex chromosome aberrations. *Journal of Mental Deficiency Research* **24**, 17–26.

Holden, E.W., Tarnowski, K.J. & Prinz, R.J. (1982). Reliability of neurological soft signs in children: reevaluation of the PANESS. (Physical and Neurologic Examination of Subtle Signs) *Journal of Abnormal Child Psychology* **10**(2) 163–172.

Holm, V.A., Cassidy, S.B., Butler, M.G., Hanchett, J.M.; Greenswag, L.R.; Whitman, B.Y. & Greenberg, F. (1993). Prader-Willi syndrome: consensus diagnostic criteria. *Pediatrics* **91**(2) 398–402.

Hoving, M.A., van Raak, E.P., Spincemaille, G.H., Palmans, L.J., Becher, J.G. & Vles, J.S. (2009). Efficacy of intrathecal baclofen therapy in children with intractable spastic cerebral palsy: a randomised controlled trial. *European Journal of Paediatric Neurology* **13**, 240–246.

Howard, H.C., Mount, D.B., Rochefort, D., Byun, N., Dupré, N., Lu, J., Fan, X., Song, L., Rivière, J.B., Prévost, C., Horst, J., Simonati, A., Lemcke, B., Welch, R., England, R., Zhan, F. Q., Mercado, A., Siesser, W.B., George, A.L., McDonald, M.P., Bouchard, J.P., Mathieu, J., Delpire, E. & Rouleau, G.A. (2002). The K-Cl cotransporter KCC3 is mutant in a severe peripheral neuropathy associated with agenesis of the corpus callosum. *Nature Genetics* **32**, 384–392.

Hyman, S.L., Shores, A. & North, K.N. (2005). The nature and frequency of cognitive deficits in children with neurofibromatosis type 1. *Neurology* **65**, 1037–1044.

Kalachnik, J.E. & Sprague, R.L. (1993). The dyskinesia identification system condensed user scale (DISCUS): reliability, validity and a total score cut-off for mentally ill and mentally retarded populations. *Journal of Clinical Psychology* **49**(2), 177–89.

Kalachnik, J., Hanzel, T., Sevenich, R. & Harder, S. (2002). Benzodiazepine behavioral side effects: review and implications for individuals with mental retardation. *American Journal of Mental Retardation* **107**, 376–410.

Kaufman, D.M. (2007). *Clinical Neurology for Psychiatrists 6th* edition, Saunders: Philadelphia, PA.

King, B.H., DeAntonio, C., McCracken, J.T., Forness, S.R. & Ackerland, V. (1994). Psychiatric consultation in severe and profound mental retardation. *American Journal of Psychiatry* **151**, 1802–1808.

Kinon, B.J., Jeste, D.V., Kollack-Walker, S., Stauffer, V. & Liu-Seifert, H. (2004). Olanzapine treatment for tardive dyskinesia in schizophrenia patients: a prospective trial with patients randomized to blinded dose reduction periods. *Progress in Neuro-Psychopharmacology and Biological Psychiatry* **28**, 985–996.

Kurokawa, T., Yokomozo, Y., Lee, S. & Kusuda, T. (2010). Clinical features of epilepsy with pervasive developmental disorder. *Brain & Development* **32**(9), 764–8.

Lann, L.A., den Boer, A.T., Hennekam, R.C., Renier, W.O. & Brouwer, O.F. (1996). Angelman syndrome in adulthood. *American Journal of Medical Genetics* **66**, 356–360.

Larbrisseau, A., Vanasse, M., Brochu, P. & Jasmin, G. (1984). The Andermann syndrome: agenesis of the corpus callosum associated with mental retardation and progressive sensorimotor neuronopathy. *Canadian Journal of Neurological Sciences* **11**, 257–261.

Lenhoff, H.M., Wang, P.P., Greenberg, F. & Bellugi, U. (1997). Williams syndrome and the brain. *Scientific American* December, 68–73.

Lerner, V., Miodownik, C., Bersudsky, Y., Kaptsan, A., Libov, I., Sela, B.A. & Witztum, E. (2007). Vitamin B6 treatment for tardive dyskinesia: a randomized, double-blind, placebo-controlled, crossover study. *Journal of Clinical Psychiatry* **68**, 1648–1654.

Lowry, M. & Sovner, R. (1991). The functional existence of problem behavior: a key to effective treatment. *The Habilitative Mental Health Care Newsletter* **10**, 59–63.

Lowry, M. & Sovner, R. (1992). Severe behavior problems associated with rapid cycling bipolar disorder in two adults with profound mental retardation. *Journal of Intellectual Disability Research* **36**, 269–281.

Madhusoodanan, S. & Bogunovic, O.J. (2004). Safety of benzodiazepines in the geriatric population. *Expert Opinion on Drug Safety* **3**, 485–93.

Matson, J.L., Fodstad, J.C. & Rivet, T.T. (2008). The Convergent and Divergent Validity of the Matson Evaluation of Drug Side-effects (MEDS). and the Dyskinesia Identification System: Condensed User Scale (DISCUS). *Journal of Intellectual & Developmental Disability* **33**(4), 337–44.

Miller E.R., Pastor-Barriuso, R., Dalal, D., Riemersma, R.A., Appel, L.J. & Guallar, E. (2005). Meta-analysis: high-dosage vitamin E supplementation may increase all-cause mortality. *Annals of Internal Medicine* **142**, 37–46.

Mount, R.H., Hastings, R.P. & Reilly, S. (2002). Behavioral and emotional features in Rett syndrome. *Disability & Rehabilitation* **23**, 129–138.

Munetz, M.R. & Benjamin, S. (1988). How to examine patients using the Abnormal Involuntary Movement Scale. *Hospital & Community Psychiatry* **39**(11), 1172–1177.

Nijhuis-van der Sanden, R., Smits-Engelsman, B. & Eling, P. (2000). Motor performance in girls with Turner syndrome. *Developmental Medicine & Child Neurology* **42**, 685–690.

O'Shea, T.M. (2008). Diagnosis, treatment, and prevention of cerebral palsy. *Clinical Obstetrics and Gynecology* **51**, 816–828.

Pappa, S., Tsouli, S., Apostolou, G., Mavreas, V. & Konitsiotis, S. (2010). Effects of amantadine on tardive dyskinesia: a randomized, double-blind, placebo-controlled study. *Clinical Neuropharmacology* **33**, 271–275.

Post, R.M., Ketter, T.A., Joffe, R.T. & Kramlinger, K.L. (1991). Lack of beneficial effects of l-baclofen in affective disorder. *International Clinical Psychopharmacology* **6**, 197–207.

Ratey, J.J., Sorgi, P. & Polakoff, S. (1985). Nadolol as a treatment for akathesia. *American Journal of Psychiatry*, **142**(5), page 640.

Reiss, S., Levitan, G.W. & Szyszko, J. (1982). Emotional disturbance in mental retardation: diagnostic overshadowing. *American Journal of Mental Deficiency* **86**, 567–574.

Rekand, T. (2010). Clinical assessment and management of spasticity: a review. *Acta Neurologica Scandinavica 122 Suppl.* **190**, 62–66.

Richardson, M.A., Bevans, M.L., Read, L.L., Chao, H.M., Clelland, J.D., Suckow, R.F., Maher, T.J. & Citrome, L. (2003). Efficacy of the branched-chain amino acids in the treatment of tardive dyskinesia in men. *American Journal of Psychiatry* **160**, 1117–1124.

Rodriguez-Revenga, L., Pagonabarraga, J., PhD, Gómez-Anson, B., López-Mourelo, O., Madrigal, I., Xunclà, M., Kulisevsky, J. & Milà, M. (2010). Motor and mental dysfunction in mother-daughter transmitted FXTAS. *Neurology* **75**, 1370–1376.

Salin-Cantegrel, A., Rivière, J.B., Dupré, N., Charron, F.M., Shekarabi, M., Karéméra, L., Gaspar, C., Horst, J., Tekin, M., Deda, G., Krause, A., Lippert, M.M., Willemsen, M.A., Jarrar, R., Lapointe, J.Y. & Rouleau, G.A. (2007). Distal truncation of KCC3 in non-French Canadian HMSN/ACC families. *Neurology* **69**, 1350–1355.

Sanders, R.D. & Gillig, P.M. (2010). Gait and its assessment in psychiatry. *Psychiatry* **7**, 38–43.

Sandman, C. (1990/1991). The opiate hypothesis in autism and self-injury. *Journal of Child and Adolescent Psychopharmacology* **1**, 237–248.

Sanger, T.D., Delgado, M.R., Gaebler-Spira, D., Hallett, M. & Mink, J.W. (2003). Classification and definition of disorders causing hypertonia in childhood. *Pediatrics* **11**, 89–97.

Saper, J.R., Winner, P.K. & Lake, A.E. 3rd. (2001). An open-label dose-titration study of the efficacy and tolerability of tizanidine hydrochloride tablets in the prophylaxis of chronic daily headache. *Headache* **41**(4), 357–368.

Schaefer, G.B. & Bodensteiner, J.B. (1992). Evaluation of the child with idiopathic mental retardation. *Pediatric Clinics of North America* **39**(4), 929–943.

Scott, B.L. (2000). Evaluation and treatment of dystonia. *Southern Medical Journal* **93**(8), 746–751.

Shamir, E., Barak, Y., Shalman, I., Laudon, M., Zisapel, N., Tarrasch, R., Elizur, A. & Weizman, R. (2001). Melatonin treatment for tardive dyskinesia: a double-blind, placebo-controlled, crossover study. *Archives of General Psychiatry* **58**, 1049–1052.

Shellenberger, M.K., Groves, L., Shah, J. & Novack, G.D. (1999). A controlled pharmacokinetic evaluation of tizanidine and baclofen at steady state. *Drug Metabolism and Disposition* **27**, 201–204.

Simpson, G.M. (2000). The treatment of tardive dyskinesia and tardive dystonia. *Journal of Clinical Psychiatry* **61** Suppl. 4, 39–44.

Simpson, D.M., Gracies, J.M., Yablon, S.A., Barbano, R. & Brashear, A. (2009). Botulinum neurotoxin versus tizanidine in upper limb spasticity: a placebo-controlled study. *Journal of Neurology, Neurosurgery & Psychiatry* **80**, 380–385.

Soares-Weiser, K., Maayan, N. & McGrath, J. (2011). Vitamin E for neuroleptic-induced tardive dyskinesia. *Cochrane Database of Systematic Reviews* **2**, CD000209.

Sovner, R. & Hurley, A. (1990). Assessment tools which facilitate psychiatric evaluations and treatment. *The Habilitative Mental Healthcare Newsletter* **9**, 91–98.

Sovner, R. & Hurley, A. (1991). Seven questions to ask when considering an acute psychiatric inpatient admission for a developmentally disabled adult. *The Habilitative Mental Healthcare Newsletter* **10**, 27–30.

Steffenburg, U. & Steffenburg, S. (1999). Epilepsy and other neuropsychiatric morbidity in mentally retarded children. In: Sillanpää, M., Gram, L., Johannessen, S.I.& Tomson, T. (eds.) *Epilepsy and mental retardation* pp. 47–59. Wrightson Biomedical, Petersfield, UK.

Sujansky, E. & Conradi, S. (1995). Outcome of Sturge-Weber syndrome in 52 adults. *American Journal of Medical Genetics* **57**, 35–45.

Tavano, A., Gagliardi, C., Martelli, S. & Borgatti, R. (2010). Neurological soft signs feature a double dissociation within the language system in Williams syndrome. *Neuropsychologia* **48**(11), 3298–3304.

Van Harten. P.N. & Kahn, R.S. (1999). Tardive dystonia. *Schizophrenia Bulletin* **25**, 741–748.

Vantrappen, G., Rommel, N., Devriendt, K., Cremers, C.W., Feenstra, L. & Fryns, J.P. (2001). Clinical features in 130 patients with the velo-cardio-facial syndrome. *Acta Oto-Rhino-Laryngologica Belgica* **55**(1), 43–48.

Villamonte, R., Vehrs, P.R., Feland, J.B., Johnson, A.W., Seeley, M.K. & Eggett, D. (2010). Reliability of 16 balance tests in individuals with Down syndrome. *Perceptual and Motor Skills* **11**(2), 530–542.

White, H.E., Durston, V.J., Harvey, J.F. & Cross, N.C. (2006). Quantitative analysis of SNRPN(correction of SRNPN) gene methylation by pyrosequencing as a diagnostic test for Prader-Willi syndrome and Angelman syndrome. *Clinical Chemistry* **52**(6), 1005–1013.

Williams, C. (2005). Neurological aspects of the Angelman syndrome. *Brain & Development.*, **27**, 88–94.

Williams, C.A., Angelman, H., Clayton-Smith, J., Driscoll, D.J., Hendrickson, J.E., Knoll, J.H. M., Magenis, R.E., Schinzel, A., Wagstaff, J., Whidden, E.M. & Zori, R.T. (1995). Angelman syndrome: consensus for diagnostic criteria. Angelman syndrome Foundation. *American Journal of Medical Genetics* **56**(2), 237–238.

Williams, C.A., Beaudet, A.L., Clayton-Smith, J., Knoll, J.H., Kyllerman, M., Laan, L.A., Magenis, R.E., Moncla, A., Schinzel, A.A., Summers, J.A. & Wagstaff, J. (2006). Angelman syndrome 2005: updated consensus for diagnostic criteria. *American Journal of Medical Genetics A* **140**(5), 413–418.

Wonodi, I., Adami, H., Sherr, J., Avila, M.T., Hong, L.E. & Thaker, G.K. (2004). Naltrexone treatment of tardive dyskinesia in patients with schizophrenia. *Journal of Clinical Psychopharmacology* **24**, 441–445.

Woods, S.W., Saksa, J.R., Baker, C.B., Cohen, S.J. & Tek, C. (2008). Effects of levetiracetam on tardive dyskinesia: a randomized, double-blind, placebo-controlled study. *Journal of Clinical Psychiatry* **69**, 546–554.

Wszola, B.A., Newell, K.M. & Sprague, R.L. (2001). Risk factors for tardive dyskinesia in a large population of youths and adults. *Experimental and Clinical Psychopharmacology* **9**, 285–296.

Zubenko, G.S., Cohen, B.M., Lipinski, J.F. & Jonas, J.M. (1984). Use of clonidine in the treatment of akathisia. *Psychiatry Research* **13**, 253–259.

5

Traumatic Brain Injuries and Co-occurring Mental Illness

Gretchen N. Foley, MD Assistant Professor,
Wright State University, Dayton, Ohio

Introduction

Traumatic brain injury (TBI) can result in a variable combination of cognitive problems and psychiatric symptoms. Cognitive dysfunction is common in the early course of TBI, and the severity and duration are largely dependent on the nature and severity of the injury. Persisting cognitive deficits are highly variable. Long-term cognitive impairment or dementia can follow TBI and may include problems with memory, attention/concentration, language and/or executive functioning. Such impairments may or may not improve with time and treatment. Both injured individuals and their families alike ascribe the persisting disability more often to impaired cognitive and behavioral functioning than actual physical problems (DeGuise *et al.*, 2008).

Psychiatric disorders may also occur secondary to TBI, and these can range from subtle changes noticeable only to close friends or family members, to blatantly abnormal behaviors that violate societal norms. Individuals with TBI may demonstrate irritability, impulsivity, aggression, childish behavior, affective instability or lability, poor judgment, lack of social awareness for appropriate behavior, apathy or frank abulia.

Psychiatry of Intellectual Disability: A Practical Manual, First Edition.
Edited by Julie P. Gentile and Paulette M. Gillig.
© 2012 John Wiley & Sons, Ltd. Published 2012 by John Wiley & Sons, Ltd.

Similarities and differences between patients with TBI as compared with patients with intellectual disability

There are similarities between individuals with TBI and those who have intellectual disability (ID). Cognitive and communication impairments may be present in varying degrees. Both populations tend to require a multifaceted treatment approach that combines both medication management and non-pharmacologic interventions. Family members and other caregivers are often integral to effective treatment. Both groups exhibit higher medication sensitivity, requiring lower doses and longer medication trials. Polypharmacy is not an uncommon practice.

ID is commonly considered a genetic or congenital disorder, often present from birth or early childhood, though it can develop through age 22 and sometimes is acquired by injury or illness. Individuals with ID are characterized by a significantly below-average score on a test of mental ability or intelligence quotient (IQ), as well as limitations in the ability to function in areas of daily life – including self-care, mobility, learning, communication or navigating social situations.

ID is sometimes referred to as a cognitive disability or, formally, as mental retardation (CDC, 2004). In contrast, patients with TBI have acquired deficits in cognitive functioning as a result of damage to the brain that can occur at any age. These individuals generally maintain a normal IQ but may have problems with attention, concentration, memory, slowed thought processing and more complex tasks involving executive functioning that impair their functional abilities. Further, while intellectual functioning is overall preserved, individuals with TBI often have communication difficulties after injury that make it difficult to express themselves coherently to others.

Both populations require mental health providers to take a patient and compassionate approach to care. These individuals may require longer appointment times, more frequent meetings and a more comprehensive treatment approach than do those without such cognitive or communication difficulties.

Overview of TBI: definitions, classification and epidemiology

Much of the knowledge regarding disability secondary to TBI has been developed as a result of evaluation and treatment of persons injured during military service, and this is currently used as a guideline for treatment of civilian injuries from falls, motor vehicle accidents and other traumas. TBI has been defined (Department of Veterans Affairs, 2010) as any traumatically induced structural injury and/or physiological disruption of brain function as a result of an external force that is indicated by new onset or worsening of at least one of the following clinical signs, immediately following the event:

1 Any period of loss of or a decreased level of consciousness.

2 Any loss of memory for events immediately before or after the injury.

3 Any alteration in mental state at the time of the injury (e.g. confusion, disorientation, slowed thinking).

4 Neurological deficits (e.g. weakness, balance disturbance, praxis, paresis/plegia, change in vision, other sensory alterations, aphasia) that may or may not be transient.

5 Intracranial lesion.

The external forces responsible for TBI may include any of the following:

- The head being struck by an object.

- The head striking an object.

- The brain undergoing an acceleration/deceleration movement without direct external trauma to the head.

- A foreign body penetrating the brain.

- Forces generated from events such as a blast or explosion, or other undefined force.

The severity of a TBI depends on a variety of factors and occurs on a continuum ranging from mild concussion with no apparent sequelae to a completely comatose states or death. TBI is generally classified based on the following factors:

1 Glasgow Coma Scale (GCS) score – scores range from 3 (coma/death) to 15 (fully conscious), based on eye opening (4 points), motor response (6 points) and verbal response (5 points).

2 Length of loss of consciousness (LOC) – defined as the period of non-responsiveness following injury.

3 Length of altered consciousness (AOC) – defined as the period of altered mental status following injury.

4 Length of post-traumatic amnesia (PTA) – defined as the time elapsed since an injured individual regains consciousness until he or she can consistently form memory for ongoing events.

These four criteria are used in conjunction with findings on neuroimaging to grade the severity of TBI. GCS scores generally are taken at the time of presentation for medical care. LOC and length of AOC can be difficult to assess with an unwitnessed event, as the injured person may be unaware whether he or she lost consciousness and may be dazed, confused, and/or disoriented. Length of PTA is even more problematic to determine reliably, as pain medications or sedatives can prolong this state artificially. Further, it is important to distinguish between what the injured individual actually remembers, versus what others may have told them happened.

The Department of Defense and Department of Veterans Affairs (DoD/DVA) consensus-based classification of closed TBI severity can be found in Table 1.

TBI remains a significant cause of morbidity and mortality in the United States. Each year, approximately 1.7 million Americans incur a TBI of some sort (CDC, 2010). Of

Table 1 Classification of traumatic brain injury severity.

Severity criteria	Concussion/mild TBI (mTBI)	Moderate TBI	Severe TBI
Neuroimaging findings	Normal structural imaging	Normal or abnormal structural imaging	Normal or abnormal structural imaging
Initial GCS	13–15	9–12	< 9
Length of LOC	0–30 minutes	>30 minutes but less than 24 hours	>24 hours
Length of AOC/AMS	1 minute up to 24 hours	>24 hours	>24 hours
Length of PTA	0–1 day	>1 but less than 7 days	>7 days

Source: adapted from Department of Veterans Affairs (2010), page 11.

these, 1.365 million (nearly 80%) are treated and released from an emergency department. Another 275,000 individuals are hospitalized and 52,000 die (CDC, 2010). These numbers are likely to underestimate the true incidence, as those with mild or military-related injuries may not seek treatment in the first place. Direct costs for hospital care, extended care, and other medical care and services, coupled with indirect costs such as lost productivity in the U.S., were estimated at $60 billion annually in 2000 (Finklestein *et al.*, 2006).

TBI can be sustained in a variety of circumstances. Table 2 shows the most common causes of TBI in the United States. Children, the elderly and men in any age group are at higher risk for TBI. Approximately 18% of all TBI-related emergency department visits involve children aged 0–4 years. Approximately 22% of all TBI-related hospitalizations involved adults aged 75 years and older. Males account for over half (59%) of those diagnosed with a TBI (Faul *et al.*, 2010). Those with alcohol or drug abuse or dependence are also at higher risk for TBI than those without substance use disorders (Vassallo *et al.*, 2007).

Table 2 Causes of TBI.

Falls (35.2%)	Most common cause overall. Responsible for 50% of TBIs among children aged 0–14 years and 61% of TBIs among adults aged 65 years and older.
Motor vehicle or traffic-related incidents (17.3%)	Responsible for the largest percentage of TBI-related deaths (31.8%).
Struck by/against events (16.5%)	The second leading cause of TBI among children aged 0–14 years (25%).
Assaults (10%)	Significantly lower rates in children aged 0–14 years (2.9%) and in adults aged 65 years old and older (1%).
Unknown/other (21%)	Important note: CDC estimates of TBI do not include injuries seen at U.S. Department of Defense or U.S. Veterans Health Administration Hospitals.

Source: adapted from Faul *et al.* (2010), page 21.

Table 3 Clinical presentation based on site of TBI.

Injury Site	Possible clinical presentation
Frontal lobe	Impaired executive functioning, apathy or disinhibition, hemiparesis, Broca's aphasia
Temporal lobe	Irritability, aggression, memory impairments, word-finding and naming difficulties
Parietal lobe	Visual-spatial impairments, difficulty understanding language (if left hemisphere involved)
Occipital lobe	Blindness, visual field deficits, inability to recognize objects
Cerebellum	Poor coordination, difficulty ambulating, nystagmus, tremors
Diffuse injury	Generalized slowing of cognitive processes, longer reaction time, difficulty completing tasks

Common mental health presentations following TBI

Presentations after TBI vary dramatically depending on the severity of injury, the affected individual's premorbid functional status and the type and site of injury. We have already discussed classification of the severity of TBI and, generally speaking, those with a more severe TBI have more significant symptomatology and greater deficits on clinical exam. Those with higher functional status prior to injury have better outcomes overall (Raymont *et al.*, 2008).

The type and location of injury has important clinical implications. Primary brain injuries are classified as focal, diffuse or mixed. Focal damage is usually the result of direct impact of the brain against the cranium, but it may also occur in penetrating or open head injuries. Focal lesions may include subdural or epidural hematomas, subarachnoid or intracerebral hemorrhage, and cortical contusion. Such lesions are often visible on neuroimaging. Table 3 demonstrates some common presentations after focal injuries. Diffuse axonal injury is caused by rotational acceleration-deceleration forces and results in more widespread damage that may be undetectable on neuroimaging. It is possible to have both focal and diffuse damage from a single traumatic event.

Following an initial TBI, mechanisms of secondary injury include cellular neurochemical and metabolic cascades, increased intracranial pressure, ischemia, hypotension, hypoxia or temperature dysregulation.

Clinical Vignette #1

Mr. Jones is a 50-year-old married Caucasian male who was involved in a traffic accident in which he was a pedestrian struck by a car. As a result of this collision, Mr. Jones sustained a head injury as well as two fractured legs. Upon the arrival of paramedics, he was found to be unconscious, with a GCS of 10; he remained non-responsive for nearly eight hours.

After transportation to the hospital, he was found to have a subdural hematoma and was determined to have sustained a moderate TBI. After appropriate neurosurgical interventions and a lengthy ICU stay, in which he developed a new-onset seizure disorder, Mr. Jones was transferred to a rehabilitation facility that specialized in head injuries. During this period of time, he was started on carbamazepine to control his seizures and to assist with mood lability. He was also started on citalopram for moderate depressive symptoms. Both improved significantly and, after his physical rehab was completed, Mr. Jones was discharged home with his family.

Meeting with a psychiatrist for ongoing outpatient care, Mr. Jones reported that things were just fine. He stopped taking the citalopram because he said he didn't feel depressed. However, his wife was particularly concerned by changes in his personality and memory difficulties. She reported that her husband was more easily irritable and very forgetful. He often got confused in the middle of tasks and became frustrated when unable to do the things he used to do. This resulted in angry outbursts and very labile emotional states.

The psychiatrist checked his carbamazepine level and determined that this medication was at a suboptimal dose. This was adjusted at the first appointment, in hopes of helping with the irritability. Later, donepezil was added at a low dose to help with cognitive deficits. Both interventions helped to some degree but, six months later, Mr. Jones reported to his primary care physician that he was again feeling depressed.

The primary care doctor restarted citalopram at the previous dose – 40 mg daily. Within two weeks, Mr. Jones became agitated and threatened to kill himself after an argument with his wife. She brought him to the emergency department for evaluation, where Mr. Jones was noted to be sobbing uncontrollably and repeatedly asking, "Doc, am I going crazy?" His carbamazepine level was found to be 0, and Mr. Jones reported that he had stopped this when he started the antidepressant. "I got confused. I thought I was only supposed to take one or the other." He was admitted for acute stabilization and the agitation and suicidality resolve, with discontinuation of the citalopram and achieving a therapeutic carbamazepine level.

This vignette illustrates several points. First, the communication between a patient's treatment providers is of utmost importance. Having multiple physicians on the case increases the risk for polypharmacy. Second, well-intentioned changes can cause unforeseen problems in patients with TBI, as they are more sensitive to medication dosages and side effects. Further, providers must be very clear in their instructions regarding a patient's treatment. Generally, providing a written list of all changes to medications and enlisting the help of family in administering these can increase treatment adherence and success.

Individuals with TBI present with varying complaints, which generally fall into three categories: physical, cognitive, or emotional/behavioral problems. Common presenting symptoms are listed in Table 4.

TBI may predispose individuals to psychiatric illness. One study looking at traumatic injuries in general – not just TBI – showed that 31% of patients reported a psychiatric disorder and 22% developed a psychiatric disorder which did not pre-exist within a year of the trauma. The most common new psychiatric disorders were generalized anxiety disorder (9%), depressive disorders (9%), post-traumatic stress disorder (6%) and agoraphobia (6%) (Bryant *et al.*, 2010).

After a TBI, mood disorders may occur secondary to the injury itself, or to changes in the affected individual's physical/emotional state and cognitive processing. In one study, major

Table 4 Common symptom presentations of TBI.

Physical	Cognitive	Emotional/behavioral
Headache	Difficulties or impairments in:	Depression
Nausea/vomiting	• attention	Apathy
Dizziness/loss of balance	• concentration	Mania
Blurred vision	• new learning	Anxiety
Sleep disturbance	• memory	Agitation
Weakness/paresis/plegia	• speed of mental processing	Anger/irritability
Sensory loss	• planning	Impulsivity
Spasticity	• reasoning	Emotional lability
Aphasia	• judgment	Aggression
Dysphagia	• executive control	Social disinhibition
Apraxia	• self-awareness	Personality change
Difficulty with coordination	• language	"Acting out"
Seizures	• abstract thinking	PTSD

Source: adapted from Department of Veterans Affairs (2010), pp. 6, 69.

depressive disorder (MDD) occurred more frequently in those with TBI than those with other trauma not involving the central nervous system (Jorge *et al.*, 2004). Another found that, of those with TBI, about half (53%) met criteria for MDD at some point during the first year of their recovery (Bombardier *et al.*, 2010).

Manic or psychotic episodes can also develop after TBI, though it is questionable whether this is more likely to occur if the brain was vulnerable prior to the injury. One study demonstrates that individuals who developed psychosis following TBI had significantly more premorbid neurological problems (previous brain injury, learning disorders, seizures, birth complications, etc.) than controls (Fujii & Ahmed 2001). Another failed to demonstrate differences in perinatal or developmental abnormalities between those who went on to develop psychosis after their TBI and those who did not. However, this study did note that having a first-degree relative with a psychotic disorder was one of the strongest predictors for developing post-TBI psychosis, perhaps reflecting a genetic vulnerability to such symptoms (Sachdev *et al.*, 2001).

Many patients with TBI suffered a traumatic event at the time of their injury (motor vehicle accident, assault, combat situation, etc.). Such traumas often cause anxiety reactions, including post-traumatic stress disorder (PTSD). The association between PTSD and TBI remains a focus of ongoing investigation, especially given the increased prevalence of TBI in military populations. Part of the difficulty in assessing these conditions is that their significant symptom overlap. Both PTSD and TBI can result in complaints of sleep disturbance, fatigue, irritability, depression and poor attention or memory. Symptoms unique to PTSD include flashbacks, avoidance, hypervigilance, nightmares and re-experiencing phenomenon. Symptoms more attributable to mild TBI or concussion (mTBI) include headaches, nausea, vomiting, visual problems and sensitivity to light or sound.

In one study, the presence of mTBI was highly associated with PTSD symptoms three to four months after returning from deployment during Operation Iraqi Freedom (Hoge *et al.*, 2008). These authors also concluded that PTSD and depression were important mediators between mTBI and physical health problems, since mTBI alone only accounted for continued complaints of headache (not other physical problems) when they controlled for those with PTSD and/or depression.

As stated earlier, cognitive dysfunction is common in the early course of TBI, and the severity and duration are largely dependent on the nature and severity of the injury. Persisting cognitive deficits are highly variable. Long-term cognitive impairment or dementias can follow TBI and may include problems with memory, attention/concentration, language and/or executive functioning. Such impairments may or may not improve with time and treatment.

Both injured individuals and their families ascribe the persisting disability more to impaired cognitive and behavioral functioning than actual physical problems (DeGuise et al., 2008). The rate of cognitive recovery tends be rapid in the early weeks after injury, but slows at one year post-injury. There is, however, some evidence that functional cognitive improvements may continue up to ten years post-injury (Draper et al., 2008). There is some debate about whether gains late in TBI recovery may be more related to increased adaptability to the environment through compensatory behaviors, rather than actual improvement in cognitive function.

Also, as mentioned earlier, personality changes may also occur secondary to TBI. These can range from subtle changes, noticeable only to close friends or family members, to blatantly abnormal behaviors that violate societal norms. Individuals with TBI may demonstrate new irritability, impulsivity, aggression, childish behavior, affective instability or lability, poor judgment, lack of social awareness for appropriate behavior, apathy or frank abulia. Others may comment that the injured individual may literally no longer seem to be the "same person" as before their TBI. Families often have unrealistic expectations for recovery or "return to normal" (Lezak, 1986). These misconceptions tend to exacerbate the situation, as the TBI-affected individual's abnormal behavior may be perceived as intentional.

Patients with traumatic brain injuries and co-occurring mental illness

Just as TBI can predispose patients to concurrent or subsequent psychiatric illness, premorbid psychiatric conditions influence the risk of sustaining TBI and affect the course of illness and recovery. Impulse control difficulties, substance abuse, family problems and previous psychiatric problems increase the risk for brain injury (Vassallo et al., 2007). Alcohol and drug withdrawal can worsen cognitive dysfunction, resulting in delirium, seizures or death. Detoxification protocols may require dose adjustments, due to reduced tolerability of many medications, including benzodiazepines, in those with TBI.

Patients with previous diagnoses of depression or anxiety tend to be less functional and more disabled after TBI than those without these comorbidities (Fann et al., 2002). They also perceive themselves to have more severe injury and cognitive deficits than controls. Those with schizophrenia or other psychotic disorders may already have dysfunction in the prefrontal cortex, temporal lobes and hippocampus, all of which are vulnerable to further injury with TBI thus worsening prognosis overall. Premorbid personality traits influence the defense mechanisms utilized to cope with TBI (Strain & Grossman, 1975).

Clinical Vignette #2

Mr. Doe is a 30-something Hispanic male who is an illegal immigrant and speaks limited English. He was admitted to the hospital after being found "down" in the street, a victim of assault. Mr. Doe had sustained a severe TBI and was comatose in the intensive care unit (ICU) for several weeks. Eventually, he emerged from the coma and was transferred to a general medical unit, where he appeared relatively non-cooperative with members of his treatment team. He was combative at times and had physically struck a nurse who was attempting to change a dressing.

The psychiatry service was initially consulted to manage insomnia and "behavioral problems." Mr. Doe was started on mirtazapine and valproate that was gradually titrated to a therapeutic level. His sleep and agitation both improved, and he was able to participate in his therapies. He remained hospitalized for an extended period of time, as a result of difficulties in determining a long-term disposition due to his immigration status.

Approximately four months after the psychiatry consult, Mr. Doe's mental health condition abruptly worsened. He was sleeping all day and refused therapy and most meals. He became very agitated whenever staff attempted to awaken him. The primary team augmented his current regimen with haloperidol and discontinued all therapy due to "patient non-participation."

Two weeks later, the psychiatry service was re-consulted because the patient was completely non-compliant with treatment, had lost an unhealthy amount of weight, and the aggressive behavior necessitated a 1:1 sitter for safety reasons. One of the therapists who spoke Spanish felt Mr. Doe was depressed and feeling hopeless about ever getting out of the hospital. The psychiatry team increased the mirtazapine dosage and provided daily supportive therapy, but improvement was minimal. During this time, Mr. Doe kept complaining about hitting his head. He was very upset about this, and everyone assumed he was referring to his initial injury. Eventually, a thorough chart review revealed that around the time his condition acutely changed, Mr. Doe had lost his balance and struck his head in the elevator during a trip off the unit for testing.

Once the staff addressed this concern, Mr. Doe was much more cooperative with therapy, and buspirone was added to address residual irritability with good response. Unfortunately, the primary team was so burnt out from caring for this patient that they were reluctant to re-engage with him. Eventually, the psychiatrist called a treatment team meeting to explain the sequence of events and to address the counter-transference that had developed. They then re-ordered the physical and occupational therapies, and careful coordination with the translator greatly benefited Mr. Doe.

This vignette demonstrates the importance of collaborating with a team of treatment providers. Everyone on the team must communicate, and often therapists have more day-to-day information that would be helpful to physician staff. This example also illustrates the value of continuing to search for potential underlying causes of depression or behavioral abnormalities in patients with TBI. In this case, there was a language barrier that contributed to the confusion; however, patients with TBI may not be aware of, or able clearly to verbalize, their emotional states, depending on their particular impairments. Medication interventions may not always be the appropriate primary intervention for behavioral problems, especially when there is a shaky therapeutic alliance between patient and providers.

Assessment and treatment options

Initial management of moderate to severe TBI focuses on medical stabilization of the injured individual, followed by early rehabilitation and careful attention to preventing complications. When patients are well enough to leave the hospital or rehabilitation facility, a transitional program to assist with community re-entry is helpful. Not all affected individuals can complete this transition, and some may require ongoing long-term or residential care. Many of those who return home will require continued mental health care in some regard. In this section, we will focus on options for long-term outpatient treatment of TBI.

Thorough assessment of the injured individual is necessary for appropriate treatment planning. This should always include a comprehensive history (to include medical and psychiatric conditions, substance use pattern, family history and social history, particularly focused on academic and/or occupational functioning) and physical examination (to include a mental status examination, a mini-mental state examination, complete neurological exam, screening lab studies, and possible radiology or neuropsychological studies), as well as collateral information (to include medical and mental health records, educational records and reports from family or close friends).

Listed in Table 5 are ten questions that the Department of Veterans Affairs recommends providers use in their initial meetings with patients. In more severe cases, the initial assessment may require an interdisciplinary approach, with expert input from multiple other health care providers. Depending on the patient, referrals for psychological testing or treatment of concurrent medical illness may be needed. Table 6 lists potential subspecialists that may be helpful in the care of patients with complicated presentations.

Interventions should be guided by the severity of the initial TBI and the patient's current clinical presentation. A symptom management approach is often utilized, and this must take into account other concurrent medical diagnoses, cognitive disability, psychological/emotional/behavioral symptoms and psychosocial considerations.

There are several non-pharmacological interventions for treatment of TBI. Cognitive rehabilitation, along with occupational, physical and language therapies, address specific cognitive and physical disabilities, with a focus on recovery when possible and developing compensatory techniques where deficits still exist. These may include practical recommendations to minimize distractions, working on one task at a time and using a calendar, organizer or "to do" lists, as well as repetitive review of information and regularly checking for mistakes or errors in activities.

Social skills training and/or group psychotherapy address the communication difficulties and resulting social problems and isolation that may arise after TBI. Individual psychotherapy, whether supportive or cognitive-behavioral, may help patients with TBI address denial of their deficits, decrease their sense of loneliness and regain their sense of self (Pollack, 2005). Because TBI never affects only the individual, family education and therapy can help caregivers grieve the loss of the affected individual's previous life and level of functioning while fostering more realistic expectations for recovery (Lezak, 1986).

There are multiple pharmacological interventions that may be of use in individuals affected by TBI. Patients with brain injuries are more sensitive to potential medication side effects than those without TBI. Monotherapy is preferred but often not possible. Many

Table 5 Clinical Pearls 1: Questions that may assist in developing a management plan for patients with TBI.

Interview questions	Potential clinical implications
1. What brings the patient to seek services at this time?	What specific issues are most bothersome to the patient? Why are they coming to see you now?
2. What was the medical severity of the initial injury?	Severity of the initial injury is a good predictor of long-term prognosis.
3. What has been the course of recovery from the event?	Generally, recovery from TBI is gradual and eventually plateaus. An acute change in the recovery course or more stepped progress may indicate medical complications or behavioral issues requiring attention.
4. What services and interventions have already been utilized?	Knowing what a patient has already tried, what worked and what didn't can lead to more efficient treatment plans.
5. What is the severity and duration of the symptom complex?	Patients with less severe symptoms may be managed through primary care, but those with more complicated or prolonged symptoms may require multiple specialists for effective care.
6. What is the global impact of the patient's current symptoms?	It is critical to assess how a patient's symptoms effect their day-to-day life. Patients may be more concerned about interpersonal, academic or occupational difficulties than their actual symptoms.
7. Is there a root cause to the current impairment?	If there is an underlying medical or psychiatric issue that is causing recovery to stall, identifying and addressing that cause is important.
8. What is the patient's readiness to change?	Establishing a good therapeutic alliance and working with the patient to address their perceived needs may improve outcomes. A motivational approach can foster readiness to change over time.
9. Are there comorbidities that add to the complexity of the presentation?	Remember, "all that is cognitive or behavioral dysfunction is not TBI". Look for underlying or concurrent issues that may be contributing to the situation.
10. How should disability compensation and status affect care?	Disability is sometimes seen as incentive not to recover. It is critical to educate patients that, despite disability determinations, most patients with TBI improve with appropriate treatment.

Source: adapted from Department of Veterans Affairs (2010), pp. 2–4.

medications used in the management of TBI have not been fully studied in terms of assessing their efficacy in this specific population. The Veterans Health Initiative on Traumatic Brain Injury lists several common-sense guidelines in regards to pharmacotherapy in patients with TBI (see Table 7).

Whenever possible, using medication to treat a specific diagnosis is preferred. However, given the complex nature of TBI and multiple symptom overlap between various medical

Table 6　Clinical Pearls 2: Possible referrals that may be helpful in the care of patients with TBI.

Clinically-directed and appropriate referrals may include consults to the following disciplines:

Physiatrist
Neurologist
Neuro-ophthalmologist
Neuro-optometrist
Neurosurgeon
Endocrinology
Audiologist
Neuropsychologist
Clinical psychologist
Speech/language pathologist
Physical/occupational therapist
Kinesiotherapist
Recreation therapist
Social worker
Vocational rehabilitation counselor
Case manager

Source: adapted from Department of Veterans Affairs (2010), p. 46.

and psychiatric issues, a symptom-based approach is often utilized. Table 8 lists various target symptoms and recommendations for medication selection. Since many patients will require multiple medications for either psychiatric or physical problems, use of a pill box to organize medications, and reminders to prompt administration, are often necessary if another individual is not available to assist the patient.

Table 7　Clinical pearls 3: Common principle for prescribing medications for patients with TBI.

Useful guidelines for prescribing medications to individuals with TBI include:
• Begin medications after non-pharmacologic interventions have been unsuccessful.
• Obtain a detailed medication profile (including over-the-counter agents).
• Start low and go slow.
• Make only one medication change at a time.
• Provide an appropriate therapeutic drug trial.
• Allow adequate time for one drug to clear out of the person's system before changing to another medication.
• Be aware of confounding comorbidities (e.g. substance abuse, PTSD).
• Individuals with TBI are at higher risk for health illiteracy-related medication issues.
• Check for medication compliance in non-responders.
• All providers and caregivers should be aware of current medications and any medication changes.
• Don't prescribe what already hasn't worked or has had negative effects.
• The following classes of medication are not generally recommended in the management of TBI-related symptoms: antihistamines, narcotics, benzodiazepines.

Source: adapted from Department of Veterans Affairs (2010), p. 74.

Table 8 Pharmacological management of symptoms associated with TBI.

Symptom	First-line	Second-line	Notes
Post-traumatic Headache: tension-Type	Acetaminophen	NSAIDs	Avoid narcotic pain relievers (cognitive impairment).
Post-traumatic Headache: migraine-type	Triptans	Daily prophylaxis	Avoid narcotic pain relievers (cognitive impairment).
Headache Prophylaxis	SSRIs, valproate	TCAs, topiramate, beta blockers, calcium channel blockers	Avoid antidepressants in those with comorbid mania.
Sleep disturbance	Zolpidem, prazosin	Trazodone	Avoid benzodiazepines (cognitive impairment).
Fatigue	Moderate caffeine use	Methylphenidate, Modafinil, Amantadine	Rule out underlying cause (i.e. pain, sleep apnea). Try sleep hygiene first.
Dizziness	Meclizine, dimenhydrinate	Low-dose benzodiazepine	Consider referral to ENT.
Depression	SSRIs, SNRIs	TCAs, MAOIs, stimulants	Avoid bupropion (seizure risk).
Mania	Valproate, quetiapine	Carbamazepine, lithium	Other atypicals can be used, balance risks, benefits and side effect profile.
Pseudobulbar affect	SSRIs	Dextromethorphan/quinidine, amantadine	
Anxiety/PTSD	SSRs	Buspirone, Moderate Half-life Benzodiazepines (lorazepam/oxazepam)	Avoid short-acting benzos (addiction potential, rebound anxiety) and long-acting benzos (cumulative side effects).
Psychosis	Atypical antipsychotics	Typical antipsychotics	Rule out delirium.
Acute Agitation	High-potency antipsychotics	Benzodiazepines	Rule out delirium.
Disinhibited Personality	SSRIs, Anticonvulsants	Atypical antipsychotics	Avoid benzodiazepines.
Apathetic Personality	SSRIs, stimulants	Bromocriptine	Avoid benzodiazepines.
Cognitive Impairment	SSRIs, stimulants	TCAs, dopaminergic agents, donepezil, rivastigmine	Limit polypharmacy. Utilize cognitive rehabilitation.

Source: adapted from Department of Veterans Affairs (2010), pp. 145–148.

Conclusion

Individuals with traumatic brain injuries have similarities to those with ID, and both populations can experience the entire range of mental health conditions. The nature and severity of the brain injury will impact both long- and short-term outcomes and prognosis. The assessment and data collection will guide the mental health clinician in formulating a comprehensive treatment plan.

Improvement over time following the brain injury is a variable course, and it is dependent on multiple factors. It is important that the mental health needs of individuals with brain injuries are appropriately diagnosed and treated, as the impact on independence, relationships, educational and occupational functioning, among other areas of life, can be significant.

References

Bombardier, C.H., Fann, J.R., Temkin, N.R., Esselman, P.C., Barber, J. & Dikmen, S.S. (2010). Rates of major depressive disorder and clinical outcomes following traumatic brain injury. *JAMA* **303**, 1938–1945.

Bryant, R.A., O'Donnell, M.L., Creamer, M., McFarlane, A.C., Clark, C.R. & Silove, D. (2010). The psychiatric sequelae of traumatic injury. *American Journal of Psychiatry* **167**, 312–320.

Centers for Disease Control and Prevention (2010). Injury Prevention and Control: Traumatic Brain Injury. Available at: www.cdc.gov/TraumaticBrainInjury/statistics.html. Accessed March 20, 2011.

Centers for Disease Control and Prevention (CDC) (2004). Developmental Disabilities: Intellectual Disability. Available at: www.cdc.gov/ncbddd/dd/ddmr.htm. Accessed February 15, 2011.

DeGuise, E., LeBlanc, J., Feyz, M., Meyer, K., Duplantie, J., Thomas, H., Abouassaly, M., Champoux, M.C., Couturier, C., Lin, H., Lu, L., Robinson, C. & Roger, E. (2008) Long-term outcome after severe traumatic brain injury: the McGill interdisciplinary prospective study. *Journal of Head Trauma Rehabilitation* **23**, 294–303.

Department of Veterans Affairs (2010). Veterans Health Initiative Traumatic Brain Injury Independent Study Course: Available at: www.publichealth.va.gov/docs/vhi/traumatic-brain-injury-vhi.pdf. Accessed March 30, 2011.

Draper, K. & Ponsford, J. (2008). Cognitive functioning ten years following traumatic brain injury and rehabilitation. *Neuropsychology* **22**(5), 618–625.

Fann, J.R., Leonetti, E., Jaffe, K., Katon, W.J., Cummings, P. & Thompson, R.S. (2002). Psychiatric illness and subsequent traumatic brain injury: a case control study. *Journal of Neurology, Neurosurgery and Psychiatry* **72**, 615–620.

Faul, M., Xu, L., Wald, M.M. & Coronado, V.G. (2010). *Traumatic brain injury in the United States: emergency department visits, hospitalizations, and deaths.* Centers for Disease Control and Prevention, National Center for Injury Prevention and Control, Atlanta, GA.

Finkelstein, E., Corso, P., Miller, T., Fiebelkorn, I. & Zaloshnja, E. (2006). *The Incidence and Economic Burden of Injuries in the United States.* Oxford University Press, New York.

Fujii, D.E. & Ahmed, I. (2001). Risk factors in psychosis secondary to traumatic brain injury. *Journal of Neuropsychiatry and Clinical Neurosciences* **13**, 61–69.

Hoge, C.W., McGurk, D., Thomas, J.L., Cox, A.L., Engel, C.C. & Castro, C.A. (2008). Mild traumatic brain injury in US soldiers returning from Iraq. *New England Journal of Medicine* **358**, 453–463.

Jorge, R.E., Robinson, R.G., Moser, D., Tateno, A., Crespo-Facorrom B. & Arndt, S. (2004). Major depression following traumatic brain injury. *Archives of General Psychiatry* **61**(1), 42–50.

Lezak, M.D. (1986). Psychological implications of traumatic brain damage for the patient's family. *Rehabilitation Psychology* **31**, 241–250.

Pollack, I.W. (2005). Psychotherapy. In: Silver, J.M., McAllister, T.W. & Yudofsky, S.D. (eds.), *Textbook of Traumatic Brain Injury*, pp 641–654. American Psychiatric Publishing, Washington DC.

Raymont, V., Greathouse, A., Reding, K., Lipsky, R., Salazar, A. & Grafman, J. (2008). Demographic, structural and genetic predictors of late cognitive decline after penetrating head injury. *Brain* **131**, 543–558.

Sachdev, P., Smith, J.S. & Cathcart, S. (2001). Schizophrenia-like psychosis following traumatic brain injury: a chart-based descriptive and case-control study. *Psychological Medicine* **31**, 231–239.

Strain, J. & Grossman, S. (1975). Psychological reactions to medical illness and hospitalization. In Strain, J.& Grossman, S. (eds.) *Psychological Care of the Medically Ill: A Primer in Liaison Psychiatry*, pp 23–36. Appleton-Century-Crofts, New York.

Vassallo, J.L., Proctor-Weber, Z., Vanderploeg, R. D, Lebowitz, B.K. & Curtiss, G. (2007). Psychiatric Risk Factors for Head Injury. *Brain Injury* **21**, 567–573.

6

Interviewing Techniques

Julie P. Gentile, MD, Associate Professor, Wright State University, Dayton, Ohio

Paulette Marie Gillig, MD, PhD, Professor, Wright State University, Dayton, Ohio

"There is universal agreement that all individuals with ID might present with behavior and interaction skills of a chronologically younger child and might maintain these characteristics throughout the lifespan. Thus, any judgment about symptom presentation must be evaluated within the context of developmental delay."

(Szymanski & King, 1999)

Introduction

Communication is the foundation of every relationship. How individuals perceive their connection with their mental healthcare providers significantly influences the success of their treatment relationships (Finlay & Lyons, 2002). Many mental health professionals lack specialized training in the field of intellectual disabilities (ID), including a lack of training in communicating with patients who have limited expressive language skills. Although, in most educational programs, the mental health assessment of patients focuses on history-taking, the mental status examination and the interview process, if an individual is nonverbal or has limited communication abilities, then the clinician may lack confidence in interviewing him or her.

Another difference is that, although emphasis normally placed during residency training on the clinical dyad, when treating patients with ID there is nearly always at least one other person in the room, whether it be a caregiver, family member, guardian or other interested

Psychiatry of Intellectual Disability: A Practical Manual, First Edition.
Edited by Julie P. Gentile and Paulette M. Gillig.
© 2012 John Wiley & Sons, Ltd. Published 2012 by John Wiley & Sons, Ltd.

party. There is an art to "managing the triangle," which means talking to the patient with ID and simultaneously collecting collateral data from others who are present. One element of this skill is that the clinician should always talk directly to the patient during the appointment, even if the patient is nonverbal or has no usable verbal communication abilities.

The psychiatric interview of patients with ID is time-consuming and can be complicated by communication deficits. However, by utilizing certain question types and avoiding others, one can gain a wealth of information and effectively develop rapport. The evaluation must be performed in the context of the patient's specific developmental framework, and all subjective information obtained from the individual must be considered within this frame-work, for reasons that will be discussed later in this chapter (Fletcher, *et al.*, DM-ID, 2007).

The interviewer also must attend closely to nonverbal communication. Of course, patients with ID are not the only ones who utilize nonverbal communication. An estimated 60–65% of all interpersonal communication among people in the general population is conveyed via nonverbal behaviors (Foley & Gentile, 2010). Therefore, a better understanding of nonverbal communication will improve our understanding of all patients – both verbal and nonverbal – regardless of their expressive language skill ability. Finally, in addition to having an awareness of various forms of communication, the interviewer must recognize that, as with any other patient, the culture, environment, socioeconomic status and education of both the interviewer and the patient all influence how a message is delivered, as well as how it is received.

Levels of intellectual disability

There is a vast difference between interviewing a patient with mild ID versus one with severe or profound ID. Patients with *mild* ID generally will be verbal, but will communicate in concrete terms. The patient with *moderate* ID will typically be verbal but may answer questions with monosyllabic or other short responses as opposed to more complete phrases or full sentences. Many patients with *severe or profound* ID have more significantly limited verbal communicative abilities.

An awareness of the level of a patient's developmental framework and communicative ability can assist not only with the interview and information collection process, but also in understanding how the person processes grief and loss, the importance of routine and structure in the patient's life, and other important areas of psychological functioning. Communicative skills are often described in three categories by speech and language therapists (Hassiotis *et al.*, 2009) and are outlined in Table 1.

Expressive and receptive language skills: disparity

Most patients with ID have better developed receptive language skills than they do expressive language skills. An individual who is nonverbal, or one with no usable or severely limited language skills, may still understand everything that others are saying in the room.

The clinician can use observational skills to make this determination. For example, if a caregiver is describing a behavior that the nonverbal patient exhibits at home, and the patient begins displaying the behavior, it is evident that receptive language skills are well

Table 1 Categories of communicative skills.

Preverbal	The individual does not have cognitive ability to understand words. Typically, individuals functioning with preverbal communication have profound and multiple learning disabilities. They can be assisted through the use of routines, tone of voice, repetition, context of situations, objects and their own experience.
Nonverbal	Individuals have the ability to understand words, but do not have the ability to express themselves through words and will use alternative means, e.g. use of signing or pictures.
Verbal	Individuals will have a variety of skills for understanding language and will have expressive capabilities, predominantly using speech.

Source: Reproduced with permission from Hassiotis, A., Barron, D.A. & Hall, I. *Intellectual Disability Psychiatry: A Practical Handbook*, page 5. © John Wiley & Sons 2009.

developed. Irrespective of the expressive language skills of the patient, all comments to anyone in the room should be delivered with the expectation that the patient understands and will immediately pick up on being disrespected or ignored.

Setting the stage for the interview

Setting the stage for an interview is important because of the interviewee's possible past experiences with clinicians, which may or may not have been positive. *Prior* to the first interface with the patient, it is very important to review medical records whenever possible. A record review allows the clinician to use time more wisely during the meeting, and to eliminate redundancy in collecting information that is easily obtained from medical records.

As mentioned in Chapter 2, collateral informants should be introduced to everyone in the room, and their role and necessity for being present during the evaluation should be described. If the individual was referred for a specific reason, the person who ordered the evaluation should be present to discuss the details.

Inquire about the patient's idea of the purpose of the interview and correct it, if necessary. If the patient is non-verbal, begin with introductions and an explanation of the purpose of the meeting. It may be helpful to point out what will *not* happen as well (i.e. the individual will not receive an injection, for example, which is a common fear when arriving at an office). The interviewer should specifically point out to the patient that some words or questions may be difficult to understand, and the interviewer should take responsibility for any miscommunication. Communicate your expectations that the individual will ask questions, then check to make sure that questions are answered periodically throughout the interview. Create the expectation that, by the end of the interview, you (the clinician) will understand the patient's story.

Interviews should begin with general questions about non-threatening issues. For example, the interview of a child with ID could begin by asking about school (if this is non-threatening to the child) and their favorite activities. For adults, the interview may start by asking about their work and living situations. Such questions allow an individual to respond accurately, facilitate the development of rapport and allow for the patient to get practice in answering (Ott, 2005). If there are sensitive questions about intimate details of the patient's life, these are best left until later in the interview or for after a therapeutic alliance has been established. The patient's consent should be obtained before talking to others and before broaching sensitive topics.

Be aware of the patient's documented level of ID. If it the patient has only *mild* ID, for example, but you observe that he or she does not respond to questions, investigate and explore this, as it does not match what would be expected from the cognitive impairment that would be expected at that developmental level. Perhaps the patient is so anxious that he or she is unable to express things verbally, or perhaps he/she has a thought disorder and is manifesting thought blocking. Consider that the patient may have very limited socialization in the community, or may not have been addressed directly in previous appointments with mental health or other professionals and does not know that an answer is expected. Patients may be taken aback by being addressed by a person viewed as an authority figure.

Cognitive processes in the context of developmental framework and how this can affect the history

Hassiotis *et al.* (2009) reviewed the cognitive processes relevant to individuals with ID, summarized below:

Magical thinking

"Magical thinking" is not due to psychotic thought process, but related to the level of cognitive development of the individual. The individual is unable to make clear distinctions between fantasy and reality and may converse with people he or she has created or imagined. These presentations must be distinguished from hallucinatory and delusional experiences (Hassiotis *et al.*, 2009).

Pre-logical thinking

Pre-logical thinking is characteristic both of preschool-aged children and most individuals with severe to moderate ID (Hassiotis *et al.*, 2009). The individual may ramble or be tangential; this is not due to psychosis but rather the inability to comprehend inter-relationships among subjects.

Concrete thinking

Concrete thinking occurs when thinking and reasoning are grounded in the here and now: what can be seen, counted, and observed (Hassiotis *et al.*, 2009). On a typical mental status exam question, "What does the saying mean, 'people in glass houses shouldn't throw stones'?," the patient with ID might answer, "Because stones would break the glass." Concrete thinking also can be seen in thought disorders, however, and it also may occur in typically developing adults with organic brain disorders, such as traumatic brain injuries.

Egocentrism

Egocentrism is the individual viewing and interpreting the world exclusively from their own perspective based on their personal experiences (Hassiotis *et al.*, 2009). Egocentrism is seen in pre-school children, and may be confused with narcissism, oppositional behavior or conduct problems. Individuals functioning at this level of cognitive function do not comprehend what others experience, nor do they typically recognize the effect they have on others.

Intellectual distortion, psychological masking, cognitive disintegration, baseline exaggeration

Other important concepts about assessment of the patient with ID (Sovner, 1986) include intellectual distortion, psychological masking, cognitive disintegration and baseline exaggeration. These also are discussed in Chapter 2. To review:

Intellectual distortion

In the case of *intellectual distortion*, psychiatric symptoms, although present, are difficult for the patient to describe because the patient has deficits in abstract thinking and/or in receptive or expressive language skills.

Clinical Vignette #1

Example of intellectual distortion A 21 year old female who was living in a group home presented for initial psychiatric evaluation after several weeks of increasingly agitated behavior at her sheltered workshop. This behavior had been initially been attributed to excitement over members of her extended family moving back into her home state. She had recently hidden under tables at work, exhibited episodic agitation and appeared scared at times when looking at walls, she but could not explain why.

During the psychiatric evaluation, she attended to the unoccupied side chair and appeared frightened while peering at the wall adjacent to the psychiatrist. Psychosis was suspected and, after a negative medical examination and normal laboratory testing, she was started on a low dose second generation antipsychotic and stabilized within two weeks. She returned to work without further incident.

Psychological masking

Psychological masking occurs when the patient's limited social experiences influence the content of psychiatric symptoms. In such cases, symptoms may be less elaborate, and sometimes they are missed because they do not, on the surface, seem "odd" or "grandiose" to the observer. For example, a delusion of grandeur may be present when a lonely patient with ID believes in the existence of a boyfriend or girlfriend when there is none.

Although it can be difficult, a delusion of grandeur must be differentiated from the developmental processes of *magical thinking* and *egocentrism*. Because patients with ID are less likely to question, introspect or attempt to interpret their psychological symptoms, they may present their mental experiences as "reality." Many patients with ID have very limited social experiences, and this fact will greatly affect both the psychological fabric of their ordinary thinking and the content of mental health symptoms. Statements which sound like delusions could simply represent magical thinking. On the other hand, a seemingly commonplace experience for a person from the general population may actually be a delusion for the patient with ID. A good interviewer will learn to distinguish between the two possibilities.

Cognitive disintegration

Cognitive disintegration refers to decreased ability to tolerate stress on the part of a person with ID that leads to reversible anxiety-induced decompensation, sometimes misinterpreted as psychosis. Most individuals with ID have deficits in executive functioning and have difficulty in determining "better from best." These cognitive difficulties can be exaggerated or may escalate during times of high stress or anxiety. In addition, when decompensated, patients may have even more problems expressing things verbally.

Finally, during a period of cognitive disintegration, patients who otherwise do not have behavioral symptoms may look psychotic or may exhibit somatization (a preoccupation with physical symptoms). They may exhibit self- injurious behavior, rocking or other repetitive movements. These symptoms may resolve spontaneously when the stress is reduced.

Baseline exaggeration

Baseline exaggeration refers to an increase in the severity or frequency of pre-existing chronic maladaptive behavior after the onset of a psychiatric illness or exposure to an acute stressor. In order to determine that a new disorder has emerged, the clinician must be familiar with the patient's baseline, or otherwise may be unable to interpret the patient's presenting symptoms. This is one of the purposes of reviewing the patient's chart prior to examining the patient. Evaluating maladaptive behavior (e.g. talking to imaginary friends, rocking, lashing out aggressively, etc.) is challenging and must be interpreted in the context of the patient's "normal" or baseline mode of functioning.

The clinician must also know what coping strategies are potentially available to the patient, and then use supportive interventions to shore up defenses. This is the time to use what functional coping skills exist and attempt to maximize or optimize these. Later, when the patient is more stable, the clinician can help the patient increase their repertoire of coping strategies in an effort to try to reduce the frequency and severity of any future decompensation and cognitive disintegration as a result of stress.

The clinician must remain aware, however, that even patients with only mild or even borderline level ID will probably retain some prominent features of early development throughout their adult lives, including self-talk, imaginary friends, out-loud monologue and fantasy play. These behaviors are not outside normal limits for the patient's developmental level, and they should not necessarily be a focus of treatment (Fletcher *et al.*, DM-ID, 2007).

Clinical Vignette #2

Assessment of increased anxiety   In the following exchange, the patient is a 22 year old man with a history of anxiety disorder not otherwise specified and mild intellectual disability, who is referred to a psychiatrist for "medication management":

Psychiatrist: Good Morning John, how are you doing today?
Patient: OK. [concrete, monosyllabic response]
Psychiatrist: How have you been since our last appointment?
Patient: OK.
Psychiatrist: Are you having any problems? [factual yes/no question]
Patient: No. [need to cross-question to make sure answer is accurate]
Psychiatrist: So you have no problems right now, is that right?
Patient: No.
Psychiatrist (to Caregiver): Can you share with me how you think John is doing?
Caregiver: John, do you want to discuss the issue we talked about on our way here this morning?
Patient: I don't remember.
Caregiver: I have been worried because when you are nervous or sad, you stay in your bedroom a lot, and the last couple weeks I have noticed you doing this a lot.
Psychiatrist: John, have you been upset about something?
Patient: I don't know.
Psychiatrist: If you have a problem, I want to be able to help you. Is there something making you sad?
Patient: At work. [looks at Caregiver]
Caregiver: John's workshop supervisor was changed a couple weeks ago. I didn't know this had affected John, but now that you mention it, this was about the same time he started staying in his room.
Psychiatrist (to Patient): How do you feel about the change at work? [open-ended question]
Patient: I don't like it.
Psychiatrist: What is it about work that you don't like? [focused open-ended question]
Patient: I don't know.
Psychiatrist: Is your new boss mean? Or hard to work with? Or different from your old boss? [multiple choice]

Patient: Different from my old boss. [possibly accurate or may be serial order/last option effect]
Psychiatrist: How is he different?
Patient: He didn't let me go to lunch.
Caregiver: I think you were supposed to go on an outing last week, but it was canceled because they didn't have transportation for everyone. Is that the lunch you missed?
Patient: Yes.

In this case, use of various question types, collateral data from a knowledgeable caregiver and some detective work allows for a productive appointment, and the psychiatrist can facilitate a solution to this misunderstanding and avoid unnecessary medication changes.

Formal mental status examination

A formal mental status examination always should be performed. It may increase accuracy to adapt a child or adolescent version of the mental status exam, or to make other adjustments that take into account the developmental framework of the patient. The formal mental status examination should include noting the patient's appearance and his or her relationship to others in the room, as well as the patient's mood and expression of affect, and it should include any other general observational findings that might suggest medical problems or neurological impairment (see Chapters 2, 3 and 4).

- Take note of the person's level of alertness and consciousness, as these will affect responses and also may indicate over-sedation.

- Observe motor movements (whether decreased or increased from baseline, and including any abnormal movements or tremors).

- Take note of communication ability.

- Note ability to follow simple commands, orientation to person, place, time and situation, any stereotypies and automatisms (Silka & Hauser, 1997).

See Table 2 for a summary of recommendations for individuals with mild/moderate ID and severe/profound ID as outlined by Levitas *et al.* (2001).

Mild ID and concrete operations: interpreting mental status examination findings

Persons with mild ID usually function at the cognitive level of "*concrete operations*." Concrete operations is the developmental stage that occurs from approximately 7–11 years for an individual in the general population. Patients with mild ID who continue to function at the level of concrete operations are able to use *inductive logic* (taking a specific concept and generalizing it) but cannot use *deductive logic* (taking a general concept and using it to

Table 2 Summary of recommendations for mental status examination alterations for mild/moderate ID and severe/profound ID.

	Mild/moderate ID	Severe/profound ID
Appearance/mannerisms	Look for self-removed nails (Smith-Magentis), numerous superficial cuts or scratches (borderline personality or drug allergy), dysmorphisms (genetic syndromes), passive gaze-avoidant (autism).	Interview should be performed with caregiver present, so as not to increase anxiety. Aloofness and gaze-avoidance (autism)
Psychomotor behavior	Note involuntary movements (tics or stereotypies, tremor, choreoathetoid movements, paresis or spasticity), inability to sit still (akathisia or mania), finger wiggling or hand flapping (autism or Fragile X).	Overactivity (mania, akathisia), hypoactivity (depression). Note involuntary movements as in mild/moderate ID. Stereotyped movements, especially of head, neck and eyes should increase suspicion of partial simple or partial complex seizures. See mild/moderate notes.
Intelligence	Review formal testing and compare actual functional level to expected level.	
Speech	Overcompliance (acquiescence), 'palatal speech' (cleft palate, as in 22q11 deletion), stuttering, cluttering (as in Fragile X), echolalia (autism or severe/profound ID), monotone or robotic speech (autism), pronominal reversal, i.e. using 'you' instead of 'me' (autism).	Patients with severely limited communication ability should not automatically be diagnosed with autism. Perseverative questioning (autism or anxiety). Echolalia and automatic phrases (autism, Fragile X, etc.).
Emotional expression	Draw faces and ask individual to identify the emotion (happy, sad, mad, fearful, etc), then ask to point to the one that shows how he/she feels today, alexithymia i.e. inability to identify emotion (autism).	Mood expression often attenuated. Dysmorphism or paresis may impede or limit facial expression. Athetoid or pseudobulbar palsy may exaggerate facial expression.
Thinking and perception	Self-talk, imaginary friends and subvocalizations (practicing speech before delivering it) may all be part of the developmental framework of the individual. Delusions are typically less elaborate and are often not questioned or interpreted by the individual. Distinguish preoccupations (recurrent thoughts to which the person returns voluntarily) from obsessions	Avoidance of visual stimuli but enthusiastic response to vibratory stimuli (autism). Observe for compulsions (e.g. picking up lint or dust, repeatedly adjusting clothes, playing stereotypically with preferred object, etc.).

	(involuntary and may be attributed to others by the person with ID). The ability of persons who actually complete suicide or harm others is easily underestimated; the assessment of safety is no different from that in the general population. Distinguish auditory input heard through the ears from that inside one's head (hallucinations versus 'auditorization of thought').	
Sensorium	Oriented to person: referral to self by name or in the third person (autism). Oriented to time; if staff navigates schedule, may be irrelevant to the individual.	Does the individual know the caregivers? Do they respond appropriately to the unfamiliar person/clinician?
Attention/memory/concentration	Concentration: consider asking individual to perform repetitive, sustained manual task. Memory: hypermnesia i.e. exact and detailed memories (autism). Verbal memory is generally limited in most mild/moderate ID. Consider hiding object with individual watching, and ask to retrieve object 20 minutes later.	Concentration and memory can be inferred from collateral data source.
Insight/judgment	Note any changes based on collateral data reports. "What do you have to do to get a job?... an apartment?... a boyfriend?"	No suggestions; difficult to ascertain.
Other	Save time for one-on-one interface with patient; utilize other techniques, e.g. paper and crayons, simple puzzles, etc.	

Source: adapted from Levitas et al. (2001).

Table 3 Examples of concrete speech.

Concrete answers to questions	"How do you sleep?" "*On my bed.*"
Concrete responses to tests of abstract thinking	"When in Rome, do as the Romans do." "*I don't want to go to Rome, I don't know anyone there.*"
	"The best things in life are free." "*I got a free coat one time.*"
	"Turn the other cheek." "*If I hit you, you should turn your cheek.*"
	"The early bird catches the worm." "*Whoever gets up first gets the worm.*"
	"People who live in glass houses should not throw stones." "*Stones break glass.*"

predict or determine the outcome of a specific event). Therefore, the person with mild ID may have difficulty understanding abstract or hypothetical concepts (Chapman, 1988, Commons & Richards 1984, Fischer, 1980).

Concrete thinking, when associated with impaired communication ability, results in several challenges. Patients have difficulty describing symptoms and providing subjective data regarding emotions. For example, patients may state that they are "scared" instead of "mad."

When making treatment recommendations for the future, proposing a chart or other pictorial representation of various emotions may be helpful in increasing this skill set, so that the patient can accurately identify and communicate emotions. Providing patients with their own take-home set of laminated pictures of faces demonstrating a variety of emotions is one way for patients to practice this skill with support from direct care staff or involved family between appointments.

Once a therapeutic alliance is established, one finds that the patient at the concrete operations developmental stage is typically able to communicate in a very genuine and authentic way. Table 3 gives some examples of concrete answers.

In order to evaluate the level of organization of thought processes (as when examining for loose associations), individuals with ID who are functioning at the level of concrete operations can be asked to describe similarities between simple items, as described in Table 4.

One of the most important developments of concrete operations is the *understanding of reversibility.* This is the awareness that actions can be reversed and that relationships between categories can be reversed. An example of an acceptable response that demonstrates an understanding of the concept of reversibility would be: "The dog is a poodle."; "*The poodle is a dog.*"

The patient with mild ID who is operating at the concrete level is less egocentric than the person with ID with more severe deficits. The patient with mild ID usually is capable of beginning to see things from others' perspectives.

Table 4 Examples of acceptable answers for patient at concrete level.

"How is a table similar to a chair?"
"*One you eat on; one you sit in.*"
"How is a boy similar to a girl?"
"*They aren't the same.*"
"How are praise and punishment different?"
"*I know what punishment is, but not the other word.*"

Table 5   Responses from patient with moderate ID.

Example of query to patient with moderate ID and typical response: A caregiver may attempt to discuss the problem of the individual's stealing money from a peer by posing the question: "How would *you* feel if John stole *your* money?" The typical individual with moderate ID who is in the pre-operational stage *will not be able to comprehend this question*.

Example of task assigned to patient with moderate ID and typical response: Using a three-dimensional display of a mountain scene, individuals with moderate ID were asked to choose a picture that shows the scene they had viewed. Next, they were asked to select a picture showing *what someone else* would have observed when looking at the mountain from a different viewpoint. They almost always chose the scene *showing their own view* of the mountain scene.

Source: Fischer (1980).

Moderate ID and the preoperational stage: interpreting mental status examination findings

Patients with moderate ID usually function at the *preoperational stage* of cognitive development (Chapman, 1988, Commons & Richards, 1984, Fischer, 1980). For individuals with typical cognitive ability, the preoperational stage occurs at approximately 2–6 years of age. Language development is a hallmark of the preoperational developmental stage, but speech is still egocentric. The typical patient with moderate ID has egocentric speech and still sees things from his or her own perspective, and does not have the ability to see things from others' viewpoints. Patients with moderate ID typically "cannot mentally manipulate information" and the patient has great difficulty drawing logical conclusions from information (Commons & Richards, 1984, Fischer, 1980). Table 5 provides some examples of possible responses from a patient with moderate ID.

In the preoperational cognitive stage of someone with moderate ID, the patient will also tend to focus attention on one aspect of an object while ignoring other facets, and will usually have difficulty ranking the importance of various aspects of a situation or experience. This is why Likert-type scales are not useful for self-report by these patients. Mental concepts that are formed are typically simple or crude and are often irreversible. Table 6 illustrates typical responses of a person with moderate ID to differing sizes and shapes:

Table 6   Example of typical response of person with moderate ID at the preoperational stage to differing sizes and shapes.

Equal amounts of liquid are poured into identical containers. The liquid in one container is then poured into a differently shaped cup, such as a tall and thin cup or a short and wide cup. Individuals with moderate ID are then asked which cup holds the most liquid.

Despite *saying* that the liquid amounts are equal, they almost always choose the cup that *appears* fuller (Commons & Richards, 1984, Fischer, 1980).

More recently, other researchers have found that there are variations in the age wherein one achieves understanding of conservation, so there is no absolute age of acquisition (Fischer, 1980).

Individuals with severe/profound ID (nonverbal communication): interpreting the mental status examination

Piaget's sensorimotor stage of development is defined as taking place from birth until the development of language. With the development of language, an individual understands the world by integrating sensory information with behavior and actions (Fisher, 1980, Commons & Richards, 1984). Patients who have severe/profound ID have limited to no development of language, and they could be considered to be operating at the sensorimotor stage of development. Observation of a patient becomes even more important when communication deficits are more significant. It is more difficult to diagnose mental illness accurately as the level of cognitive deficit becomes more severe, but it is important to do so because the ID patient population is probably at a higher risk for developing mental illness than is the person with typical cognitive development.

While the history is being taken from caregivers or others, the severe to profound ID patient can be observed for appearance, relatedness to others, impulse control, activity level (including both voluntary and involuntary motor movements), expression of affect, attention span, any unusual, ritualistic, stereotypic or repetitive behaviors and external signs of anxiety (diaphoresis, rapid breathing, tremulousness). The patient with severe or profound ID may appear stable at the initiation of the interview, but may decompensate as the interview goes on, depending on the severity of mental health symptoms and degree of social skills.

Clinical Vignette #3

Behavior change   Patty is a 27 year old female with history of mild intellectual disability, Williams syndrome and post-traumatic stress disorder, who presents to her psychiatrist's office for a medication management appointment accompanied by her mother, following an increase in dose of antidepressant medication after she began refusing to attend the workshop.

Psychiatrist: Hello Patty, it's good to see you.
Patty: Yes.
Psychiatrist: How are you doing?
Patty: OK.
Psychiatrist: Are you taking your medicine every day?
Patty: Yes. [check for acquiescence]
Psychiatrist: Are you having any problems with your medicine?
Patty: No.
Psychiatrist: What have you been doing since our last appointment? [open-ended question]
Patty: I watch TV and I saw a movie.
Psychiatrist: What else?
Patty: I go to work every day and I eat lunch there too.

Psychiatrist: What else?

Patty: I got a paycheck and I went to shopping with my Mom.

Psychiatrist: That sounds great. What do you like to buy when you go shopping?

Patty: New shoes and clothes.

Psychiatrist: That sounds great. Is it OK if I ask your Mom some questions, too?

Patty: Yes.

Psychiatrist to Mom: How do you think Patty is doing?

Mom: I think she's doing well. The medication change from last appointment has really been helpful. I see no problems at this point.

Nonverbal communication

Nonverbal communication is especially important in patients with no usable language. Table 7 provides for examples of nonverbal behavior as diagnostic criteria for several common psychiatric disorders (DSM-IV-TR 2000).

Universal facial expressions

Insight can be gained into the emotions and mental health status of the patient with limited expressive language skills through knowledge of universal facial expressions (see Table 8). The clinician with acute observational skills, attention to detail and familiarity with patients with ID will be more successful in attaining accurate diagnoses and providing higher quality care.

Although verbal communication is partly subjective and influenced by culture, attitudes, and emotions (Foley & Gentile, 2010) in all languages and cultures, emblems and

Table 7 Examples of nonverbal behavior as diagnostic criteria.

Autistic disorder	Marked impairment in eye-to-eye gaze, facial expression, body postures and gestures; stereotyped, repetitive motor mannerisms.
Attention deficit/ hyperactivity disorder	Does not appear to listen when spoken to; easily distractible; fidgeting; inability to remain seated.
Substance intoxication or withdrawal states	Conjunctival injection with cannabis intoxication; miosis in opiate intoxication; lacrimation, rhinorrhea, yawning in opiate withdrawal.
Schizophrenia	Flat affect, poor eye contact, avolition (negative symptoms); disheveled appearance, unpredictable agitation, rigid or bizarre postures (grossly disorganized or catatonic behaviors).
Major depressive disorder	Psychomotor agitation or retardation; restricted or blunted, dysphoric affect; tearfulness.
PTSD	Hypervigilance; exaggerated startle response; restricted range of affect.

Source: adapted from American Psychiatric Association (2000), p. 40.

Table 8 Universal facial expressions of emotion.

Surprise	Jaw drops, opening the mouth without tension; eyes open widely; brows are raised, high and curved; forehead wrinkles horizontally throughout.
Fear	Lips tense, stretch and draw back; eyes open with lower lid tense and upper lid raised; brows are raised, drawn close together; forehead wrinkles horizontally in the center only.
Disgust	Upper lip raises and nose wrinkles; lower eyelid moves upward; brows are lowered.
Anger	Lips tightly closed; eyelids tense; brows are lowered and drawn close together; wrinkling appears vertically between the brows.
Happiness	Corners of the lips draw upward and nasolabial folds become prominent; lower eyelid raises and wrinkles appear around the eyes.
Sadness	Lips tremble or corners draw downward; eyes may tear; inner brows are raised and often drawn together.

Source: Ekman & Friesen (1975), p. 42.

illustrators supplement verbal expression (Ekman, 1977). *Emblems* have well-defined and specific meaning; for example, a head nod usually (but not always) indicates an affirmative response. *Illustrators* are less specific and may be interpreted differently by others, depending on their own personal experiences. An example of an illustrator would be where an individual creates a "drawing" in the air while speaking.

Some nonverbal behaviors tend to be universal (Ekman, 1977), such as rapid raising of eyebrows when one is ready for interpersonal contact, while some nonverbal behaviors, such as personal space, vary dramatically from culture to culture. The interviewer should be aware of his/her own culture and be prepared to interface with individuals with ID from other cultures.

Beginning in their early years, the majority of patients with ID also display more nonverbal behaviors – referred to as "*body manipulators*" – which counterbalance some of the shortcomings in their development of expressive language skills (Ekman, 1977). Body manipulators are movements that communicate information over and above verbal expression (i.e. fidgeting, rocking, tapping fingers, gyrating legs, and rubbing feet against each other). Body manipulators can also provide the clinician with valuable information to better understand the patient's emotional status and mental state. Emblems, illustrators and body manipulators should be considered in the context of the patient's past psychiatric history, psychosocial functioning, current circumstances and presenting symptoms (Ekman, 1977).

Individuals with ID should be observed when they are interacting with their caregivers and others who attend appointments with them. It is typical for most individuals to protect more personal space with others with whom they are unfamiliar, or with those whom they fear or have conflict. If the individual with ID appears agitated, fearful, restless or hyperactive, it may relate to feelings about their relationships with persons in the room (Ekman, 1977). Individuals tend to turn away from those with whom they have conflict, and a "closed posture" is more typical under these circumstances (i.e. folding arms across their chest or turning their head away). The individual with ID may also demonstrate some of these behaviors if others in the room are discussing an uncomfortable topic and this should be addressed directly with the patient (Ekman, 1977).

Personality traits that can influence interview behavior

The personality traits and style of the patient are important to consider when conducting the interview. If a patient is an extrovert, they may be more likely to be a "yea-sayer" or agree with the interviewer (Finlay & Lyons, 2002). This may be related to acquiescence or social desirability. Such patients will typically be more forthcoming with their conversation and more expressive. A patient who is more introverted will typically be more reserved, less expressive and internally oriented (Finlay & Lyons, 2002). Such a person may be more difficult to interview and is more likely to respond with one- and two-word answers. The degree of impulse control that a patient has also will have a considerable impact of the interview.

Another consideration regarding communication strengths and weaknesses in the person with ID is that there are syndrome-specific language and communication strengths and weaknesses.

Three disorders with syndrome-specific language and communication strengths and weaknesses

Down syndrome

Language is the most well researched behavioral domain in Down syndrome (DS) (Dykens *et al.*, 2000). There appear to be significantly impaired grammatical abilities in DS, with a large number of individuals failing to progress beyond the three year old level linguistically. Dykens *et al.* (2000) also state that "*acquiring adult formations of negatives, 'wh-' questions, irregular past tense, embedded sentences, passives, and other more complicated sentence types are all difficult for individuals with DS.*"

Typically developing children reach mature levels of language communication at approximately age 5 years but, even as adults, individuals with DS will not reach the same level. Expressive language skills in children with DS are typically less developed than receptive skills (Dykens *et al.*, 2000). In addition to difficulty with "wh-" words, including "who," "where," "why" and "when," DS patients also have difficulty with irregular past tense questions (saying "go" instead of "went"; saying "say" instead of "said"), and embedded sentences (i.e. instead of "I can see that Anne is running," they might say "Anne is running."). Language of the individual with DS also is often difficult to understand, due to impaired pronunciation combined with mid-face abnormalities and a high prevalence of impaired hearing. The high prevalence of mid-face abnormalities often results in recurrent upper respiratory infections, which can leave the patient congested and even more difficult to understand. These upper respiratory conditions frequently affect their hearing ability, further affecting their ability to communicate. In fact, 60–80% of individuals with DS have inner ear problems (Dykens *et al.*, 2000).

Fragile X syndrome

Individuals with Fragile X Syndrome (FXS) are often hypersensitive to light and sound. They will avoid eye contact; for example, they may wear dark glasses, or they may close

Table 9 Examples of indirect responses by patient with Fragile X syndrome.

"How do you feel about your new job?"
"The van picks me up, John sits by me, the van needs gas too."
"Would you like a new coat?"
"I want to pick it out, pick it up at the place you where you shop, the store, but I don't have the time to make, oh, the money to get it for me, uh, for you."

---

their eyes until the interviewer breaks eye contact and looks in another direction. The interviewer should be aware of what has been called the "Fragile X handshake" where the individual will stand at a 45° angle to the interviewer, shake the interviewer's hand but will avoid eye contact until the interviewer looks away, at which time the patient will look at the interviewer's eyes.

Patients with FXS also commonly respond to questions with echolalia, repeating the last two or three words of the interviewer's question as opposed to a suitable response. Many males show uneven and unpredictable rates of speech, alternating between short, rapid bursts of speech (called "staccato speech"), intermixed with longer pauses (Dykens *et al.*, 2000). Speech is also characterized by whole and part word repetitions, i.e. repeating sounds and words, substitutions or omissions of sounds, and "cluttering," which is an indirect style of verbal expression involving a type of verbal clumsiness or difficulty in controlling the sequence of complex motor movements required in speaking. Table 9 provides examples of typical indirect responses by patients with FXS.

Delays are consistently found in both receptive and expressive language skills of males with FXS, as well as in their syntax abilities. Expressive language delays in young boys are the most frequent cause for the family to seek evaluation by a medical professional. Later as they age, both receptive and expressive vocabulary words become very well developed and become a consistent cognitive adaptive strength.

There are several uses of language which are characteristic of FXS and are of great interest to researchers. For example, individuals with FXS are often tangential and will develop several phrases or terminology which they will overuse in social conversation, and often in the form of a question. There also is a tendency to perseverate, or repeat a word, phrase, or idea over and over. These automatic or "routinized" phrases are often utilized when they don't know the answer to the question posed to them, or when they are anxious or talking to an unfamiliar person. This is an effective adaptive mechanism, since it turns the conversation back to the interviewer or a nearby familiar person. The automatic phrase may consist of something like: "Isn't that right?" or "What do you think?" or "Does that make sense?"

Clinical Vignette #4

Examples of typical responses from a patient with fragile X syndrome   Bobby is a 42 year old man with history of moderate intellectual disability and Fragile X syndrome, who presents for a mental health appointment. The psychiatrist angles the chairs so that the patient is not directly facing anyone in the room and does not make extended eye contact with the patient during the appointment. The patient is wearing sunglasses despite being inside the building, possibly to shield his eyes from the lights.

Psychiatrist: Bobby, how are you doing today?
Bobby: OK.
Psychiatrist: What have you been doing lately? [open-ended question]
Bobby: I have some music and I went to a party. I played the music. I got a new radio and the car has a radio too. [cluttering]
Psychiatrist: The party sounds fun. I have a few questions for you today. Is that OK?
Bobby: Sure.
Psychiatrist: Do you know what the date is today?
Bobby (to Caregiver): Now what do you think about that, Ben? [routinized or automatic phrase used when unsure of answer or when anxious]
Caregiver: Do you know what the date is today, Bobby?
Bobby: What do you think about that, Doc?
Psychiatrist: Today is March 23, 2011. Do you know what day of the week it is, Bobby?
Bobby: I don't know now. Is it Tuesday? What do you think, Ben? [Automatic phrase]
Caregiver: You are correct. It *is* Tuesday, Bobby.
Psychiatrist: What city and state are we in?
Bobby: Dayton, Ohio. We are in Dayton.
Psychiatrist: That's correct, Bobby. Thank you. Can you repeat some numbers back to me? Let's try 4-6-2.
Bobby: 3-3-7-4-6. What do you think about that Ben? [Responds with his zip code, which is a number committed to memory, and follow with an automatic phrase]
Psychiatrist: Let's try another one. Can you repeat this number? 5-2-9.
Bobby: 3-3-7-4-6
Psychiatrist: 0-3-9.
Bobby: 3-3-7-4-6.
Psychiatrist: Bobby, what are your plans for this weekend?
Bobby: What do you think about that, Ben?
Caregiver: You have plans, Bobby. Do you remember where we go every Saturday morning?
Bobby: Saturday – I don't know about that. What do you think, Ben?
Caregiver: Bobby, remember on Saturday mornings we pick your friend up, and where do we go?
Bobby: Bowling!
Caregiver: That's right, and last week you had a great score. Do you remember?
Bobby: I got a great score, Doc. I'm good at bowling.

Imaging studies of the central nervous systems of individuals with FXS reveal an increase in volume of the caudate nucleus. This is thought to be a result of inadequate pruning (reduction of the total number of neurons or connections in an area of the brain during normal development of the structure, leaving more efficient synaptic connections).

This finding may be associated with abnormalities in frontal lobe circuits regulating cognitive and emotional functioning, including the ability to inhibit verbal responses. With less inhibitory activity in place, the result may be perseveration, or repetition of words, phrases or gestures (Dykens *et al.*, 2000).

Williams syndrome

Many individuals with Williams syndrome (WS) have abnormally high levels of affect in their expressive language (Dykens *et al.*, 2000). There are several ways in which they tend to engage people in conversation, including frequent use of exclamatory words and narrative that is rich with descriptive words and phrases. In general, they can be described as hyperverbal. Early in the developmental years, this can precipitate positive social inter-actions, but later it may cause issues with social boundaries.

Individuals with WS tend to exhibit rather complicated syntax, including embedded clauses and excessively long mean length of utterance, exceeding that of their peers of the same age (Dykens *et al.*, 2000). The degree of expressive language ability may create unrealistic expectations in others – for example, in teachers and, caregivers. The language nuances of individuals with WS are of great interest to researchers, as findings will have profound implications for understanding their cognition and language.

Useful guidelines for speaking with patients with ID

The following are guidelines for use when speaking with the person with ID. They take into consideration the developmental level of the patient and serve to (a) increase the amount of valuable and accurate information, and (b) assist in building rapport and the therapeutic alliance:

1. Avoid hypothetical or abstract future-oriented questions and "why" questions. Avoid abstract questions such as "What did you think might happen when you stayed home from work?" or "Why did you decide to stay home from work?"

2. Avoid jargon or slang, as well as other technical language. Use concrete descriptions and avoid figurative language. For example, avoid terms like "spread eagle," "blown away" or "busy as a bee."

3. Avoid conversational punctuations such as "really" and "you know," because these may be taken literally (Modell, 2006).

4. Frequently check understanding of conversation with the individual with ID. Ask what particular words mean to the individual, and use *their* words when possible.

5. Match questions and answers with the individual's expressive language. Avoid double negatives. Use words that patient uses for body parts. Let the patient's abilities drive the interview.

6. Avoid abstract concepts. Avoid "why" questions, "how" questions and "if" questions whenever possible. If possible, concretize the abstract. Instead of saying "recreational activities," the interviewer may say "bowl" or "watch TV," for example (Modell, 2006, Ott, 2005, Finlay & Lyons, 2002).

7. Use alternative language systems, e.g. picture and line drawings, etc. as an adjunct when needed.

8. A colloquialism is a phrase that is common in everyday, unconstrained conversation, rather than in formal speech (Modell, 2006, Ott, 2005). Monitor your own speech for colloquialisms and avoid these whenever possible. For example, do not say "y'all" instead of "all of you." Do not say "wanna" instead if "want to."

9. Match the interviewee's mean length of utterance; use "plain language" or language less than 6th grade level. Use single clause sentences. Use active verbs rather than passive ones. Use present tense whenever possible, and use time anchors when discussing the past.

10. Avoid idioms. Do not say "You can't teach an old dog new tricks." Do not say "Kill two birds with one stone".

11. Avoid direct comparisons. Comparisons should be divided into two parts. For example, a less effective comparison would be: "Do you like your new home and job?" More effective questions would be: "How do you like your new job?", "How do you like your new home?"

12. Avoid judgments of frequency and quantity. Avoid perceptions of third parties. Posing these questions will be low-yield with most patients.

13. Awareness of echolalia is important. Tactful and appropriate interventions by yourself or caregivers can be made to attempt redirection of the patient who responds with echolalia. For example: If, to "How are you today?," the patient responds: "you today," the interviewer might add "you feeling...?"

14. Yes/no questions are higher-yield when used regarding activities and events, but they are not as accurate with feelings and emotions. Avoid confrontational or potentially embarrassing yes/no questions, e.g. "Do you smoke pot?" "Do you sleep with your girlfriend?" Avoid double-barreled questions: "Do you like your home and your staff?" Avoid long and multiple questions: "Do you like your job and your home, and what you think about your supervisor and your staff?" Avoid leading questions: "You knew what you were doing was wrong, didn't you?"; "You know better than that, right?" Avoid random probing and coercive: "You wouldn't want to lose your job, would you?" Avoid embarrassing or accusatory questions: "How often do you hit other people at work?" Use caution with "why" questions: "Why did you hit your roommate last week?" Specifically but tactfully address dishonesty and confabulation, and make the option of not responding acceptable. Extra caution should always be exercised with the use of humor.

Perseveration

Patients with ID may repeat words, phrases or topics, and the etiology may be related to either acute or chronic psychiatric symptoms or a known developmental syndrome (i.e. Fragile X syndrome), or to anxiety related to the interview itself, among other factors. Eliminate irrelevant stimuli, including distractions whenever possible. This includes objects in the office such as books or games, which may steal the attention of, or create a distraction for, an individual with ID.

Some patients are told by caregivers that if they comply with the interview or appointment, they will receive a drink or meal afterward, but this may sabotage the interview if that becomes the focus of the patient. Refocus the attention of the patient at regular intervals. Set up transitions from one part of the interview to the next. Acknowledge anxiety. If a patient is responding to every question with "yes," for example, cross-questioning can be very effective to discern this from true affirmative responses. An example of cross-questioning that demonstrates a "yes" answer to all questions would be: "Do you sleep well?" "Yes." "Do you have trouble sleeping?" "Yes."

Subvocalizations

Patients with ID may "practice" before verbalizing their thoughts, or may vocalize a thought process ("hearing" the words) prior to delivery (Modell, 2006). A subvocalization is a strategy that a patient might use to "mentally rehearse" what the patient will say or is planning to do. It may appear to others that the individual is stalling or confused, being evasive or equivocal, or attempting to avoid the question (Modell, 2006). A subvocalization is not a hallucination or other internal stimulus, and it should be differentiated from a mental health issue. If a person regularly takes long pauses, thought blocking (from psychosis or related to severe anxiety) should be ruled out.

Many individuals in the general population also frequently "practice" or rehearse what they will say, but they typically do this silently and more quickly. Individuals with ID may practice by whispering or verbalizing in a quieter voice, which may appear to be mumbling or experiencing psychotic symptoms (Modell, 2006).

Acquiescence

Acquiescence refers to the tendency to agree with any statement the interviewee is given, and this is relatively common in individuals with ID (Finlay & Lyons, 2002). It is especially important to avoid leading questions, e.g. "You knew that was wrong, didn't you?" The presence of acquiescence is directly correlated with a higher intelligence quotient; in other words, the patient with more severe cognitive deficits is *less* likely to acquiesce. Acquiescence is more common if the interviewer is viewed as an authority figure, if the patient wants to gain the approval of the interviewer ("social desirability"), or if there are comprehension problems.

The tendency toward acquiescence makes it a challenge for the interviewer to determine whether a patient's responses are truthful and constitute real information. The patient may

Table 10 Twelve ways to ask the question.

1. Are you happy about living where you live?
2. Are you Unhappy about living where you live?
3. Do you wish you had a better place to live?
4. Where would you like it better?
5. Do you wish you were happier with your home?
6. Would you rather live somewhere Else or where you live Now?
7. Would you rather live where you live Now or somewhere Else?
8. Do you see these faces? [SAD FACE ON LEFT]
   This one has a big smile because he is very happy.
   This one has a little smile because he is a little happy.
   This one is in between; not sad and not happy
   This one is a little sad.
   This one is very sad.
   Please point to the face that shows how you feel.
9. Do you see these faces? [HAPPY FACE ON LEFT]
    Please point to the face that shows how you feel about your home where you live.
10. Would you like to spend more time at home?
11. Do you wish you had a different home?
12. Most of the time do you like your home?

Source: Heal & Sigelman (1995), p. 337.

fear consequences, or a negative response, or disappointment from the interviewer. If information is questionable, the interviewer can use the interview techniques described above, including cross-questioning, to clarify the response. Most importantly, although acquiescence may represent a desire to please or increased submissiveness, it should also be seen as a possible response to questions that are grammatically too complex, or which require complicated judgment beyond the cognitive ability of the patient (Finlay & Lyons, 2002). See Table 10 for alternate ways to ask the same question.

Managing acquiescence when interviewing a patient with ID

Using either/or, yes/no or multiple-choice question formats can assist in deciphering whether or not acquiescence is a factor in the patient's responses (Finlay & Lyons,

Table 11 Four techniques to detect acquiescence in interviews.

1.	Questions where the correct answer should be "no," e.g. "Does it snow in the summer here?"; "Can you fly an airplane?"
2.	Pairs of questions that are opposite in meaning, e.g. "Are you happy? Are you sad?"
3.	Pairs of questions in which the same question is asked in different formats, i.e. yes/no and either/or.
4.	Informant checks.

Source: Finlay & Lyons (2002), p. 16.

2002). See Table 11. Pay attention to "serial order" or "last option" effects, and use cross-questioning to help clarify as needed. Check answers with reliable informants. When developing questions for patients with ID:

- manipulate inquiries to utilize reverse wording;

- include "don't know" options or other expressions of indecision;

- simplify question wording and sentence structure;

- be aware of questions which require the individual to make judgments;

- recognize the type of content that makes acquiescence more likely;

- ask for examples (Finlay & Lyons, 2002).

Caution should be used when there is inconsistent information, because this might be caused by memory failure or lack of attention, both of which are common problems in individuals with ID. When questions are too long, or when the sentence structure is too complex, the patient may only focus on some of the words or phrases within the question, as opposed to the concept as a whole. Most individuals with ID are taught to get along with other people and to respect those in authority so, as a result, they may give socially desirable responses or they may acquiesce. Expect to take more time to investigate and explore this if it is in question.

Decreased attention span

Individuals with ID often experience difficulty in initiating and maintaining attention and/or eye contact for several reasons, including the co-occurrence of ADHD. The prevalence rate for ADHD among children without ID is approximately 5% (Habler & Reis, 2010), but in children with ID it co-occurs at rates between 8.7–16%. Response rates for psychostimulants in children with ID are 10–30% lower, relative to response rates in the general population (see Chapter 12).

Even if the patient with ID is not formally diagnosed with ADHD, it is likely they will still have attentional problems related to cognitive deficits. Patients with ID also commonly have problems with frontal lobe functioning, and therefore they often have difficulty filtering or controlling changes in their attention to topics other than those at hand.

Inattention during the psychiatric evaluation

It is important and helpful to frequently review and summarize what has been discussed. This helps to refocus the interviewee on the topic at hand. It also provides an opportunity for the individual to add detail and to clarify what is being discussed and to agree or disagree with the interviewer's interpretations (Modell, 2006; Ott, 2005). Multiple sessions, rather than one long interview, should be considered; the plan should be based on the needs of the individual. Multiple trials increase the consistency of results when gathering information from any patient with attention deficits (Modell, 2006; Ott, 2005).

Serial order effects/last choice responses

Serial order refers to different options posed to the individual with ID in a question, as in multiple-choice or either/or question types. The option offered *last* tends to be chosen by patients with ID because it may be the only one they are able to recall, as opposed to the one which truly represents their thoughts or wishes. Response biases are less of a problem for either/or questions, although there is still a tendency for last choice responding/serial order effects. Finlay & Lyons (2002) argued that either/or questions are more successful when they involve short or single-word options. Multiple-choice questions will be even more problematic in patients with autistic spectrum disorders, or in patients who exhibit echolalia.

Examples of managing serial effect would be:

- "Is it A or B or C?" (if serial effect is an issue, patient will choose C.) Therefore, rephrase the question: "Is it C or B or A?"

- "Are you sad or happy?" Rephrase: "Are you happy or sad?"

- "Do you get to work by bus or car?" Rephrase: "Do you get to work by car or bus?"

One strategy to eliminate serial order effect during the psychiatric evaluation is to repeat the question and vary the order in which the alternatives are presented. Follow up responses to either/or questions with requests for examples or further elaboration. The greatest problem with yes/no responses is serial order effects, so extra caution should be used with this question type. Utilizing pictures or line drawings greatly decreases serial position effects.

Memory issues

Memory is the ability to store, retain and recall information. There are various types of memory; receptive memory is the "ability to note the characteristics of a given stimulus and recognize it later" (Mandler, 1967; Danziger, 2008). Sequential memory is the "ability to recall stimuli in order of observation or presentation." Rote memory is the "ability to learn certain information as a habit formation, such as the alphabet." Short term memory lasts from a few seconds to a minute, such as in recalling a phone number or the name of a person just introduced (Mandler, 1967; Danziger, 2008).

Individuals with ID may have memory difficulties, and this can be complicated by attention span difficulties, comprehension difficulties and acute mental health or medical symptoms, among other factors. Because of their difficulty with recalling past events, it may take longer or require different techniques, but it is definitely possible. As with individuals in the general population, this difficulty is increased in the presence of anxiety, depression or other mental health symptoms. On the other hand, very short term and short term memory in individuals with ID is comparable to that of persons without ID (Modell, 2006, Henry & Gudjonsson, 1999).

Retrieval requires pulling information from memory. Recognition requires identifying something that is named and represents a simpler form of recall (Mandler, 1967; Danziger, 2008; Modell 2006). Individuals with ID will be more successful with interview questions containing multiple choice questions, as opposed to questions requiring full sentence responses, and the use of line drawings and/or pictorial expressions can greatly increase accuracy of information obtained.

Persons with ID have difficulty in describing past events in an unambiguous fashion. This is particularly true when retelling or creating a story (Ott, 2005). Individuals are often asked to do this during mental health appointments, e.g. "What happened last week at work when you were upset?" Recall of past events generally is without order or a sense of relationships between events. The use of anchor events may help in these situations. The interviewer can facilitate by clarifying, summarizing and recapping; all three strategies are highly effective. Meeting with the patient several times to review and add details is also a high-yield technique (Ott, 2005).

Saliency

"Emotional strength or pull" of a piece of information or an event has a considerable impact on whether the information will be retained (Modell, 2006). If something was emotionally charged for an individual (whether positive or negative) or has personal relevance, it is much easier for the individual to recall details surrounding it. Most people can effortlessly recall times when they received terrible news as well as the most precious moments in their lives. These events are "salient" or noteworthy, and they made an impression at the time they occurred. Similarly, patients with ID are much more likely to recall details of events that were important to them, such as celebrations or other memorable activities.

The saliency of common events (e.g. eating at a restaurant, bowling) may be increased in patients with ID (Modell, 2006). During the interview process, it is important to be aware of the salient activities and events for a given individual, so the interviewer can use them as anchor events or otherwise link them to the situations of interest.

The same applies to exploring information that is important to mental health clinicians, versus that which is personally relevant to an individual. For example, a patient may not be aware of the location of their swimming class, since they aren't required to drive themselves to the event. Their involvement may be to prepare a bag with their swimming suit and a towel; they do not navigate to the location of the pool or sports club. The patient with ID may not know how many bedrooms are in their group home, for example, because they do not enter others' areas. The portions of the floor plan that are personally relevant are their bedroom and common areas. Therefore, when informally testing memory or other parts of the mental status examination, the interviewer should take into account the saliency of both personally deemed and mental health deemed relevance.

Memory issues when interacting with the patient during treatment process

Formal neuropsychological testing should be considered at baseline and whenever mental status changes are noted. The interviewer can assess memory informally by asking questions about information for which the answer is known. When requesting that patients recall events from the past, whether one day ago or a month ago, the interviewer must understand that memory generally declines for all individuals as the time since the event increases.

Use time anchors whenever possible; e.g. birthdays, holidays, significant life events. Interview third parties who can help with accuracy whenever possible. This should be done with the patient's permission and with appropriate release of information in place. Another strategy is to pose the question "What else?" to the patient several times, to prompt them for additional information.

For example: "What do you like to do in your spare time?" "Bowling." "What else?" "Watching TV." "What else?" "Listening to music." "What else?". . .

Responsiveness

Sigelman *et al.* (1982) reviewed the responsiveness of persons with ID to questions in an interview situation. Responsiveness (measured by the percentage of questions answered appropriately) was a stable individual behavior among the subjects, was positively correlated with IQ and was comparable across the three samples. Responsiveness varied as a function of question type, with yes/no questions and those calling for pictorial choices yielding greater responsiveness than either/or questions (Sigelman *et al.*, 1982). All of these were easier to answer than verbal multiple choice and open-ended questions.

When the question was revised each time, it increased accurate response rate (Sigelman *et al.*, 1982). For example, 73% of patients with ID correctly answered the question, "How do you get to work most days?" In contrast, when the question was revised to: "Do you get to work by car? Or by bus? By walking? Or by some other method?" patients with ID were able to answer 94% of the time. When pictures were used with the above questions, 100% of patients with ID were able to answer accurately.

Social skills

Social skills and interpersonal experiences make significant differences in a patient's level of adaptive functioning and communication abilities. For example, consider a patient with mild ID who has been isolated from the community, who has not attended formal educational programming or who has not experienced regular interface with people in their community. This patient may have a vastly different presentation than a patient with mild ID who was socialized from the very beginning of life, who attended school with an individualized educational program in place and who has had regular interface with the community. Two individuals may have an identical intelligence quotient per neuropsychological testing, but they may have vast differences in social skills and adaptive functioning.

The role of open-ended questions

Despite a person's possible cognitive difficulties, open-ended questions are always worth a try with patients who have any degree of verbal capacity. Be aware that they require a higher level of linguistic and cognitive ability. If a patient struggles with an open-ended question, there are interventions that may be helpful and may improve productivity and output. A therapeutic alliance and establishing a rapport will assist in the process, and therefore the success of utilizing open-ended questions will typically increase over time as a treatment relationship is firmly established. If a patient is initially hesitant in responding, or if they are asked for a list of things and they respond with one item, a useful intervention is to respond by asking "What else?," which will typically prompt the individual to provide additional information (Modell, 2006; Finlay & Lyons, 2002).

Finlay & Lyons, (2002) reported that even though open-ended questions produced fewer details, the responses contained more accurate information and fewer errors than did yes/ no questions posed to individuals with ID. For testimony from a person with ID in a judicial case, the use of cognitive interviews (wherein the individual is asked a variety of open-ended questions regarding the same incident) has shown increased levels of recall (Modell, 2006).

When formulating open-ended questions for a patient with ID, it is recommended to ask the patient to explain in their own words what they think the problem is and how it has affected their life. When ending an appointment or interview, the mental health professional should explain one's own thinking process, how one came to that conclusion, the specific treatment recommendations and their rationale. After giving instructions, a summary or a treatment plan, the interviewer can ask the patient to explain it back (depending on their expressive language ability) in order to confirm understanding.

Medical problems

Many patients with ID have medical conditions which may be undiagnosed or under-treated. Depending on which organ system is affected, this can greatly affect the patient's comfort, communication ability, quality of life and psychological functioning. It is also common for patients with ID to experience "white coat syndrome" when interfacing with physicians or other people who are viewed as authority figures. This may be very intimidating and may be a product of previous treatment relationships. The patient may be accustomed to being ignored, not addressed or talked about as if they are not present. They might find the appointment a boring experience and will likely be offended by this type of behavior. Chapter 3 discusses various behavioral presentations of commonly undiagnosed or under-treated medical conditions in patients with ID.

Clinical Vignette #5

Co-occurring medical problems; saliency of questions to patient and caregiver   Sue is a 48 year old woman, with a history of moderate intellectual disability and obsessive compulsive disorder, presents for psychiatry appointment following a hospitalization for medical illness (for acute exacerbation of her insulin-dependent diabetes mellitus):

Psychiatrist: Hello, Sue. I know you just got home from the hospital a couple days ago. How are you doing?

Sue: I'm OK now.

Psychiatrist: I heard that you had some problems with your blood sugar.

Sue: I have to eat healthy. I am going swimming every week, too.

Caregiver: We have been trying to encourage exercise, so we take Sue and her house-mates swimming a couple times a week.

Psychiatrist: That's great. I'm so glad to hear about that. Do you like swimming, Sue?

Sue: Yes, a lot.

Psychiatrist: Where do you go to swim? [Question is not salient to the patient; only salient to the caregivers who transport her there]

Sue (pause): *She* knows. [Pointing to caregiver]

Caregiver: We have memberships for everyone at the local health club. It's about ten minutes from the house, so it's very convenient. We are also planning our grocery list more carefully and making very healthy meals, since everyone needs to be more active and lose weight.

Sensory deficits

It is common for individuals with ID to experience sensory deficits – in particular, visual and auditory. This can greatly affect their ability to interface with others. A patient with hearing impairment, for example, may appear confused or may not understand conversation, merely because they are unable to hear others in the room. A patient with an untreated hearing impairment may also become frustrated and angry, and will be vulnerable to develop secondary depression or anxiety. Chapter 3 reviews sensory deficits in greater detail.

Sensory hypersensitivity

Many patients with ID and in particular patients with autistic disorder and Fragile X syndrome may be hypersensitive to light, noise, tactile stimulation or other sensory perception experiences (Dykens *et al.*, 2000). Being alert to this fact can be the difference between the patient being comfortable and willing/able to share information, or refusing to interact with the interviewer or clinician.

Baranek *et al.* (1997) studied sensory defensiveness in persons with ID. Sensory defensiveness is "a tendency to over-react or respond adversely toward specific sensory stimuli that are non-threatening." People with sensory defensiveness will either avoid or overreact to certain types of touch, sounds, lights, smells, tastes, or movements. These behaviors are more evident in special populations, such as those with ID. Baranek *et al.* reported that all subjects with ID demonstrated marked and atypical behaviors in reaction to sensory stimuli. Two of the behaviors, including "being upset by noise" and "general hypersensitivity," were more common in children with ID than in adults. It was hypothesized that the behaviors may diminish over time with increasing developmental maturity and social experience. Researchers suggest that there are two separate and distinct subtypes of sensory defensiveness: tactile defensiveness and auditory/general hypersensitivity (Baranek *et al.*, 1997).

Assistive devices

Incorporate assistive devices as part of the patient's personal space whenever needed. Employ professional interpreters when needed, and utilize collateral informants familiar with the patient wisely. It will serve the interviewer well to learn the basics of sign language, i.e. common words such as "thank you," "bathroom," "please," "sad," "happy," "good," "bad." This will help establish rapport and formation of a therapeutic relationship. If the patient is nonverbal, utilization of yes/no questions may be helpful. Learning some of the basics directly from the individual with ID will certainly help in establishing an alliance.

Expressed emotion

The concept "expressed emotion" refers to the degree of certain affects in relationships between people, and it is characterized by "criticism, hostility and emotionally over-involved attitudes" (Hastings & Lloyd, 2007). Researchers have specifically quantified the use of critical comments and dominance in relationships. In the general population, expressed emotion (EE) is a marker that explains some of the deviation and severity and/or course of a number of psychiatric disorders (Hastings & Lloyd, 2007). In the general population, there is an association established between the degree of expressed emotion in parents and their children's behavior issues.

Hastings & Lloyd (2007) reviewed eleven studies of expressed emotion in families with a child or adult with ID. They concluded that the existence of behavior problems in individuals with ID may have a relationship to high-EE parents, with some limited data consistent with a causal relationship of high EE maintaining or exacerbating behavior problems as the individual with ID progresses through the developmental years.

EE is best conceptualized as the affect in an interpersonal relationship between the individual with ID and a caregiver. EE may be more prevalent in conflicted or stressful relationships, as is quite common in instances where someone has significant dependency requirements, such as an individual with ID. The families and caregivers of persons with ID are often highly stressed and should not be held responsible or blamed. The appropriate interventions may include psychoeducation of the caregiver and respite for the caregivers and/or family members. In some cases, a recommendation for psychotherapy may be in order.

Cultural awareness and sensitivity

Culture is "a system of shared beliefs, values, customs, behaviors, and artifacts that members of society used to cope with their worlds in with one another." Culture is threaded throughout family structure and is inherently passed on through the generations (Jackson, 2000).

Communication affects our verbal as well as nonverbal expressive language. Culture is fundamental to all of our internal and external experiences and, most importantly, to how we navigate relationships (Jackson, 2000, Department of Developmental Services, 1997). It is important for the clinician to be aware of his or her own cultural background, as well as being familiar with the culture of their patients. We can learn the general principles of other cultures, but we should never make assumptions about any individuals based on their cultural background. The interviewer should have the ability to alter his/her own communication style, based on the needs of the patient (Jackson, 2000, Department of Developmental Services, 1997).

Understanding an individual's cultural or ethnic background plays a significant role in connecting with patients and in building rapport. Being aware of personal space, gestures, eye contact or broaching sensitive topics can all be handled very differently, depending on the culture, as alluded to previously. Jackson (2000) described cultural competence as valuing "diversity with the goal to manage the dynamics of difference." This transcends accommodating assistive devices or providing an interpreter when indicated; it speaks to respecting the individual (Developmental Disabilities and Bill of Rights Act, 2000). It is a commitment to hear the patient's story on his or her own terms.

The effectiveness of a psychotherapist will increase with the level of their self-awareness. Understanding one's own culture is important, because of the tendency to regard one's own cultural group as the standard to which all others are compared (Jackson, 2000, Department of Developmental Services, 1997). The effective interviewer will communicate with persons with ID in a professional, thoughtful, and nonjudgmental manner (Jackson, 2000), including nonverbal communication.

Showing (and experiencing) respect for the individual with ID is especially important in constructing a strong therapeutic alliance, because some of these persons have had bad experiences within their culture or in previous treatment relationships. Unfortunately, some cultures have critical or judgmental interpretations of the causes of disabilities, and in particular intellectual disabilities (see Table 12). A patient's self-esteem may have been seriously affected by experiencing behavior from others that was based on these beliefs.

Attitude of the interviewer

Tone of voice and attitude of the interviewer has a significant impact on the productivity of an interview (Antaki, 1999). For example, in Antaki's study, when patients were asked "Well?" using differing tones of voice, they interpreted some interviewers as disagreeing with their previous responses or irritated with pauses, and this greatly impacted their future responses. This effect was greater if the interviewer was seen as an authority figure. It is important to be aware that patient responses can inadvertently be biased by the tone of a question, making any information thus obtained be less useful or factually inaccurate.

Table 12 Summary of cultural beliefs about disabilities.

• Result of bad conduct by an individual or family member in this life or in a previous existence.
• Caused by disobeying God.
• Source of family embarrassment and shame.
• Caused by supernatural or natural causes.
• Public display of disability or weakness is discouraged.
• Cause of significant stigma.
• Justification for abandonment of a child.

See also: Department of Developmental Services (1997), p. 6.

Interviewing the victim, witness or suspect with ID
(see also Chapter 15)

Individuals with intellectual and other disabilities are disproportionately criminally victimized (Henry & Gudjonsson 1999). In fact, they are four to 12 times more likely to become crime victims than persons without a disability (Sobsey & Doe, 1991). The victimization rate is not correlated with residential placement or location.

The rate of sexual assault is more than 12 times the rate of the general population (Sobsey *et al.*, 1995). Victimization rates for persons with disabilities is highest for sexual assault (more than ten times as high) and robbery (more than 12 times as high) (Sobsey *et al.*, 1995). Balderian (1991) reports that increased victimization rates are related to the following factors:

* Longstanding barriers to reporting and prosecution.

* Physical vulnerability of the victim.

* The abuser taking advantage of a position of trust (97–99% of abusers of victims with ID are known and trusted by the victim).

Prior to meeting the person, it is important to determine if the individual uses an interpreter or a communicative aid. The same interventions for calming an individual from the general population work well for those with ID, but the interviewer should be prepared to take more time. The interviewer should speak naturally, and questions should be concretized or simplified as needed, in order to meet the needs of the developmental framework of the individual. In addition to the allotment of extra time, multiple interviews may be necessary. Before concluding the interview, the interviewer should make some summary statements to the person and ask the individual if the statements are accurate, e.g. "Let me review what you've told me, and you tell me if it is right."

Cognitive interviewing techniques can be helpful when interviewing a victim, witness, or suspect. Modell (2006) summarizes cognitive interviewing techniques as follows:

1. Report everything.

2. Reconstruct the circumstances.

3. Recall the events in a different order.

4. Change perspective.

The interviewer should focus initially on having the interviewee report everything, as opposed to reconstructing the entire event from start to finish. The details can be filled in throughout the meeting or in subsequent meetings.

Such statements as "Tell me everything you think is important" should be avoided (Modell, 2006). Individuals with ID have executive functioning deficits; areas affected include the frontal lobe processes, wherein an individual decides "good" versus "bad" or "better" versus "best." This filtering process is used to determine what is important or salient and what is not. The individual will usually not be able to distinguish between a minor problem and a major problem in terms of seriousness. Do not ask the person to edit information, but communicate to them that everything is important and you can sort through the details later. Make it clear that a "don't know" response is acceptable. Whenever possible, use time anchors or other information that is salient to the individual.

Putting a detailed sequence of events together will be difficult – something that is true for everyone and is not limited to individuals with ID. When attempting to reconstruct the circumstances, "focused open-ended questions" will be useful. An example of a "focused open-ended question" might be: "When you opened your purse at the movie theater, what was missing?" or "At work yesterday, who made you mad?"

There is a difference between recognition and word finding. Retrieval requires recalling information from memory (Findlay & Lyons, 2001). Recognition is more straightforward, since it only requires identifying something that is named. Keeping these principles in mind should facilitate the interview.

If you become familiar with the person's normal daily routine, you will be able more easily to place the event of interest before or after happenings well known to the individual. Whenever possible, use the person's own words and build on the information they provide to you. Having reliable collateral data sources available to facilitate can be invaluable.

Some authors recommend the use of two interviews, the first being used for free recall, utilizing carefully worded open-ended questions (Findlay & Lyons, 2001, Henry & Gudjonsson, 1999). In the second interview, a variety of question types should be employed and information from the first interview can be confirmed and clarified.

Conclusion

The best way to get experience is to get experience! Educate yourself by interviewing as many individuals with ID as possible. This not only increases your experiential knowledge base, but also your confidence and comfort level. Be a detective and investigate the core issue. Be aware of the commonalities within each category of ID, and study the principles of the developmental framework of the patient while keeping in mind that each person is an individual with a unique personality. Be honest when you do not understand the individual's speech or communication, and feel free to ask the individual to repeat the response – or enlist the assistance of a collateral source in the room when appropriate. When discussing intimate or sensitive topics, keep in mind that you can always request one-on-one time with the individual. See Table 13 for clinical pearls.

Use "who," "what" and "where" questions rather than "when," "how" and "why" questions (Dykens *et al.*, 2000). Be respectful of all assistive and communicative devices and treat these devices as if they are part of the individual's personal space. Attend to a patient's individual communication style or format.

With regard to question types, remember that the high-yield accurate information will most likely be gained from use of pictorial multiple-choice and factual yes/no questions, closely followed by subjective yes/no questions. Question types that tend to be lower-yield (although individually dependent on the person with ID) include either/or questions, and the least consistent are verbal multiple-choice and open-ended questions. It is always worth-while to add either focused or general open-ended questions in the mix, whether or not they

Table 13 Clinical Pearls: interviewing persons with intellectual disability.

- Ask permission to involve collateral data sources.
- Do your homework/review medical records (know what to expect).
- Collect collateral data/manage the triangle.
- Asked for repetition as needed; do not pretend you understand the patient's verbalizations if this is not the case.
- Concretize the abstract.
- Be respectful.
- Ask the individual to repeat something if you did not understand.
- Take responsibility for miscommunication
- Match mean length of utterance.
- Gesturing/animation.
- Use time anchors.
- Eliminate distractions and unnecessary noise/movements and other environmental considerations.
- Be aware of sensory deficits.
- Do not use slang or figurative speech.
- Allow more time and consider multiple meetings if needed.
- Recapping/summarizing/clarifying.
- Cultural awareness and sensitivity.
- Keep trying/persistence.

are answered accurately; they can still provide the interviewer with new insight and valuable information.

Remember to recap, summarize, clarify, paraphrase and use time anchors. Above all, establish an alliance with the patient. When you are able to collect important diagnostic data from the patient while making them feel at ease, there is more potential to diagnose accurately. This patient population is most gratifying and genuine to work with. Each individual with ID, whether verbal or nonverbal, has an important story to tell.

References

American Psychiatric Association (2000). *Diagnostic and Statistical Manual of Mental Disorders*, (4th ed. text revision) Washington, DC.

Antaki, C. (1999). Interviewing Persons with a Learning Disability: How Setting Lower Standards May Inflate Well Being Scores. *Qualitative Health Research* **9**(4), 437–454.

Balderian, N. (1991). Sexual abuse of people with developmental disabilities. *Sexuality and Disability* **9**(4), 323–335.

Baranek, G.T., Foster, L.E. & Berkson, G. (1997). Sensory Defensiveness in Persons with Developmental Disabilities. *Occupational Therapy Journal of Research* **17**(3), 173–185.

Barnette, J.J. (2000). Effects of Stem and Likert Response Option Reversals on Survey Internal Consistency: If you feel the need, there is a better alternative to using those negatively worded stems. *Educational and Psychological Measurement* **60**(3), 361–370.

Booth, T. & Booth, W. (1994). The Use of Depth Interviewing with Vulnerable Subjects: Lessons from a Research Study of parents with Learning Difficulties. *Social Science and Medicine* **39** (3), 415–424.

Chapman, M. (1988). *Constructive Evolution: Origins and Development of Piaget's Thought*. Cambridge University Press, New York.

Commons, M.L. & Richards, F.A. (1984). "A general model of stage theory" and "Applying the general stage model." In Commons, M.L., Richards, F.A. & Armon, C. (eds.). *Beyond formal operations: Vol.1: Late adolescent and adult cognitive development*, pp. 12–140, 141–157). Praeger, New York.

Danziger, K. (2008). *Making the Mind: A History of Memory*. Cambridge University Press, Cambridge, UK.

Department of Developmental Services (1997). *How To Be Culturally Responsive*. Services and Supports Section, Sacramento, CA.

Developmental Disabilities and Bill of Rights Act (2000). PUBLIC LAW 106-402 (October 30, 2000). 114 STAT. 1677. www.acf.hhs.gov/programs/add/ddact/DDACT2.html. Access Date 05/17/11.

Dykens, E.M., Hodapp, R.M., & Finucane, B.M., (2000). *Genetics and mental retardation syndromes: A new look at behavior and interventions*. Paul H Brookes Publishing, Baltimore, MD.

Ekman, P. (1977). Biological And Cultural Contributions To Body And Facial Movement. In: Blacking, J. (ed) *Anthropology of the Body*, pp. 34–84. Academic Press, London.

Ekman, P. & Friesen, W.V. (1975). *Unmasking the Face*. Prentice-Hall Inc., Englewood Cliffs, NJ.

Finlay, W.M.L. & Lyons, E. (2001). Methodological Issues in Interviewing and Using Self-Report Questionnaires with People with Mental Retardation. *Psychological Assessment* **13** (3), 319–335.

Finlay, W.M.L. & Lyons, E. (2002). Acquiescence in Interviews With People Who Have Mental Retardation. *Mental Retardation* **40**(1), 14–29.

Fischer, K.W. (1980). A theory of cognitive development: The control and construction of hierarchical skills. *Psychological Review* **87**(2), 477–531.

Fletcher, R., Loschen, E., Stavrakaki, C. & First, M. (eds.), (2007). *Diagnostic Manual – Intellectual Disability (DM-ID): A Textbook of Diagnosis of Mental Disorders in Persons with Intellectual Disability*. NADD Press, Kingston, NY.

Foley, G.N. & Gentile, J.P. (2010). Nonverbal Communication in Psychotherapy. *Psychiatry* **7** (6), 38–44.

Habler, F. & Reis, O. (2010). Pharmacotherapy of Disruptive Behavior in Mentally Retarded Subjects: A Review of the Current Literature. *Developmental Disabilities Research Reviews* **16**, 265–272.

Hassiotis, A., Baron, D.A. & Hall, I. (2009). *Intellectual Disability Psychiatry: A Practical Handbook*. Wiley Publishing, UK.

Hastings, R.P. & Lloyd, M.R. (2007). Expressed Emotion in Families of Children and Adults with Intellectual Disabilities. *Mental Retardation and Developmental Disabilities Research Reviews* **14**(4), 339–345.

Heal, L.W. & Sigelman, C.K. (1995). Response biases in interviews of individuals with limited mental ability. *Journal of Intellectual Disability Research* 39 Part 4, 331–340.

Henry, L.A. & Gudjonsson, G.H. (1999). Eyewitness Memory and Suggestibility in Children with Mental Retardation. *American Journal of Mental Retardation* **104**(6), 491–508.

Individuals with Disabilities Education Act 1975 (IDEA). www.law.umaryland.edu/marshall/crsreports/crsdocuments/RS20366_01112002.pdf Access Date 05/17/11.

Jackson, W. (2000). *Cultural Communication* (*PowerPoint* presentation). Interpretation and Translation Services (ITS): Florida Dept. of Health, Bureau of TB and Refugee Health. The Office of Minority Health website at: www. hhs. gov/ocr/lep.

Levitas, A.S., Hurley, A.D. & Pary, R. (2001). The Mental Status Examination in Patients with Mental Retardation and Developmental Disabilities. *Mental Health Aspects of Developmental Disabilities* **4**(1), 1–16.

Mandler, G. (1967). Organization and memory. In: Spence, K.W. & Spence, J.T. (eds.) *The psychology of learning and motivation: Advances in research and theory*. Vol. 1, pp 328–372. Academic Press, New York.

Modell, S.J. (2006). Interview Techniques and Considerations for Victims with Developmental Disabilities. (*PowerPoint* presentation), Elder Abuse Conference (NAPSA) San Francisco, CA.

Ott, D. (2005). *Interview Techniques: Working With Persons With Co-Occurring Developmental Disabilities & Mental Illness* (*PowerPoint* presentation). Ohio Coordinating Center of Excellence in Mental Illness/Developmental Disabilities Annual Conference, Zanesville, OH.

Sigelman, C.K., Budd, E.C., Spanhel, C.L. & Schoenrock, C.J. (1981). Asking Questions of Retarded Persons: A Comparison of Yes-No and Either-Or Formats. *Applied Research in Mental Retardation* **2**(4), 347–357.

Sigelman, C.K., Budd, E.C., Winer, J.L., Schoenrock, C.J. & Martin, P.W. (1982). Evaluating Alternative Techniques of Questioning Mentally Retarded Persons. *American Journal of Mental Deficiency* **86**(5), 511–518.

Sigelman, C.K., Winer, J.L., Schoenrock, C.J. (1982). The Responsiveness of Mentally Retarded Persons to Questions. *Education & Training in Mental Retardation* **17**, 120–24.

Silka, V.R. & Hauser, M.J. (1997). Psychiatric Assessment of the Person with Mental Retardation. *March. Psychiatric Annals* **27**(3) 162–169.

Smith, P. & McMarthy, G. (1996). The Development of a Semi-Structured Interview to Investigate the Attachment-Related Experiences of Adults with Learning Disabilities. *British Journal of Learning Disabilities* **24**, 154–158.

Sobsey, D. & Doe, T. (1991). Patterns of sexual abuse and assault. *Sexuality and Disability*, **9**(3), 243–260.

Sobsey, D., Wells, D., Lucardie, R.,& Mansell, S. (eds.). (1995). *Violence and disability: An annotated bibliography*. Paul H. Brookes, Baltimore, MD.

Sovner, R. (1986). Limiting factors in the use of DSM-III criteria with mentally ill/mentally retarded persons. *Psychopharmacology Bulletin* **22**(4), 1055–9.

Szymanski, L. & King, B.H. (1999). *Practice Parameters for the Assessment and Treatment of Children,Adolescents and Adults with Mental Retardation and Comorbid Mental Disorders*. American Academy of Child and Adolescent Psychiatry, Washington, DC.

7

Mood Disorders

Ann K. Morrison, MD, Associate Professor,
Wright State University, Dayton, Ohio
Christina Weston, MD, Associate Professor,
Wright State University, Dayton, Ohio

Introduction

In the past, it was incorrectly believed that people with intellectual disabilities (ID) experienced lower rates of mood disorders than did the general population. Indeed, this view was common enough that Sovner & Hurley (1983) titled an early literature review "Do the mentally retarded suffer affective illness?" However, more recent studies indicate that unipolar depression is common in this population (Cooper, 2007). Some (Hurley *et al.*, 2003), but not all (Cooper, 2007) studies suggest that a milder degree of intellectual impairment is even more likely to be associated with depression than is more severe disability.

One factor contributing to the lack of appreciation of depression in persons with ID is that the usual diagnostic criteria for depressive disorders (for example) require historical detail and subjective report of distress that might exceed the individual's ability to report. As a result of this under-recognition of depression, the frequency with which the two primary modalities of treatment – antidepressants and psychotherapy – have been offered to people with ID has not been well studied.

The existing literature consists of studies of treatment approaches that have been mainly case series, focused on pharmacologic treatments (Antonacci, 2008). Antipsychotics, on

Psychiatry of Intellectual Disability: A Practical Manual, First Edition.
Edited by Julie P. Gentile and Paulette M. Gillig.
© 2012 John Wiley & Sons, Ltd. Published 2012 by John Wiley & Sons, Ltd.

the other hand, although historically not seen as playing a major role in the treatment of non-psychotic depression in the general population, have often been widely used to treat people with ID for a variety of disorders (Spreat *et al.*, 1997).

To improve recognition of depressive disorders in the ID population, experts in the field of ID advise modifying the usual diagnostic criteria in existing manuals to include more objective data (Fletcher *et al.*, 2007). For example, depressed mood could be described by the observations of others, such as an observed change from usual behavior, and irritable mood may be recognized by its association with agitation, stereotypies, ritualistic or repetitive behaviors.

Bipolar disorder prevalence rates in individuals with ID in more recent studies have been reported at 2.4% (Merikangas, 2011) and 2.5% (Cooper, 2007). The assessment of symptoms of mania (such as euphoria, grandiosity, increased goal-directed or pleasure-seeking behavior and disruption of neurovegetative patterns) has also been difficult in persons with ID, because they may have difficulty in verbalizing changes in their thought processes or mood.

In the past, persons with ID were more likely to reside in very structured environments, where more subtle changes in mood or behavior may not have been readily expressed or appreciated. Subtle symptoms of hypomania or mania such as irritability, dysphoria and impulsivity may have been difficult to interpret, because affective lability and behavioral disinhibition were common.

In contrast to the argument that unipolar depression may be more common in persons with *mild* ID, Cooper *et al.* (2007) noted an increase in the diagnostic frequency of bipolar disorder as the degree of ID became *more severe,* and speculated that this was because mania was less often overlooked in these persons by caregiver informants.

While antidepressants have likely been underused due to under-diagnosis of depression, mood stabilizers/anticonvulsants are quite commonly prescribed for people with ID, not only when there has been a formal diagnosis of bipolar disorder or epilepsy, but also for aggression, self-injurious behavior, and impulsivity (Antonacci *et al.*, 2008; Antonacci & Attiah, 2008). There has been recent controversy as to whether bipolar disorder may now be over-diagnosed in the general population (Zimmerman, 2010; 2008). Whether this is also the case in individuals with ID is unknown at this time but, given the added difficulty of assessment in the ID population, the possibility exists.

However, the essential feature of bipolar disorder, the existence of episodes of behavior change, is often overlooked when the patient has chronic mood lability and affective instability. Just as the differential diagnosis of borderline personality disorder, among other causes of these behavioral disturbances, may be missed in the general population (Zimmerman, 2010), one should be alert to this possibility in individuals with ID (see Chapter 10).

When evaluating a patient with ID for the presence of an affective disorder, knowledge of family psychiatric history, caregiver informants, and a review of old records for past presenting symptoms and treatment responses are all useful. Assessment scales may also be helpful. The diagnostic nuances of intellectual distortion, psychosocial masking, cognitive disintegration and baseline exaggeration should be acknowledged when assessing patients with ID for affective disorders (see Chapters 2 and 6 for a further discussion of these concepts, as well as Sovner, 1986).

Major depressive disorder in ID

Prevalence and predisposing factors

Among persons with ID, the prevalence rate of major depressive disorder is 4.1%, which is about the same as in the general population (Cooper *et al.*, 2007). People with ID appear to be as susceptible to life events as other people. Hastings *et al.* (2004) found that stressful life events occurring in the prior 12 months were associated with a higher risk of developing depression in persons with ID. Natural losses, such as grief when a parent has died, may be experienced more acutely than in the general population. This is perhaps in part because people with ID often reside with their parents well into adulthood and do not have the number and intensity of relationships which the general population develops with which to buffer them from a parent's death.

Other stressors and losses include changes in supervisors and staff at occupational, habilitation and housing programs, peers moving on to other positions or other housing; and the deaths of peers. Although mortality for the general population has improved through the years, the mortality rates for individuals with ID, although improved, still exceeds the rate for the general population (Tyrer *et al.*, 2007; Decoufle & Autry, 2002; Singer & Strauss, 1997). Since it is more likely that individuals with ID will die during their work life than those in the general population, the person with ID is at a higher risk of losing peers earlier in life.

It is known that people in the general population experience more stress when they have more events occurring that are outside of their external locus of control (Wiersma *et al.*, 2011). People with ID have many more activities and decisions about their lives that are outside of their control, either formally through guardianships and payees, or informally through the structure and supervision that may be required to ensure their well-being. Even the more recent efforts to emphasize self-determination do not eradicate the sometimes limited options available to people with ID.

Maladaptive behaviors and personality traits also may place patients at higher risk for depression. For example, reassurance-seeking and subsequent episodes of rejection seem to be linked to depression in people with ID (Hartley, 2008). Personality traits such as introversion, submissiveness, passivity, increased interpersonal dependency and neuroticism may also increase risk for onset or persistence of depression in some groups (Akiskal *et al.*, 1983; Hirschfeld *et al.*, 1983, 1986, 1989). Hartley & MacLean (2009) found that depressed adults with mild ID reported a greater frequency of stressful social interactions, as well as a greater impact of the stress on their mood. They tended to internalize rejection, to have more difficulty overcoming their negative feelings and thoughts and to generalize the feelings of rejection to other relationships. They also made fewer efforts to cope, had fewer active coping strategies and used more avoidant coping strategies.

Major depressive disorder also may be caused, or co-occur with, medical conditions in a person with ID. As in the general population, chronic medical conditions as varied as arthritis, heart disease, epilepsy, stroke, Parkinson's disease and cancer are often comorbid with depression. Some of these conditions, such as epilepsy, are more common in people with ID, and some (e.g. hypothyroidism and dementia) can mimic and complicate treatment of depression. Individuals with Down syndrome are at increased risk for both hypothyroidism and dementia, and they present special challenges in differential diagnosis. Medical conditions such as gastro-esophageal acid reflux and sleep apnea are also common, and may cause sleep disruption and mood changes such as depression and irritability. As in the general population, chronic pain may lead to poor sleep, low energy, depressed mood and irritability. Individuals with ID may be less able to articulate pain, and making correct diagnoses is even more difficult. See Chapter 3 for more information on Medical Assessment.

Differential diagnosis

Identifying general medical conditions as either a cause or contributing factor is essential. Being able to identify signs and symptoms of depression with information from both the individual and informants is the next step. Since patients may lack the verbal skills to identify feelings adequately, pictorial tools for mood states may help. However, sometimes asking persons if they feel sad is a first step in arriving at an accurate diagnosis of major depression. Affective observation by the psychiatrist in the interview should also be carried out.

Another essential part of assessment is observation by family and caregivers. It is important to get these informants to describe the person's affect as objectively as possible, rather than simply relating an inference or conclusion. For instance, ask them to report the specific behavior (e.g. crying, smiling, sitting quietly, withdrawal from others, decreased eye contact, wringing of hands or other excessive behaviors), rather than concluding the person is "sad," "anxious," or "angry." When possible, quantitative measures of sleep, appetite, energy, social or work activity are helpful, especially when multiple informants are interacting with the person.

Beyond depressive symptoms themselves, assess the severity of mood disorder, including whether psychotic symptoms are present and whether the person represents a threat to him/ herself or others. Again, as the degree of ID becomes more severe, the ability of the person to report psychotic symptoms (particularly elaborate delusions) becomes diminished. Sometimes, getting the person to grasp the concept of "hallucinations" can be challenging. Take into account the person's developmental age, because some ideas and experiences may represent normal, albeit "magical" thinking for the individual, rather than psychopathology (see Chapter 6). Sometimes, the person may only be able to convey ill-formed ideas of fearfulness that seem in excess of the situation.

As in the general population, normal perceptual disturbances that commonly occur during periods of grief (transiently hearing or seeing a deceased loved one) and those due to organic causes (such as medication toxicity or seizures) need to be considered. When considering self-harm and harm to others, one needs to ascertain the person's expectation of the dangerousness of the act (intent), as well as objectively whether the idea or plan is feasible and likely to be harmful. Keep in mind that someone who really *intends* to kill themselves can come up with a more lethal plan later in the day – especially if their previous plan was debunked during the assessment.

It is often stated that patients with ID have atypical symptoms of depression. However, one needs to be aware that sometimes, rather than the symptoms being atypical or sub-syndromal, it is possible that the person is not depressed and that the symptoms are developing for some other reason. This is especially true of symptoms that are not the well-recognized atypical symptoms of depression (e.g. hypersomnia, hyperphagia and psycho-motor agitation), but rather less specific symptoms such as irritability. Conversely, even when the patient with ID is able to provide a history and good informants are available, the patient may still fall short of meeting strict DSM-IV TR criteria. In this case, the clinician should use his or her expertise and judgment in finalizing a diagnosis and treatment plan. Hurley (2008) notes that the symptoms of sad mood, crying and anhedonia are quite typical of depression in individuals with ID, and are the most useful in distinguishing unipolar depression from anxiety and bipolar disorder.

Another important disorder that should be included in the differential diagnosis is dementia. Individuals with Down syndrome (DS) develop Alzheimer's type dementia at an earlier age and with a prevalence rate that exceeds the general population (Ball *et al.*, 2008). Pathologic changes typical of Alzheimer's are almost universally found in patients with DS (Mann & Esiri, 1989).

Initial presentation of dementia in individuals with DS usually involves more personality and behavioral changes than memory complaints. Other causes of dementia in people with ID include higher than expected rates of frontotemporal and Lewy body type dementia, which exceed vascular dementia rates in this population (Strydom *et al.*, 2007). As in the general population, it is sometimes helpful to treat the depressive symptoms empirically, even if there is suspicion that some of the cognitive and behavior complaints may be manifestations of a dementing illness.

Treatment

In the general population, treatment for depression includes psychotherapy and antide-pressant medications. Other adjunctive medications and electroconvulsive therapy are also employed. In general, these same treatments should be offered to people with ID who have depression, although some modifications may be necessary.

Psychotherapy for people with ID may need to be modified to accommodate lower verbal abilities (see Chapter 13). Receptive language may be better developed than expressive language, so some individuals may be able to understand and make use of skills taught in psychotherapy to a greater degree than one anticipates. As in the interview, the use of pictures and role play may also be appropriate in understanding the individual's emotional life (see Chapter 6).

Esbensen & Benson (2007) reviewed whether Beck's cognitive triad (Beck, 1976) was a valid construct for people with ID. The cognitive triad refers to negative views of self, the world and the future, which give rise to depression. They concluded that the cognitive triad could be measured among individuals with mild and moderate ID and is related to depression and depressed mood in these patients, as well as in the general population.

When cognitive behavioral therapy (CBT) is instituted for individuals with ID, it is sometimes thought that the primary work is really behavior therapy, with very little emphasis on changing cognitions or dysfunctional thoughts. Modification in the cognitive approach, particularly in setting up reasonable homework, may be needed in order to change dysfunctional thoughts. As with CBT for the general population, one may enlist the help of significant others in homework outside of the therapy (see Chapter 13).

Perhaps the best studied area, and the field with the most evidence for successful behavior change in people with ID, is in the area of more classic behavioral therapy (see Chapter 14). While it is often focused on "challenging behaviors," there is no reason not to utilize behavior therapy to assist someone suffering from the negative behaviors typical of depression, such as disrupted sleep, lack of pleasurable activity and social withdrawal. Working on social skills may help diminish the risk for depressive relapse if some of the depressogenic social stressors can be diminished. Concrete, non-verbal ways of learning new skills may be needed in this population. Role-playing, practicing and rehearsal and over-learning may be useful. Management of the environment by formal behavior plans may also help.

Not to be overlooked, although without much research base at present, would be other standard psychotherapeutic approaches to depression, such as interpersonal therapy. Commonly, the precipitating factor or perpetuating event for depression in this population has been a breach in relationships. Romantic turmoil or breakups, or strife with a peer or a supervisor at work, are quite often the identified problem from the point of view of the individual experiencing depression. In some cases, couples psychotherapy may be appropriate. It may be challenging for the psychotherapist, when working with people with ID, to avoid simply giving advice, but instead to ascertain what the patient wishes and what the conflicts are.

Antidepressant medications are another treatment option. As there has not been a wealth of clinical trials in the use of antidepressants in the ID population, recommendations are mainly extrapolations from treatments used in the general population (American Psychiatric Association Practice Guidelines, 2010). Usually, serotonin re-uptake inhibitors such as fluoxetine, sertraline or citalopram, or newer dually acting medications such as venlafaxine or duloxetine, are common agents with which to start. In general, older medications with anticholinergic and sedating side effects, such as the tricyclic antidepressants (e.g. amitriptyline, nortriptyline, imipramine, desipramine or doxepin) are usually avoided; their sedating and hypotensive side effects can be especially problematic in people with cognitive impairment, and their anticholinergic effects can cause urinary retention and constipation, which can evolve to become medical emergencies in people with ID. However, some individuals who either do not respond to, or are unable to tolerate newer antidepressants may benefit from a carefully monitored tricyclic antidepressant trial. Since many people with ID have epilepsy, use of bupropion may be more limited than in the general population, as it can decrease seizure threshold.

Shorter-acting medications and ones with fewer drug interactions should be selected for those individuals who are medically fragile and/or are taking other medications. Starting at the lower end of standard dosing and advancing cautiously through the standard range until benefit is achieved is recommended. Maximizing one medication before moving onto another, or adding a second medication, will help avoid polypharmacy.

When considering adjuvant therapy, other target symptoms, the person's medical history and the possibility of other comorbid conditions should be considered. Factors favoring one choice over another might include comorbid attention deficit hyperactivity disorder (ADHD), or a history of the same (consider a psychostimulant), generalized anxiety disorder (consider buspirone), suspicion of bipolar disorder or impulsivity (consider lithium or another mood stabilizer).

STAR*D (Nierenberg et al., 2006) suggested that thyroid augmentation is better tolerated than lithium augmentation, so one might consider this strategy earlier, especially for individuals with higher likelihood of developing hypothyroidism. Atypical (or second generation) antipsychotics can be used, but their use should be weighed against their metabolic, extrapyramidal, cardiac and other side effects, especially because patients with ID may have subtle cardiac anomalies and conduction defects. Adjuvant drug therapies used in the general population, such as two antidepressants, lithium, thyroid hormone and buspirone, as outlined in the STAR*D trials (Rush *et al.*, 2006; Trivedi *et al.*, 2006; Nierenberg *et al.*, 2006) and the American Psychiatric Association Practice Guidelines (2010) provide some guidance in treating resistant depression in patients with ID as well.

Electroconvulsive therapy (ECT) also is an effective treatment for major depressive disorder (American Psychiatric Association, 2010), and it should not be ignored as an option for a person suffering from depression simply because they have ID. The literature on ECT spanning the last four decades is limited primarily to reviews, case reports and series. The consistent finding is that ECT is an effective treatment for treating some psychiatric illnesses in people with ID (Reinblatt *et al.*, 2004; Friedlander & Solomons 2002; Aziz *et al.*, 2001). Reinblatt's group (2004) noted that symptoms often not associated with ECT responsiveness such as hyperactivity and irritability, improve in patients with ID experiencing treatment-resistant mood and psychotic disorders. Unfortunately, Little *et al.* (2002) described significant delays in the choice of ECT for people with ID who have psychiatric illness.

Chapter 15 discusses legal issues for treatment providers and evaluators, and may provide some guidance when considering ECT treatment for persons with ID.

Clinical Vignette #1

Mr. C. is a 27 year old Hispanic male with Down syndrome. He had been successfully attending a vocational setting since his completion of school at age 22. About six months earlier, an older male peer, whom he worked beside and socialized with outside of work, retired. A younger female, Ms. A., replaced him at the next workstation.

Initially, Mr. C. seemed to adapt to the change quite well. In December, other staff began to hear from Ms. A, her family and others that Mr. C. had been frequently talking about asking Ms. A to the annual Valentine's Day dance. However, Ms. A. was not interested in a romantic relationship with Mr. C., and her family also discouraged his interest.

In January, when everyone returned from the holidays, a team meeting was held in which Mr. C. was asked about this behavior. He confirmed that he would like Ms. A. to accompany him to the dance, and he reported saving his money in order to go to dinner before the dance. He was upset that his peers had not kept his confidence about his intentions, but he attributed this to their jealousy. He noted that Ms. A. had invited him to attend a holiday concert prior to the New Year, and he took this as evidence of their special relationship. The team informed Mr. C. that he and Ms. A. had a work relationship only, and that he needed to end his plans.

While Mr. C. verbalized an understanding of these roles and guidelines, over the next couple of weeks he persisted in asking if Ms. A. would eat lunch and take breaks with him. He also began bringing in small gifts, such as candy. As a result, Mr. C. was reassigned to a different room. The job to which he was assigned was much less challenging, and additionally was less lucrative, as it was a slower part of the shop.

Over the next month, he became much more withdrawn, joked less with staff and peers, was at times short-tempered at work, and episodically appeared to abruptly run to the men's room.

At home, his mother reported that she was having increased problems getting him up and ready for work in the morning, noted that he seldom ate breakfast any more (cereal had been a favorite food), picked at his dinner and was sometimes bringing home his lunch half-eaten. She also noted that at night she sometimes heard him awaken and he seemed to be crying at times. However, he would not comment on his feelings to her.

During psychiatric evaluation, Mr. C. had difficulty in describing his feelings, but he did admit that he no longer felt he was a good worker. He also viewed the relationship with his female co-worker as something that had been interfered with by others. He believed that she was in love with him and that they would be in a romantic relationship, were it not for the actions of others. He seemed angry and defiant regarding this issue. It was only when he was asked about his retired friend that he took on a more depressed appearance, cried and admitted feeling sad and missing him. He did not show any psychotic symptoms and, while he was clearly irritated at not being able to pursue his female co-worker, he made no threats to harm others or himself.

Mr. C. was diagnosed with major depressive disorder. Treatment options, including psychotherapy and antidepressant medications, were presented to Mr. C. and his mother. Both were reluctant to have him start on a medication (this seemed at least in part due to mother's view that the patient's father had "never been the same" after he was treated with medication for what seemed to have been a depressive illness). They did, however, agree to counseling, so psychotherapy was initiated on a weekly basis.

Additionally, routine labs, including complete blood count with differential, complete metabolic panel, lipid panel and thyroid function (TSH) were obtained. Mr. C did have a slight elevation in TSH, and he was referred to his primary care physician for treatment.

After about six weeks, the psychotherapist reported that, while Mr. C. faithfully attended the sessions, he seemed to do little but ruminate about the unrequited relationship. He had also begun to miss about two days of work a week. There was little improvement in his neurovegetative symptoms. At the next psychiatric appointment, Mr. C. was again offered, and this time accepted, antidepressant therapy. Sertraline was initiated at 50 mg daily.

After a month, Mr. C. was showing some improvement in his work performance and was sleeping and eating better, but he still seemed to decline activities he enjoyed and he made negative comments about himself. Similarly, his psychotherapist reported some improvement in his ability to process the work problems, but felt he still seemed pessimistic and expressed feelings of guilt and poor self-esteem. Sertraline was titrated to 100 mg daily and he continued in psychotherapy.

After three months, Mr. C. seemed to be back to his usual self. However, he still remained somewhat dissatisfied with his assignment at work. Plans were made that if Mr. C.'s work performance remained high over the next three months, consideration would be given to returning him to his old job – but with less proximity to Ms. A.'s station.

This vignette illustrates the interactions between Mr. C.'s environment (rejection and loss experiences), his biological vulnerability and comorbid medical illness, which can contribute to affective instability. For successful treatment all of these contributors needed to be addressed.

Clinical Vignette #2

Mr. R. is a 55 year old male with intellectual disability and diabetes, with neuropathic pain and chronic back pain from an old injury from a car accident 20 years ago. Over the previous year, he had increased the frequency with which he went to his family physician. Indeed, sometimes, if more than two weeks had elapsed, he would complain of increasing pain and demand that the physician be called.

On some of these occasions, despite the physician instructing him to come to the office the next morning to be evaluated, he would escalate his demands and complaints, resulting in the last three months in near-weekly trips to the emergency room. In addition to his pain complaints, when the patient became upset he would also report shortness of breath, palpitations, and dizziness.

Interview with Mr. R. revealed that his sister, his main family support, had opted for early retirement about a year before, and she was planning to move to Florida before the next winter. Medical staff noted that sometimes he would also ask that his sister be called during his times of increased pain and anxiety symptoms. They were also concerned that Mr. R. was becoming increasing aggressive toward both staff and himself when his demands were not met. He would sometimes throw items at them, bite himself, or slap himself on the head.

During the evaluation, staff noted Mr. R. wanted to sleep from the moment he got home. He refused weekend outings and was no longer interested in his favorite movies. He was up briefly for dinner, and they were having more problems getting him to adhere to his diabetic diet. In addition, he would frequently bring food home from work and eat voraciously but secretly. His old injuries were evaluated radiographically, and no acute changes were noted. However, his inactivity and increased appetite were leading to increased weight gain, worsening the control of his pain and diabetes.

Mr. R. was diagnosed with depression. His family physician had previously prescribed sequentially fluoxetine and citalopram, but he had refused antidepressant medication in the last month, demanding something for pain and his nerves. He declined counseling. He did agree to try another antidepressant. Duloxetine was initiated and titrated, resulting in resolution of symptoms of depression, anxiety and aggression, and improvement in his pain.

Bipolar disorder in ID

Prevalence and predisposing factors

The incidence of bipolar disorder (BD) in the ID population can be difficult to determine, because prevalence estimates vary, depending on the population studied and the criteria used to make the diagnosis. As with young children, it can be difficult to determine the internal mood state of adults with ID.

In a review of the literature of the prevalence of psychiatric disorders in individuals with ID, the diagnosis of BD was rarely identified as a category (Whitaker & Reed, 2006). In ten childhood studies, the diagnosis of BD was not identified. In 14 adult studies, the diagnostic category of BD or mania was found in only three studies. One study found rates of mania in elderly adults with ID of 0.7%, while young adults with ID had no mania (Cooper, 1997). Corbett *et al.* (1979) identified BD in 2.2% of an ID population over 15 years old. Another, more recent, study found the incidence of BD to be 0% when ICD-10 criteria were applied, but they did find that 2.2% of the population had BD when a shorter screening method was used (Deb *et al.*, 2001).

The review found that a number of studies used the indistinct category of "behavioral problems," which elevated the overall rates of psychiatric illness (Whitaker & Read, 2006). It is unclear if behavioral problems represent individuals who have a true psychiatric disorder (possibly BD) or problems that can be a focus of intervention, which should not be considered true psychiatric illness.

As cognitive deficits become more severe, individuals are less able to verbalize symptoms of racing thoughts, euphoria or grandiosity. Some have noticed that it is easier to make the diagnosis with higher levels of ID, because symptoms of mania are observed by others as being less typical of the individual's baseline behavior. In a chart review of 300 patients, evenly divided between mild, moderate/severe and profound ID, the authors compared the incidence of psychiatric disorders in this sample with 100 adults from a clinic population who did not have ID (Hurley *et al.*, 2003). They found that BD was more likely to be diagnosed in persons with ID, and was more likely to be diagnosed in moderate to profound ID than in those with mild ID. Those with more severe ID were likely to have caregivers who monitored their behavior and recognized the excessive motor activity and decreased need for sleep characteristic of mania. Since the study reviewed a clinical sample, higher overall rates of BD would be expected. BD was seen in 16% of the non-ID population and 29.5% of the ID population in this study (Hurley *et al.*, 2003).

A more extensive, population-based study of 1,023 individuals with ID was conducted by Cooper *et al.* (2007). In their study, the diagnosis was made by a psychiatrist with ID expertise, utilizing a clinical interview, a review of case notes and completion of two standardized rating scales. The Vineland Scale (survey form) and results of previous IQ tests were used to determine the level of intellectual ability (Sparrow *et al.*, 1984).

The Present Psychiatric State for Adults with Learning Disabilities (PPS-LD) is a semi-structured psychopathology schedule designed for use with adults with ID. It allows for clinical classification by Diagnostic Criteria-Learning Disorders, ICD-10-DCR and DSM-IV TR criteria (Moss, 1998). The PPS-LD and a clinical interview with a psychiatrist were used, along with other information, to establish a diagnosis. In this study, BD was found to have a point prevalence of 2.5% of the population (Cooper, 2007). Among individuals with BD, 0.5% were categorized as having a bipolar depressive episode, 0.6% having a manic episode, 1.2% with bipolar disorder with euthymia at the time of assessment, and 0.3% had cyclothymic disorder.

This more rigorous study found the incidence of BD in individuals with ID to be slightly higher than that described in DSM-IV-TR in the general population, which lists the lifetime prevalence of bipolar disorder I in community samples as 0.4–1.6% (APA, 2000).

A recent study of the worldwide prevalence of BD found that the overall prevalence of bipolar spectrum disorders was 2.4%. The prevalence of bipolar disorder I was 0.6%, bipolar disorder II was 0.4% and subthreshold bipolar disorder was 1.4% (Merikangas *et al.*, 2011). Although the Merikangas study did not report the comorbidity of ID and BD, it appears that the incidence of BD in the ID population is similar to that in the general population when rigorous examination is conducted.

Diagnosis of bipolar disorder in persons with ID

When evaluating an individual with ID for BD, it is important to understand the unique issues regarding this specialized population. Foremost are communication deficits; depending on developmental level, individuals are most likely unable to read or fill out standard rating instruments. They may be unable to communicate verbally to some varying degree. It is also critical to rely on caregivers for observations of an individual's activity level and mood states if they are unable to communicate well.

The DM-ID describes several adaptations of DSM-IV-TR criteria for use in the ID population (Charlot *et al.*, 2007). When diagnosing mania, no adaptation for the criteria of a seven-day period of elevated, expansive or irritable mood is suggested; however, it is noted that observers may report loud, inappropriate laughing or singing, excessive giddiness or silliness, intrusiveness or getting into another's space, and excessive smiling or laughing which is not appropriate to the social context. According to the DSM-IV-TR (2000) criteria, three or more (of seven) mood symptoms must be present to meet manic criteria, or four symptoms if the mood is only irritable. The DM-ID authors suggest that for individuals with limited expressive language skills, the period of mood disturbance needs only two mood symptoms (or three if the primary mood is irritable) to meet the criteria.

The DM-ID gives several examples of how manic symptoms would appear in patients with ID, and these examples are helpful for clinicians not familiar with this population.

- For the symptom of inflated self-esteem or grandiosity, no adaption is necessary, but the authors note that common observations are claims of a skill the patient does not have (e.g. driving) or exaggerating social events (e.g. getting married when they are not in a relationship, or claims of a relationship with a famous person).

- For the symptoms of decreased need for sleep, no adaptation is suggested, but it is important to recognize that the sleep change is a departure from an individual's baseline, and that they do not sleep during the day or have a roommate making noise which keeps them up at night.

- For the more talkative than usual (or pressure to keep talking) criteria, no adaptation is needed. Common symptoms seen in the ID population reported by observers include increases over baseline in screaming, noise-making, vocalizing or talking. Rapid speech can occur, as in repetitive questions, decreased ability to listen, frequent interruptions, increased perseveration, engaging in frequent monologues or singing loudly.

- For the symptoms of flight of ideas or subjective experience that thoughts are racing, no adaptation is needed. Observers can report that individuals with ID jump rapidly from topic to topic, and the DM-ID authors note that it is important to establish that this is a change from an individual's baseline.

- For the symptom of distractibility, no adaptation is needed. The DM-ID authors suggest that this can be seen in individuals with ID as a reduced productivity at workshop, diminished self-care skills and an inability to complete tasks previously mastered. It is noted that concentration difficulty or inability to complete tasks represents a change from baseline, and that the latter is secondary to distractibility.

- For the symptoms of increased goal-directed activity, no adaptation is needed. The DM-ID authors suggest that it is frequently reported by observers that an individual with ID will engage in activities with a "sped up" manner, have difficulty sitting down, will walk rapidly, pace, become very intrusive or are significantly more physically active than their usual behavior.

- For the symptoms of increased involvement in pleasurable activities that have a potential for painful consequences, no adaptation is needed. Observers may report that individuals with ID engage in more sexual behavior or talk, may masturbate more frequently, may expose themselves in public and/or touch others in a sexual manner.

- For the DSM-IV-TR criterion which requires marked impairment in occupational or social functioning, the DM-ID authors note that residential or vocational program placement can be lost when an individual has an acute mood episode.

The DM-ID authors also note that it is important to screen for physical problems that may cause pain, which can secondarily impact attention and sleep, and may cause agitation which can appear to be a manic episode. This is especially important in individuals with severe/profound ID, who have more significantly limited expressive language skills and cannot report the source of physical distress. It is also advised that added caution is necessary in patients who are prescribed selective serotonin reuptake inhibitors (SSRIs); this medication class may cause manic-like symptoms (such as agitation) that may appear to be related to BD when in fact this may not represent a true diagnosis (Charlot *et al.*, 2007).

When making a diagnosis of hypomania, DSM-IV-TR requires a period of elevated, expansive or irritable mood lasting throughout four days that is different from the usual non-depressed mood (American Psychiatric Association, 2000). As with mania, the authors of DM-ID suggest that, during the period of mood disturbance, only two (instead of three) symptoms are required to meet criteria for individuals with limited expressive skills (Charlot *et al.*, 2007). When the primary mood is irritable, they recommend that hypomania be diagnosed if three symptoms, instead of four, are present. For the diagnosis of other bipolar spectrum disorders, cyclothymia, bipolar disorder II, and bipolar disorder NOS, the DM-ID authors do not recommend any additional diagnostic modifications.

As has occurred with the diagnosis of BD in children, when there is significant behavior disturbance and chronic, nonepisodic affect and behavior dysregulation that does not meet DSM-IV duration criteria, a diagnosis of Bipolar Disorder NOS is given (Leibenluft & Rich, 2008). It is likely that clinicians treating individuals with ID are using the diagnosis of bipolar disorder NOS when significant irritability and mood disturbance occurs, but full DSM-IV-TR or DM-ID criteria are not met, if symptoms cause significant impairment and disturbance in function that treatment is warranted.

When making the diagnosis, clinicians must rely on clinical interview with the patient, in addition to collateral data from reliable sources, especially in individuals with more severe cognitive impairment. Ideally, caregivers who participate in the mental health evaluation should have knowledge of an individual's baseline, as well as how their current symptomatology contrasts to the baseline functioning, as this will be vital in the clinician's ability to make a diagnosis. Detailed guidelines for addressing the issues related to assessment of individuals with ID are described in Chapter 2.

Clinical Vignette #3

Part 1   JR is a 45 year old single white male with moderate ID and a variety of psychiatric diagnoses, characterized by mood disorder NOS and obsessive compulsive disorder. Caregivers and family gave a history of previously agitated behaviors, but were unable to describe any psychosis or clear manic symptomatology. He has been under the care of a psychiatrist, which began subsequent to a hospitalization due to seizure activity.

This was the patient's first seizure, and it occurred following an episode of excessive water intake by the patient. JR lives in a group home and is well known to his caretakers and staff. He had been frequently known to drink water to the point of intoxication when stressed, and his behavior plan allowed his staff to limit the amount of water he consumed. During his medical hospitalization, all of his psychotropic medications were discontinued by a hospitalist, including: carbamazepine (Tegretol) 200 mg at bedtime, lithium carbonate (Lithium) 300 mg daily, haloperidol (Haldol) 4 mg at bedtime, risperidone (Risperdal) 3 mg twice daily, thioridazine (Mellaril) 150 mg at bedtime, sertraline (Zoloft) 50 mg daily, ramelteon (Rozerem) 8 mg at bedtime. He had been prescribed essentially the same medication regimen for many years.

He was started on divalproex sodium (Depakote) for seizures and was discharged home after a short stay. Upon returning to his group home, his staff noticed behaviors that they had not ever previously seen in JR. He would pace excessively – so much so that he began to wear a hole in the carpet in his room. He was also agitated when staff would attempt to redirect him, and he continued to drink large amounts of water. In the days that followed, he was noted to have multiple days of hyperactivity, elevated mood, giggling, and agitation. He was sleeping a maximum of three hours at night. This would alternate with periods where he would sleep during the day and be up at night for several days without his elevated mood.

The case outlined in part 1 of Clinical Vignette #3 illustrates some of the diagnostic difficulties with individuals with ID; prior history does not give a clear diagnosis of BD or schizophrenia. The patient's previous medications included two mood stabilizers, three antipsychotics, an antidepressant and a sedative hypnotic. Presumably he was being treated for a bipolar illness, but his history makes the diagnosis unclear. As his behavior was monitored carefully, with divalproex sodium as his primary and exclusive psychotropic medication, it appears more likely that he had a form of BD. His behaviors did not meet the full criteria for mania, but it is likely that the divalproex sodium prescribed helped to prevent a manic episode. His current working diagnosis is bipolar disorder NOS.

Clinical Vignette #3 (continued)

Part 2 Given his significant change in mental status and decline in functioning, JR's previous medications were gradually restarted. He was prescribed risperidone (risperdal) and an increased dose of valproic acid initially. However, his agitated mood and episodic sleep disturbance continued and it was decided to restart a typical (first generation) antipsychotic. Fluphenazine (prolixin) was chosen in place of thioridazine (Mellaril) to avoid cardiac conduction abnormalities.

His symptoms improved and he returned to his previous baseline functioning. Laboratory evaluation eventually revealed that his AST and ALT were mildly elevated at 75 and 70. After consultation with his primary care physician, it was decided that his seizure was likely due to water intoxication and hyponatremia, and his divalproex sodium was gradually tapered without any worsening of his behavior. He has remained seizure-free for several years and, on his current medications, has been free of sleep disturbance, excessive giddiness, agitation or increased physical activity.

Treatment

When an individual with ID is diagnosed with BD, there is little research in the ID population available to guide treatment decisions, so clinicians are often left to utilize research for the general adult population. A Cochrane Collaborative review of antipsychotic medication for behavior problems in the ID population concluded that of 71 citations, only nine were relevant, and that they provided little evidence that antipsychotic medication helps or harms adults with learning disability and challenging behaviors (Brylewski & Duggan, 2004). To address the lack of research data, Expert Consensus Guidelines for the treatment of psychiatric and behavioral problems in individuals with ID were created and updated in 2004 (Aman *et al.*, 2004).

As with the general population, medications are necessary for the treatment of BD.

- For the manic episode of bipolar disorder I with classic euphoric mania, the consensus guidelines recommend divalproex or lithium alone, or combined with newer, atypical antipsychotic medications.

- When an individual with ID has mixed/dysphoric or rapid cycling mania, divalproex alone or combined with newer antipsychotic is recommended.

- For individuals with bipolar disorder II, in a hypomanic episode divalproex or lithium is preferred.

- For individuals with BD having a non-psychotic depression, lithium and/or lamotrigine; lithium + antidepressant, or divalproex + antidepressant or lamotrigine is recommended.

- When an individual has BD and a psychotic depressive episode, medications recommended are second generation (atypical) antipsychotic + mood stabilizer (i.e. lithium, divalproex or lamotrigine) + antidepressant (Aman, 2004).

It is useful to keep in mind that all the second generation antipsychotics, (i.e. risperidone, olanzapine, quetiapine, aripiprazole and ziprasidone) are approved by the Food and Drug Administration for the treatment of mania in BD.

In our review of the medication treatment literature, more articles describe the use of medications for behavioral problems or "problem behaviors" in ID rather than for use in the diagnosis of BD. Deb *et al.* (2008) reviewed the use of mood stabilizers and antiepileptic drugs for the management of behavior problems; they found three studies which showed some benefit for use of lithium, and four which showed benefit from different antiepileptic medications – topiramate (Topomax), valproate (Depakote) (two studies), and carbamazepine (Tegretol). It is important to realize that these studies did not examine individuals with a diagnosis of BD, but rather behavior problems described as aggression, hyperactivity and destructive behavior.

A similar review of antipsychotic medication for treatment of behavior problems with individuals with ID concluded that there were randomized controlled trials showing efficacy of risperidone (Risperdal) for adults and children, as well as evidence for the efficacy of other atypical (second generation) antipsychotics in non-controlled case studies (Deb *et al.*, 2007). An open trial of valproic acid (Depakote) in the treatment of affective symptoms found that 14 of 21 positively responded to treatment for two years. It was reported that individuals with ID with possible epilepsy were more likely to have a favorable response, as their behavioral cycling may have responded to anticonvulsant treatment (Kastner *et al.*, 1993).

In a review of 14 studies of rapid cycling BD in the ID population, Vanstraelen & Tyrer (1999) found several case reports which used mood stabilizers. Their analysis showed a poor treatment response overall in this population. Lithium was beneficial in nine of 25 patients, only three out of 15 patients treated with carbamazepine (Tegretol) improved and three of six patients showed improvement with sodium valproate (Depakote). The few patients treated with a combination of mood stabilizers also had poor response (Vanstraelen & Tyrer, 1999).

In a pilot study Verhoeven & Tuiner (2001) treated 28 individuals with ID presenting with rapid mood fluctuations with valproic acid (Depakote). They noted that the subjects did not have symptoms of hypomania or major depression, so could not be diagnosed with BD, but all had history of episodic changes in mood and behavior. Subjects were started on valproic acid (Depakote) and titrated to a level between 60 and 80 mg/l for up to one year. After taking valproic acid for 12, weeks their previous psychotropic medications (primarily antipsychotics) were discontinued without any significant change in response. The authors found that 19 of 28 showed moderate to marked improvement in the Clinical Global Improvement Scale (Verhoeven & Tuiner, 2001).

Carta *et al.* (2001) studied the use of adjunctive gabapentin (Neurontin) in the treatment of individuals with ID with bipolar spectrum disorders. They identified ten individuals in a residential rehabilitation center – six with a diagnosis of BD and four with schizoaffective disorder. They selected individuals who had a clinical history of two or more episodic declines in response to the same predictable life event, such as birthday, Christmas holiday or advancement of the work program.

All of the individuals were on psychotropic medications as follows: risperidone (Risperdal) ($n = 2$), haloperidol (Haldol) ($n = 7$), clozapine (Clozaril) ($n = 1$), paroxetine (Paxil) ($n = 2$), carbamazepine (Tegretol) ($n = 2$), phenobarbital ($n = 1$) and benzodiazepines ($n = 7$). They were observed before and after their critical life event, and then adjunctive therapy with gabapentin at doses from 600 to 900 mg/daily was initiated. The subjects were observed until the next critical event and reassessed. The authors reported that with gabapentin treatment, subjects lost 6.6% of their rehabilitation days during the stressful event, whereas previously they had lost 31.6%. Their psychopathology scores were also improved during the stressful event time, when they were treated with gabapentin. Symptoms which improved included physical aggressiveness, destructiveness, screaming or other noises, temper tantrums, verbal abuse, overactivity, wandering, running away and attention- seeking. This study suggests that gabapentin may have a role in the adjunctive treatment of individuals with ID and co-occurring BD.

Given the lack of research on pharmacologic treatments in BD for individuals with ID, clinicians are advised to use their clinical judgment and to continue to use evidence-based principles that have proven effective in the general population. With the ID population, it is important to consider some of their unique treatment issues. They may have difficulty swallowing pills, so therefore liquid medication, transdermal, injectable or dissolvable formulations may be needed. In some instances, higher-functioning individuals may not have caregivers available to ensure medication administration, so long-acting depot medications may be necessary. In other instances, individuals have caregivers present all the time and are actually better able to follow complicated medication regimens than the general population.

It is also important to be vigilant that individuals with ID may be sexually active, so attention to the possibility of birth defects with use of valproic acid or lithium in females of child-bearing age is imperative. In addition to medications, psychosocial treatment inter-ventions should be recommended and instituted in all comprehensive treatment plans. Those with higher cognitive levels may benefit from psychotherapy, as described in Chapter 13. It is important to educate caregivers on the nature of BD, and to assist the individual with ID with sleep hygiene practices in order to avoid sleep disturbance and unnecessary stressors which can contribute to the destabilization of their mood.

Clinical Vignette #4

AB is a 34 year old male with mild ID seen for psychiatric evaluation. He was diagnosed with cerebral palsy at two years old. His mother has bipolar disorder and, after his parents' divorce in AB's infancy, he went to live with his father and stepmother until he was 14 years old, when he was aggressive towards his stepbrother. He subsequently went to live with his mother, but he became depressed shortly thereafter and had his first psychiatric hospitalization following a suicide attempt. He was started on an antidepressant.

He was eventually placed in a therapeutic foster home. Two years later, however, he had difficulty in this placement, exhibiting aggression toward his foster parents and developing decreased sleep. He was found masturbating in the front lawn of his neighbor's house. At 18 years old, he was placed in a group home.

He was brought in for mental health evaluation after spending the past 16 years in his current home. His father was still involved, but his mother had been placed in a nursing home due to her mental illness and deteriorating medical health. AB's caregivers reported that he had a diagnosis of bipolar disorder and had a pattern of severe manic behavior, which occurred every 4–6 years despite his being maintained on mood-stabilizing medications.

His most recent episode had just ended and had lasted 4–5 months. During this period, he had become excessively religious and would shower three times a day so that he could 'be saved.' He would attempt to put water in his penis to clean it. He also believed that a prominent female pop star was his girlfriend, and he would talk about her and plans that they made together. Before the most recent episode occurred, staff noted that he became giddier, overly friendly and had an increase in masturbation. He would masturbate to such an extent that he required treatment for penile injuries.

His current medications, as prescribed by the previous psychiatrist, included lithium carbonate (Lithium) 300 mg twice daily, carbamazepine (Tegretol) 400 mg twice daily, divalproex sodium (Depakote) 500 mg twice daily, risperidone (Risperdal) 3 mg at bedtime, quietapine (Seroquel) 200 twice daily and venlafaxine (Effexor) XR 75 mg once daily. Staff reported that he was doing fairly well. However, the venlafaxine, which had been stopped by his previous psychiatrist during a manic episode, was inadvertently restarted. It was discontinued when the medication error was discovered, to avoid induction of mania. Laboratory values were checked and his depakote serum level was 55, tegretol serum level was 8 and lithium level was 1.0.

He did well for six months, then staff observed an increase in giddiness and he became infatuated with a movie star, who he believed was his girlfriend. His divalproex sodium was increased to 1,500 mg total/day and his depakote serum level increased to 80 and his mood improved. He continued to do well until he developed medical complications, which resulted in cervical cord compression, and he experienced a decrease in ability to ambulate without assistance. He underwent surgery and made significant progress with physical therapy without any alteration in his mood. His lithium was decreased by his primary care physician, but he began to get giddy and again became fixated with a movie star. His level was 0.4; it was increased to the previous dosage and his symptoms improved.

Clinical Vignette #4 describes a young man with classic manic symptoms, which were easy for his caregivers to identify. Unfortunately, his mania was difficult to control, requiring three mood stabilizers and two antipsychotic medications. While most patients with BD do not require inter-class or intra-class polypharmacy, it is occasionally necessary to control residual symptoms in intractable mental illness in a minority of patients.

Conclusions

In this chapter, we have described the symptoms of affective illness in individuals with ID and have reviewed the available treatment literature. It is important to be aware to monitor individuals with ID for mood disturbance, as it can be a significant source of impairment and is often responsive to treatment. Hopefully, more rigorous studies into effective treatments in this population will be conducted and will lead to a better understanding of affective disorders and treatment options.

References

Akiskal, H.S., Hirschfeld, R.M.A. & Yerevanian, B.I. (1983). The relationship of personality to affective disorders. A critical review. *Archives of General Psychiatry* **40**, 801–810.

Aman, M.G., Crismon, M.L., Frances, A., King, B.H. & Rojahn, J. (eds.) (2004). *Treatment of psychiatric and behavior problems in individuals with mental retardation: an update of the expert consensus guidelines for mental retardation and developmental disability populations*. Postgraduate Institute for Medicine, Englewood, CO.

American Psychiatric Association (2000). *Diagnostic and Statistical Manual of Mental Disorders*, 4th ed, Text Revision. American Psychiatric Association, Washington, DC.

American Psychiatric Association (2010). *Practice Guidelines for the Treatment of Patients with Major Depressive Disorder*, 3rd edition. *American Journal of Psychiatry* **167**(10) (supplement).

Antonacci, D.J. & Attiah, N. (2008). Diagnosis and treatment of mood disorders in adults with developmental disabilities. *Psychiatric Quarterly* **79**, 171–192.

Antonacci, D.J., Manuel, C. & Davis, E. (2008). Diagnosis and treatment of aggression in individuals with developmental disabilities. *Psychiatric Quarterly* **79**, 225–247.

Aziz, M., Maixner, D.F., DeQuardo, J., Aldridge, A. & Tandon, R. (2001). ECT and mental retardation: A review and case reports. *Journal of ECT* **17**(2), 149–152.

Ball, S.L., Holland, A.J., Treppner, P., Watson, P.C. & Huppert, F.A. (2008). Executive dysfunction and its association with personality and behavior changes in the development of Alzheimer's disease in adults with Down syndrome and mild to moderate learning disabilities. *British Journal of Clinical Psychology* **47**, 1–29.

Beck, A.T. (1976). *Cognitive Therapy and the Emotional Disorders*. International Universities Press, New York.

Brylewski, J. & Duggan, L. (2004). Antipsychotic medication for challenging behavior in people with learning disability. *Cochrane Database of Systematic Reviews* **2004**(3), CD000377.

Carta, M.G., Hardoy, M.C., Dessi, I., Hardoy, M.J. & Carpiniello, B. (2001). Adjunctive gabapentin in patients with intellectual disability and bipolar spectrum disorders. *Journal of Intellectual Disability Research* **45**, 139–145.

Charlot, L., Fox, S., Silka, V.R., Hurley, A., Lowry, M. & Pary, R. (2007). Mood Disorders. In: Fletcher, R., Loschen, E., Stavrakalaki, C. & Fist, M. (eds.) *Diagnostic Manual –Intellectual Disability (DM-ID): A textbook of Diagnosis of Mental Disorders in Persons with Intellectual Disability*, pp. 272–316. NADD Press, Kingston, NY.

Cooper, S.A. (1997). Psychiatry of elderly compared to younger adults with intellectual disabilities. *Journal of Applied Research in Intellectual Disabilities* **10**, 303–311.

Cooper, S.A., Smiley, E., Morrison, J., Williamson, A. & Allan, L. (2007). An epidemiological investigation of affective disorders with a population-based cohort of 1023 adults with intellectual disabilities. *Psychological Medicine* **37**, 873–82.

Corbett, J.A. (1979). Psychiatric morbidity and mental retardation. In: Games, F.E. & Snaith, R.P. (eds.) *Psychiatric Illness and Mental Handicap*, pp. 11–25. Gaskill Press, London.

Deb, S., Thomas, M. & Bright, C. (2001). Mental disorder in adults with intellectual disability. 1: Prevalence of functional psychiatric illness amount a community based sample population between 16 and 64 years. *Journal of Intellectual Disability Research* **45**, 495–667.

Deb, S., Sohanpal, S.K., Soni, R. Unwin, G. & Lenôtre, L. (2007). The effectiveness of antipsychotic medication in the management of behaviour problems in adults with intellectual disabilities. *Journal of Intellectual Disability Research* **51**, 766–777.

Deb, S., Chaplin, S., Sohanpal, G., Unwin, G. Soni, R. & Lenôtre, L. (2008). The effectiveness of mood stabilizers and antiepileptic medication for the management of behavior problems in adults with intellectual disability: a systematic review. *Journal of Intellectual Disability Research* **52**, 107–113.

Decoulfle, P. & Autry, A. (2002). Increased mortality in children and adolescents with developmental disabilities. *Paediatric and Perinatal Epidemiology, 16*, 375–382.

Esbensen, A.J. & Benson, B.A. (2007). An evaluation of Beck's cognitive theory of depression in adults with intellectual disability. *Journal of Intellectual Disability Research 51*(P1) 14–24.

Fletcher, R., Loschen, E., Stavrakalaki, C. & Fist, M. (eds.) (2007). *Diagnostic Manual–Intellectual Disability (DM-ID): A textbook of Diagnosis of Mental Disorders in Persons with Intellectual Disability.* NADD Press, Kingston, NY.

Friedlander, R.I. & Solomons, K. (2002). ECT: use in individuals with mental retardation. *Journal of ECT 18*(1), 38–42.

Hartley, S.L., Lickel, A.H. & MacLean, W.E. Jr., (2008). Reassurance seeking and depression in adults with mild intellectual disability. *Journal of Intellectual Disability Research 52*(11), 917–29.

Hartley, S.L. & MacLean, W.E. (2009). Depression in adults with mild intellectual disability: Role of stress, attributions and coping. *American Journal on Intellectual and Developmental Disabilities 114*(3), 147–160.

Hastings, R.P., Hatton, C., Taylor, J.L. & Maddison, C. (2004). Life events and psychiatric symptoms in adults with intellectual disabilities. *Journal of Intellectual Disability Research 48*(P1) 42–46.

Hirschfeld, R.M., Klerman, G.L., Clayton, P.J. & Keller, M.B. (1983). Personality and depression. *Archives of General Psychiatry 40*, 993–998.

Hirschfeld, R.M., Klerman, G.L., Andreasen, N.C., Clayton, P.J. & Keller, M.B. (1986). Psychosocial predictors of chronicity in depressed patients. *British Journal of Psychiatry 148*, 648–654.

Hirschfeld, R.M., Klerman, G.L., Lavori, P., Keller, M.B., Griffith, P. & Coryell, W. (1989). Premorbid personality assessments of first onset of major depression. *Archives of General Psychiatry 46*(4), 345–350.

Hurley, A.D. (2008). Depression in adults with intellectual disability: symptoms and challenging behavior. *Journal of Intellectual Disability Research 52*(11), 905–16.

Hurley, A.D., Folstein, M. & Lam, N. (2003). Patients with and without intellectual disability seeking outpatient psychiatric services: diagnoses and prescribing pattern. *Journal of Intellectual Disability Research 47*, 39–50.

Kastner, T., Finesmith, R. & Walsh, K. (1993). Long term administration of valproic acid in the treatment of affective symptoms in people with mental retardation. *Journal of Clinical Pschopharmacology 13*, 448–451.

Leibenluft, A. & Rich, B.A. (2008). Pediatric bipolar disorder. *Annual Review of Clinical Psychology 4*, 163–87.

Little, J.D., McFarland, J. & Ducharme, H.M. (2002). ECT use delayed in the presence of comorbid mental retardation: A review of clinical and ethical issues. *Journal of ECT 18*(4), 218–222.

Mann, D.M.A. & Esiri, M.M. (1989). The pattern of acquisition of plaques and tangles in Down's Syndrome patients under 50 years of age. *Journal of Neurological Science 89*, 169–179.

Merikangas, K.R., Jin, R., He, J-P., Kessler, R.C., Lee, S., Sampson, N.A., Viana, M.C., Andrade, L.H., Hu, C., Karam, E.G., Ladea, M., Medina Mora, M.E., Ono, Y., Posada-Villa, J., Sagar, R., Wells, J.E. & Zarkov, Z. (2011). Prevalence and correlates of bipolar spectrum disorder in the world mental health survey initiative. *Archives of General Psychiatry 68*, 241–251.

Moss, S., Prosser, H., Costello, H., Simpson, N., Patel, P., Rowe, S., Turner, S. & Hatton, C. (1998). Reliability and validity of the PAS-ADD checklist for detecting psychiatric disorders in adults with intellectual disability. *Journal of Intellectual Disability Research*, **42**, 173–183.

Nierenberg, A.A., Fava, M., Trivedi, M.H., Wisniewski, S.R., Thase, M.E., McGrath, P.J., Alpert, J.E., Warden, D., Luther, J.F., Niederehe, G., Lebowitz, B., Shores-Wilson, K. & Rush, A.J. (2006). A comparison of lithium and T(3) augmentation following two failed medication treatments for depression: a STAR*D report. *American Journal of Psychiatry* **163**(9), 1519–1530.

Reinblatt, S.P., Rifkin, A. & Freeman, J. (2004). The efficacy of ECT in adults with mental retardation experiencing psychiatric disorders. *Journal of ECT* **20**(4), 208–212.

Rush, A.J., Trivedi, M.H., Wisniewski, S.R., Stewart, J.W., Nierenberg, A.A., Thase, M.E., Ritz, L., Biggs, M.M., Warden, D., Luther, J.F., Shores-Wilson, K., Niederehe, G. & Fava, M. (2006). Bupropion-SR, sertraline or venlafaxine-XR after failure of SSRIs for depression. *New England Journal of Medicine* **354**(12), 1231–1242.

Singer, R.B. & Strauss, D. (1997). Comparative mortality in mentally retarded patients in California, with and without Down's syndrome, 1986–1991. *Journal of Insurance Medicine* **29**(3), 172–184.

Sovner, R. (1986). Limiting factors in using DSM-III criteria with mentally ill/mentally retarded persons. *Psychopharmacology Bulletin* **22**, 1055–1059.

Sovner, R. & Hurley, A.D. (1983). Do the mentally retarded suffer from affective illness? *Archives of General Psychiatry* **40**, 61–67.

Sparrow, S.S., Balla, D.A. & Cichetti, D.V. (1984). *The Vineland Adaptive Behavior Scales: A revision of the Vineland Social Maturity Scale by Edgar A. Doll*. American Guidance Service, Circle Pines, MD.

Spreat, S., Conroy, J. & Jones, J. (1997). Use of psychotropic medication in Oklahoma: a statewide survey. *American Journal of Mental Retardation* **102**, 80–85.

Strydom, A., Livingston, G., King, M. & Hassiotis, A. (2007). Prevalence of dementia in intellectual disability using different diagnostic criteria. *British Journal of Psychiatry* **191**, 150–157.

Trivedi, M.H., Fava, M., Wisniewski, S.R., Thase, M.E., Quitkin, F., Warden, D., Ritz, L., Nierenberg, A.A., Lebowitz, B.D., Biggs, M.M., Luther, J.F., Shores-Wilson, K. & Rush, A.J. (2006). Medication augmentation after the failure of SSRIs for depression. *New England Journal of Medicine* **354**(12), 1243–52.

Tyrer, F., Smith, L.K. & McGrother, C.W. (2007). Mortality in adults with moderate to profound intellectual disability: a population-based study. *Journal of Intellectual Disability Research* **51**, part 7 520–527.

Vanstraelen, M. & Tyrer, S.P. (1999). Rapid cycling bipolar affective disorder in people with intellectual disability: a systematic review. *Journal of Intellectual Disability Research* **43**, 349–359.

Verhoeven, W.M.A. & Tuiner, S. (2001). Cyclothymia or unstable mood disorder? A systematic treatment evaluation with valproic acid. *Journal of Applied Research in Intellectual Disabilities* **14**, 147–154.

Whitaker, S. & Read, S. (2006). The prevalence of psychiatric disorders among people with intellectual disabilities: an analysis of the literature. *Journal of Applied Research in Intellectual Disabilities* **19**, 330–345.

Wiersma, J.E., van Oppen, P., van Schaik, D.J., van der Does, A.J., Beekman, A.T. & Penninx, B.W. (2011). Psychological characteristics of chronic depression: a longitudinal cohort study. *Journal of Clinical Psychiatry* **72**(3), 288–294.

Zimmerman, M., Ruggero, C.J., Chelminski, I. & Young, D.J. (2008). Is bipolar disorder overdiagnosed? *Journal of Clinical Psychiatry* **69**(6), 935–94.

Zimmerman, M., Ruggero, C.J., Chelminski, I. & Young, D.J. (2010). Psychiatric diagnoses in patients previously overdiagnosed with bipolar disorder. *Journal of Clinical Psychiatry* **71**(1), 26–31.

8

Anxiety Disorders

Kelly M. Blankenship, MD, Assistant Professor of Psychiatry, Indiana University, Indianapolis, IN

Introduction

Anxiety is a common emotion that is experienced by every individual. Pathologic anxiety is also commonly experienced by many individuals. Individuals with intellectual disabilities (ID) are diagnosed with the same range of anxiety disorders as are individuals with typical cognitive abilities. However, there are many factors inherent in the assessment of persons with limited cognitive abilities that make diagnosis of an anxiety disorder difficult.

Anxiety causes increased arousal. It is produced by an amalgamation of biochemical changes within an individual in combination with the person's history, memories and social environment. Abnormal anxiety deviates from the typical anxiety experienced when there is a known threat, in that it is vague and triggered in response to a non-threatening situation. Individuals with ID can exhibit all types of anxiety disorders similar to persons with normal cognitive abilities. Cognitive and semantic difficulties in persons with ID can make the disorder more difficult to recognize (Fletcher, 2007).

Prevalence rates of anxiety disorders

Overall, mental disorders in individuals with ID are found at rates three to four times higher than the general population (Masi *et al.*, 2002). In cognitively intact individuals, anxiety ranks among the most prevalent mental health conditions (Cooray & Bakula, 2005). However, individuals with ID are considered to be at an even higher risk for anxiety (Masi *et al.*, 2002), as well as for depression.

Psychiatry of Intellectual Disability: A Practical Manual, First Edition.
Edited by Julie P. Gentile and Paulette M. Gillig.
© 2012 John Wiley & Sons, Ltd. Published 2012 by John Wiley & Sons, Ltd.

Most people who are experiencing high levels of anxiety center their thought processes on themes of danger, threats, unpredictability and uncertainty (Glenn *et al.*, 2003). Individuals with ID frequently are given little choice in decisions that are made for them, increasing the lack of predictability and uncertainty in their lives. Many of these decisions, such as housing, spending money, employment, leisure time, roommates and interactions with family are ones that cause significant anxiety, even in cognitively intact individuals. Individuals with ID often have fewer learned coping skills and are often given limited say in the decision-making process. Because of their limited ability to remove themselves from situations, they are also at high risk for abuse and/or neglect, which can also increase anxiety levels. Fragile self-esteem, fear of failing and loss of caregivers can also contribute to the high levels of anxiety found in this population (Szymanski & King, 1999).

Although limited, the available data suggest that anxiety disorders are under-diagnosed in the ID population (Gentile & Jackson, 2008). The prevalence of anxiety disorders has been recorded at extreme variations, depending on the diagnostic criteria utilized and the ID population studied. Prevalence rates have ranged from 0.63–57.3% in institutionalized populations, while other studies have recorded rates from 6–31% (Bailey & Andrews, 2003; Glenn *et al.*, 2003).

Complicating determination of the prevalence rate is the difficulty of diagnosing anxiety disorders in individuals with severe and profound ID. Matson *et al.* (1997) found that only "behavioral symptoms associated with anxiety could be reliably assessed" in that population. Another complicating factor is that anxiety and depression can present similarly in persons with ID, making it difficult to determine which symptoms should be attributed to which disorder (Glenn *et al.*, 2003). Some individuals with ID cannot communicate verbally, and those who can will often answer affirmatively regardless of the actual presence of symptoms (Hurley *et al.*, 2003; see also Chapter 6). Also, patients may have multiple medical or psychiatric disorders. For example, if a patient has significant anxiety but is also psychotic (Arnold, 1993), anxiety is sometimes misinterpreted as delusional paranoia.

Sometimes anxiety disorders are undiagnosed in persons with ID because of their limited ability to self-report anxiety or worry (Hurley *et al.*, 2003). Sources of information are frequently caregivers, family members, or staff who may or may not be familiar with the individual and that person's behavior.

"Diagnostic overshadowing," where clinicians accept psychiatric symptoms as normal behavior in those with ID, may also interfere with accurate psychiatric diagnosis of anxiety and other disorders (Vitiello & Behar, 1992); see also Chapters 2 and 6. Finally, many patients with ID are receiving psychotropic medications that can modify the presentation of anxiety symptoms through the drugs' sedating effects (Fletcher, 2007).

The Diagnostic and Statistical Manual of Mental Disorders – IV Text Revision (DSM-IV-TR), the *Diagnostic Manual – Intellectual Disability* (DM-ID), and the *Diagnostic Criteria for Psychiatric Disorders for Use with Adults with Learning Disabilities* (DC-LD) are resources, among others (e.g. the *International Classification of Diseases*) for making psychiatric diagnoses. Although there is consensus that anxiety disorders in those with ID exists, it is difficult to apply DSM-IV criteria to the ID population. It has been suggested that if the DSM-IV criteria were applied rigidly to the ID population, those with severe or profound ID would be exempt from many types of anxiety diagnoses.

The DM-ID suggests modifying the DSM-IV criteria to be more appropriate for the individual's developmental, cognitive and emotional level (Fletcher, 2007). The DM-ID provides a "framework" by which the DSM-IV criteria can be modified to allow diagnoses of the different categories of anxiety disorders. The DSM-IV discusses the importance of utilizing clinical judgment when making diagnosis, and to use diagnostic criteria as "guidelines" for which to form diagnoses (DSM-IV, Work Group, 1994). The DM-ID suggests that the criteria for anxiety disorders can be used for mild to moderate ID, but that there is limited data suggesting the use for it in those with severe ID, and no data to suggest its validity in those with profound ID (Fletcher, 2007).

The DM-ID includes some helpful hints that can be used for diagnosis when timelines are important. For example, in individuals with mild to moderate ID who have difficulties with the concept of temporal sequencing, it would be helpful to identify important dates (e.g. birthdays or trips) and have the individual describe the timing around that date (i.e. before or after – see Chapter 6).

The *Diagnostic Criteria for Psychiatric Disorders for Use with Adults with Learning Disabilities* (*DC-LD*: Royal College of Psychiatrists, 2001) suggested removing complex conceptual frameworks such as "depersonalization/derealization" and replacing them with "increased irritability and restlessness" (Bailey & Andrews, 2003).

Presentation of anxiety disorders in the ID population

Typically, hearing a person's subjective complaint of "anxiety" or "worry" is used by the clinician to aid in the diagnosis of an anxiety disorder. However, a certain level of cognitive ability and communication level is required to articulate signs and/or symptoms of anxiety (Cooray & Bakala, 2005). Since many individuals with ID are not able to communicate effectively with words, diagnosing anxiety in this population may depend upon clinical impressions, observations or information from caregivers (Williams *et al.*, 2007). It is easier to diagnose anxiety disorders in those with mild to moderate ID as they tend to have better communication skills (Campbell & Malone, 1991).

Observation of behavior is one of the most useful tools for diagnosis of anxiety in the ID population. Avoidant behaviors, especially when they represent a change from typical behavior patterns, may indicate anxiety. Vague, inconsistent or multiple somatic complaints may occur. Anxiety may contribute to an individual's refusal to leave a physician's office (Malloy *et al.*, 1998). Sleep disorders and brooding are commonly seen in individuals with ID who have generalized anxiety disorder (Masi *et al.*, 2000).

Obsessional thinking may be present. This is more difficult to identify in the severe to profound ID population (Bodfish & Madison, 1993), who cannot articulate their thoughts. In patients who have mild to moderate ID, obsessional thinking and rumination may appear as repetition of the same ideas in their conversation and speech.

Compulsive behavior in the population is easily observed (Bodfish & Madison, 1993), but compulsions should be distinguished from stereotypies. An individual who insists on sameness or displays simply repetitive behaviors such as hand-flapping may be at baseline and not necessarily displaying evidence of anxiety (King *et al.*, 1994). Typically, compulsions in the ID population consist of excessive washing, rearranging, hoarding and rituals.

Avoidance behaviors, such as avoiding work or school, may indicate an anxiety disorder (Szymanski & King, 1999). Other signs of anxiety can include intense rocking, an inability to sit still or suddenly sitting down (Jackson & Gentile, 2008). Episodic outbursts and irritability can also be indicators of an anxiety disorder (Vitiello & Behar, 1992; Blankenship *et al.*, 2001). Sometimes an apparent change in "mood" can represent the emergence or worsening of an anxiety disorder. Individuals might suddenly display fearful anticipation, difficulties with concentration or memory, or repetitive worry or fears. More specific symptoms of anxiety include agitation, screaming, crying, withdrawal, regressive/clingy behavior or freezing (Cooray & Bakala, 2005).

Physiologic signs that are consistent with anxiety include difficulty in swallowing, dry mouth, flushing, sweating, palpitations, tremor, headache, pallor, fatigue, hyperventilation, muscle tension, diarrhea, increased urinary frequency, paraesthesias and insomnia. These symptoms can be seen episodically or continuously (Cooray & Bakala, 2005).

All types of anxiety disorders can be diagnosed in individuals with ID (Arnold, 1993). Panic disorder, generalized anxiety disorder (GAD), obsessive compulsive disorder (OCD) and post-traumatic stress disorder (PTSD) are some of the commonly diagnosed anxiety disorders.

Panic disorder

There are only two published case reports which specifically discuss panic disorder in the ID population. The first one, by Malloy *et al.* (1998), described a patient who would on occasion call 911 with a complaint of "I feel bad." This escalated over time to more frequent complaints and calls with, at times, threats of committing suicide. After being given the Structured Clinical Interview for DSM-III-R (SCID) questionnaire, the patient was diagnosed with panic disorder and treated accordingly (Malloy *et al.*, 1998). This case report discussed the need for clinicians to be aware of avoidant symptoms and vague somatic complaints that could be signs or symptoms of panic disorder, because persons with ID may not be able to describe detailed somatic complaints such as racing heart or nausea.

A second case report was published by Khreim & Mikkelsen (1997), describing an individual with mild ID and panic disorder. The authors discuss the fact that subjective panic sensations can be both difficult to articulate and confusing for individuals with ID. Vitiello & Behar (1992) suggested that panic disorder in the ID population may cause episodic outbursts and may be difficult to diagnose using conventional interviews.

The DM-ID lists no adaptation for those with mild to moderate ID. It is recommended that, when assessing those persons with severe to profound ID, recurrent panic attacks should be diagnosed when they are observed by others, rather than waiting for them to be reported by the individual. The persistent concern that one might have future panic attacks is not likely to be communicated verbally by this population. Instead, observe whether the individual displays increased anxiety, a need for reassurance or an increase in clinginess. In addition, look for gasping for breath, difficulty in breathing, weak cry or cough, clutching or rubbing of the chest, retching, staggering, chills and hot flashes (Fletcher, 2007).

Clinical Vignette #1

Panic disorder   David is a 33 year old Caucasian male with moderate intellectual disability. He has been living in the same group home for the past five years. He has always exhibited intermittent bouts of aggression. About eight months ago, staff reported an increase in the intensity and frequency of the outbursts. They reported that he would appear highly agitated "out of nowhere." They reported that sometimes, during these episodes, he would rub his chest and appear short of breath. The outbursts would last about 5–10 minutes.

Between outbursts, he was described as compliant and considerate. There were no behavior issues or aggression outside of the isolated outbursts. The staff and behavioral therapist had tracked the outbursts and had not been able to find a consistent trigger. In fact, staff reported that they seem to "come out of the blue." He was evaluated by his primary care physician because of the rubbing of his chest and appearing short of breath. A medical cause for the outbursts was ruled out.

Due to the increase in intensity and frequency of the outbursts, a psychiatric consultation was requested. David reported feeling out of control during these episodes. He described feeling that he could not control his behavior during the attacks and feeling very "scared." He told the psychiatrist that his heart would beat "real fast" and that he sometimes had difficulty breathing during the bouts.

The psychiatrist diagnosed him with panic disorder and started him on citalopram. The behavioral therapist educated David about panic attacks. She discussed with him that during times of increased agitation, he was experiencing a panic attack. She helped him put his feelings into words and taught him relaxation techniques to use during the panic attacks. Within four months staff had noted a significant decrease in outbursts and aggressive behavior. David reported that he no longer felt out of control and "scared" during the episodes. Staff also reported a decrease in the frequency of the panic attacks.

Obsessive compulsive disorder (OCD)

The DM-ID reports that to make the diagnosis of OCD in persons with ID, the presence of either obsessions or compulsions is required. However, the DM-ID also notes that *obsessions* may not detectable because of difficulties in communication. It is not required that the obsession experienced by a person with ID be interpreted as ego-dystonic. Also, for individuals with mild to moderate ID, it may not be possible to interpret an individual's attempt to ignore or suppress the obsession. Those with severe to profound ID may not attempt to suppress the obsession or may be unable to communicate attempts to suppress the obsession. For those with mild to moderate ID, it may not be possible to determine if they understand that the obsessions are part of their own mind; and for those with severe or profound ID, the understanding of the obsession is not considered (Fletcher, 2007).

According to the DM-ID, those persons with mild or moderate ID who exhibit *compulsions* frequently have signs of ordering, hoarding or rubbing. Their "mental compulsions" may be difficult to elicit. The function that the compulsion may serve also may not be accessible or obtainable. It is important to distinguish stereotypies and insistences on sameness from compulsions in this population. Behaviors such as pacing, stealing, humming, overeating or drinking, masturbating and verbal perseveration have been studied in individuals with ID and excluded from a diagnosis of OCD (Fletcher, 2007).

In those with severe to profound ID, their compulsions will typically center on acts (and thoughts) such as insisting on fixed sequences, compulsive ordering or filling/emptying. Again, the purpose of the compulsion may not be obtainable. Those with mild to moderate

ID are often unable to recognize that the compulsion is unreasonable; and those with severe or profound ID do not (Fletcher, 2007). In those with all forms of ID who have obsessions or compulsions, anxiety or distress may occur. Self-injury and/or aggression may occur if the individual is prevented from performing the compulsion.

There are multiple difficulties that are encountered when diagnosing OCD in the ID population. The concept of obsessions may be difficult for the person with ID to describe. Individuals with ID have significant difficulty with the abstract concept of ego-dystonic thoughts and the act, or thought, of trying to resist them (Bailey & Andrews, 2003). For example, it can be difficult to differentiate stereotypies from compulsions in the nonverbal population, when they are not able to describe obsessions or identify that they are performing a compulsion in response to an obsessive thought. Certain common compulsions are more easily identified, such as hoarding, cleaning and arranging, and these are suggestive of OCD in the ID population (Szymanski & King, 1999).

Research on OCD in the ID population

In one residential setting, compulsions could be diagnosed and distinguished from stereotypies in 6% of the population (Vitiello *et al.*, 1989). In another study of 302 institutionalized ID individuals, 3.5% had compulsions that were significantly interfering with daily functioning (Lund, 1985). Resistance to compulsions is not commonly seen in the ID population (Vitiello & Behar, 1992).

There maybe neurochemical differences between stereotypies and compulsions (Bodfish, 1995). In one study, blink rate was recorded as an indicator of central dopamine function and recorded in three groups of ten individuals with ID. One group of individuals had a body-rocking stereotypy, another group had been diagnosed with compulsions and the third group had neither. The group with stereotypy had a significantly lower blink rate (and, presumably, reduced central dopamine function) than the other two groups (Bailey & Andrews, 2003).

In two separate studies, "ordering" was found to be the most common compulsion in individuals with ID. Cleaning, checking/touching, completeness and grooming were the next most common compulsions, respectively. Hand-washing appeared to be less frequently seen in individuals with ID than in other patients with OCD (Bailey & Andrews, 2003).

Attempts at modifying DSM-IV criteria to become more consistent with cognitive abilities in the ID population have been made in some research studies. In a small study by Bodfish & Madison (1993) regarding the use of fluoxetine to treat compulsions in the ID population, they used the following criteria to identify OCD:

- Engagement in one or more compulsive behavior, including ordering, hoarding, touching, checking, cleaning, arranging, etc.

- Staff impression that the compulsion interfered with training and or socialization efforts.

- The individuals were resistant to change.

Of the ten adults that fulfilled their criteria, nine had self-injury behavior as the primary focus of treatment (Bodfish & Madison, 1993).

In an open study of clomipramine performed by Barak *et al.* (1995) with 11 adults with ID, the DSM-IV criteria were modified by deleting the specifier of "poor insight" (Bailey & Andrews, 2003).

Clinical Vignette #2

Obsessive compulsive disorder   Samuel was a 54 year old African American male with mild intellectual disability. He had a long history of asking questions or making statements four times and would become upset if others tried to prevent him from asking the fourth time or repeating himself. He had always lived with his mother, who had never felt that his compulsion interfered with his life and had always tolerated it. She would at times indicate that she found it "cute" and did not want him to receive treatment or therapy to help him discontinue it.

Samuel did not exhibit other compulsions or obsessions until his mother passed away when he was 53 years old. After this significant loss, he moved into a group home with 24-hour supervision. He was not given any counseling or allowed to attend his mother's funeral. Immediately following the death of his mother and the move to the group home, he become very schedule-oriented. If his schedule were changed in the slightest manner, he would become very upset. He started to close doors and repeat tasks four times.

During the months following the death of his mother, these behaviors increased. It became difficult for him to leave the house, as his compulsion to repeating things four times became very time-consuming. If staff tried to interrupt his compulsions, he would become physically aggressive.

The staff requested a psychiatry referral due to the physical aggression. Once evaluated by a psychiatrist, Samuel was diagnosed with obsessive compulsive disorder. He was started on sertraline, and it was also recommended that he be allowed to visit his mother's grave and have a psychotherapist work with him regarding bereavement.

Three months later, the compulsions had improved some but were still present. The psychotherapy transitioned to exposure therapy. The therapist helped Samuel to create a "worry thermometer," placing the compulsions that caused his anxiety to "rise" at the top. With the therapist's help, he was able to stop performing compulsions that caused less anxiety. Eventually, he was able to prevent himself from performing the compulsions at the top of the thermometer or the compulsions that caused him the most anxiety.

Post-traumatic stress disorder (PTSD)

Persons with ID are very vulnerable to abuse and neglect as they are dependent on others, face communication barriers, want to please caregivers and often do not understand their rights. In general, The American Academy of Child and Adolescent Psychiatry regards PTSD in children and adolescents, as well as persons with ID, to be "significantly under-diagnosed" and "should routinely be considered" (Szymanski & King, 1999).

Literature regarding the identification and treatment of PTSD in the ID population is sparse, although it has been observed that the symptoms of PTSD are frequently mis-diagnosed as "problem behaviors" (Turk *et al.*, 2005). McCarthy (2001) reported that individuals with ID who were suffering PTSD commonly complained of anxiety, insomnia, aggression and irritability. She described the need to consider PTSD within the context of developmental, cognitive and emotional levels (Turk *et al*., 2005). The signs and symptoms of PTSD in adults with ID can closely resemble those of children in the general population who have PTSD.

The finding that children can exhibit symptoms of PTSD when significant caregivers die seems likely to extend to adults with ID (Mitchell & Clegg, 2005). Hollins & Esterhuyzen (1997) reported that, following the death of a parental figure, individuals with ID were more likely to exhibit irritability, anxiety, adjustment difficulties and depression than were those without ID. However, nearly 75% of the caregivers failed to attribute the behavioral changes to the parental deaths. Arrangements were made for only half of the individuals with ID to attend the funeral of their deceased parent (Hollins & Sinason, 2000).

Harper & Wadsworth (1993) have argued that caregivers of this population often inadvertently inhibit coping and expression of grief by individuals with ID. This may be due to the assumption that individuals with ID are unaware about the process of death and the finality of it (Harper & Wadsworth, 1993). While the death of a loved one is traumatic, not being allowed to grieve and learn to cope with the loss can further intensify the traumatic effect. Other symptoms noted by Harper and Wadsworth in those individuals with ID bereaving a lost loved one were breathing difficulties, disorientation, hyperactivity, increased sexual behavior, suicidal statements, loss of body function and pretending to be dead (Mitchell & Clegg, 2005).

The criterion in the DSM-IV requiring that the individual has been exposed to a traumatic event, in which the person witnessed or experienced a threatening situation, has no adaptation for individuals with ID. In those with ID, there appears to be a greater range for "traumatizing" events. In this population, seemingly benign experiences, such as developmental milestones or residential placements, have led to "post-traumatic reactions." Those with younger developmental ages frequently respond to the traumatic event with disorganized or agitated behaviors (Fletcher, 2007).

There is also no adaptation in the DSM-IV for the re-experiencing of traumatic events by those with mild to moderate ID; in those with severe to profound ID, however, behavioral re-enactment of the traumatic event has been reported. Recurrent dreams of the event are commonly replaced by dreams with frightening content that is not recognizable (Fletcher, 2007).

Clinical Vignette #3

Post-traumatic stress disorder   Stephanie is a 20 year old Caucasian female with a mild intellectual disability. She lived with both of her parents until she turned 19 years old and she then moved into a group home. Initially, she did very well at the group home; she socialized well with the other housemates and was compliant with requests from the staff. She was well liked by everyone. She did not exhibit any behavioral issues or concerns.

During a weekend visit at her parent's home, the house was robbed. She awoke during the robbery and was held at gunpoint. No one was injured during the robbery, but the robbers were never apprehended.

Over the following weeks, Stephanie developed nightmares and insomnia. She would become very anxious at night and would lock her bedroom door and barricade the door with furniture. She became more anxious regarding strangers. Her staff reported her to be extremely "jumpy" and "paranoid" at night. Staff reported that she had become very irritable and would "snap" for no apparent reason.

A psychiatric examination was requested due to her increased agitation since the robbery. During the psychiatric appointment, Stephanie reported being afraid at night and worrying "all the time" that somebody would attempt to break into her home. She also reported trying to "push" the thoughts of the robbery "out of my head" but finding it very difficult. She said she felt unable to return to her parents' home, as this made her anxiety intolerable.

She was diagnosed with post-traumatic stress disorder. The psychiatrist initiated treatment with a selective serotonin reuptake inhibitor (SSRI) and consulted with the behavioral therapist. The behavioral therapist started a modified form of trauma-focused cognitive behavioral therapy.

Five months after initiating treatment, Stephanie noted an improvement in nightmares and anxiety. Her sleep significantly improved. She reported feeling a general decrease in arousal. She resumed making visits to her parent's home and tolerated this well.

There is no adaptation for the avoidance of stimuli associated with the trauma and numbing of general responsiveness in individuals with ID, with the exception of sensing the future foreshortened. The DM-ID discusses that the assessment process can be complicated in those with severe to profound ID, because of difficulties in communication.

The avoidance of reminders of the traumatic event is sometimes misinterpreted as non-compliance by caregivers (Fletcher, 2007). There is no adaptation for individuals with ID for symptoms of persistent increased arousal (Fletcher, 2007).

Generalized anxiety disorder (GAD)

A study by Deb *et al.* (2001) found that a community-based sample population of individuals with ID ages 16–64 years exhibited GAD at a rate of 2.2% (Deb *et al.*, 2001). Masi *et al.* (2000) published a study comparing clinical features of GAD in adolescents and young adults with ID, compared with children and adolescents of normal IQ. They found that the symptomatology was similar, with the exception of a higher rate of brooding, somatic complaints and sleep disorders in the ID population. They found a high rate of comorbidity with depression in both populations. Khreim & Mikkelsen (1997) have postulated that perhaps individuals with ID and excessive worry present more similarly to children matched to their developmental age (Bailey & Andrews, 2003).

The DM-ID lists no adaptation for those with mild or moderate ID. Individuals with severe ID only require *one* of the following six symptoms – restlessness, tiring easily, trouble concentrating, irritability, muscle tension or disturbance in sleep – instead of the usual three required for other individuals. According to the DM-ID, difficulty concentrating in individuals with severe ID is difficult to detect and is not applicable in those with profound ID (Fletcher, 2007).

Clinical Vignette #4

Generalized anxiety disorder Sally is a 23 year old Caucasian female who lives with her parents. She was diagnosed with mild intellectual disability when she was a young child. Six months ago, her father was involved in a car accident. He was hospitalized for one week but has fully recovered.

Sally's parents started to notice that, in the course of those six months, she had become more irritable and had started to perseverate regarding the health of her family members. She had also begun to complain about her stomach hurting. Her family had her examined by her primary care physician, who could not find a medical explanation for the complaints of stomach pain and reported that she was healthy. She has never had medical problems that required more than a single course of antibiotics.

Her family assumed that the agitation was likely a response to her father's car accident, and they hoped it would wane over time. However, six months after the car accident, her symptoms had worsened. She started to perseverate over subjects other than her family's health. When she did this, her family would find her pacing. When they confronted her regarding the pacing and tried to prevent her from continuing, she became more agitated and started crying.

Her primary care physician referred her to a psychiatrist. She told the psychiatrist that she has trouble "getting thoughts out of my head" and that after her father's car accident she started to worry it would happen again. She reported that she started to worry about her father and her mother and then "everything," and she described pacing as a way of trying to "get the thoughts out of my head."

The psychiatrist diagnosed her with generalized anxiety disorder. He prescribed sertraline and referred her to a behavioral therapist to provide her with cognitive behavioral therapy. Three months after starting therapy and medication, she reported having a much easier time "getting the thoughts to stop." Her parents reported that she was no longer pacing and that she was less agitated and rarely perseverated on topics.

Treatment: pharmacologic interventions and psychotherapy

The general psychopharmacological and psychotherapeutic treatment of individuals with anxiety disorder is fundamentally the same, independent of their cognitive ability. However, modifying treatment and techniques are important with regard to the individual's needs, circumstances, communication abilities and cognitive status. The goal of treatment is to decrease symptoms and to help the individual improve their quality of life (Szymanski & King, 1999).

Pharmacologic interventions

There is a dearth of controlled, evidence-based research in the ID population with which to guide prescribers in pharmacologic interventions regarding medication choices and dose modifications. Case studies that have been reported include that of Khreim & Mikkelsen (1997), who described an individual with mild ID and panic disorder. This individual responded well to a combination of sertraline, clonazepam and cognitive therapy (Bailey & Andrews, 2003). Malloy *et al.* (1998) described a patient diagnosed with panic disorder and ID who experienced remission of her symptoms after treatment with paroxetine and clonazepam.

Ratey *et al.* (1991) reported on eight individuals diagnosed with GAD and ID, who also had other psychiatric diagnoses. All eight of these individuals responded to buspirone at 15–45 mg a day. Ratey *et al.* (1991) also reported on six other patients with ID, four of whom were diagnosed with GAD. Of the four individuals who had GAD, all exhibited a reduction in anxiety after treatment with buspirone.

Khreim & Mikkelsen (1997) reported an individual with GAD and moderate ID who responded to a combination of buspirone and cognitive therapy (Bailey & Andrews, 2003). May *et al.* (2008) reported an individual with OCD and mild ID who responded to citalopram. However, this individual was taking clonazepam, haloperidol, quetiapine, and valproic acid concomitantly (May *et al.*, 2008).

A retrospective case analysis was performed by Branford *et al.* (1998) on reports of 37 individuals with perseverative and maladaptive behaviors, treated with fluoxetine or paroxetine. Forty percent of the patients derived no benefit from treatment, 25% exhibited deterioration and 35% exhibited a reduction in behaviors. There was no difference in response to paroxetine and fluoxetine (Branford *et al.*, 1998).

Bodfish and Madison (1993) studied adults with ID and "compulsive behavior disorder." Compulsive behavior disorder was defined by a set of diagnostic research criteria created to potentially indentify OCD in people with ID and aberrant behaviors. Ten individuals who met criteria for compulsive behavior disorder, and six who did not, were prescribed fluoxetine. Seven of the ten individuals with compulsive behavior disorder experienced a reduction in symptoms with fluoxetine. None of the comparison individuals experienced an improvement in behaviors (Bodfish & Madison, 1993).

Lewis *et al.* (1995) performed a randomized controlled crossover trial with clomipramine in ten individuals with severe to profound ID who exhibited stereotyped, repetitive self-injurious behavior and repetitive compulsive behaviors. Three individuals exhibited significant side effects. Six of the seven individuals who were able to continue the study exhibited a clinically significant decrease in one or more repetitive behavior, as judged by a 50% reduction in the aberrant behavior checklist (ABC) scale (Sohanpal *et al.*, 2007).

An open trial of fluoxetine was performed in individuals with autism or ID and perseverative behaviors (Cook *et al.* 1992). Fifteen of the 23 autistic individuals responded to fluoxetine, and ten of the 16 individuals with ID responded. Six of the autistic and three of the individuals with ID exhibited side effects that caused an interference with their ability to function. Side effects in these groups included restlessness, hyperactivity, agitation, a decrease in appetite and insomnia.

Although there are no double-blind controlled studies in this population, recommended psychopharmacologic treatment for individuals with ID and anxiety disorders is currently similar to those without ID. Medications typically used include selective serotonin reuptake inhibitors (SSRIs), serotonin noradrenalin reuptake inhibitors (SNRIs), buspirone, beta-blockers and benzodiazepines. In general, first line agents are SSRIs. There is some limited evidence for buspirone and antipsychotics (Cooray & Bakala, 2005).

There is controversy regarding the use of benzodiazepines in this population. Individuals with ID are more likely to become disinhibited with benzodiazepines. There is evidence that a combination of stereotypy and self-injurious (SIB) behaviors may be a significant risk factor for disinhibition with benzodiazepines. Benzodiazepines can also cause hyperactivity, SIB or withdrawal-induced manic symptoms in these individuals (Blankenship *et al.*, 2010).

Psychotherapeutic interventions

There has been some controversy regarding the use of psychotherapy in those with ID. In the past, it has been argued by some that normal intelligence is required for psychotherapy to be effective. Sternlicht (1965) argues that it a significant error to believe that psychotherapy requires normal intelligence. He points out that there are techniques that can be used that do not require verbal skills (Gentile & Jackson, 2008).

One psychotherapeutic technique that has been studied in individuals with ID who have been diagnosed with an anxiety disorder is progressive relaxation. Lindsay *et al.* (1989) studied behavioral relaxation and abbreviated progressive relaxation in 50 individuals with moderate to severe ID. They found that behavioral relaxation was more effective than abbreviated progressive relaxation, which was more effective than no therapy (Lindsay *et al.*, 1989).

Other literature also supports the use of relaxation techniques in those with mild, moderate and severe ID. Martin *et al.* (1998) supported the use of multisensory stimulation to accomplish relaxation in those with severe to profound ID. There is evidence to support the use of cognitive behavioral therapy in those with borderline or mild ID (Cooray & Bakala, 2005). Recently cognitive behavioral therapy has been developed to help parents teach their children with ID to change negative thoughts and to improve coping skills (Hollins & Sinason, 2000).

Summary

Anxiety disorders are common disorders that are experienced by all individuals, regardless of cognitive ability. Prevalence rates of anxiety disorders in individuals with ID have been recorded at extreme variations. This is likely to be due in part to the inherent difficulties in diagnosing anxiety disorders in the ID population because of limited verbal skills and an inability to interpret signs and symptoms of autonomic arousal. Clinicians should be alert for vague, inconsistent somatic complaints, avoidant behaviors, sleep disorder, brooding, repetition in conversation or speech, intense rocking, inability to sit still, episodic outbursts and compulsive behaviors. The DM-ID suggests modifications to the DSM-IV that can be helpful when evaluating individuals with ID, as some of the criteria set forth in the DSM-IV are not applicable to some individuals with ID.

Treatment for individuals with ID and anxiety is similar to those without cognitive limitations. However, it is important to modify the treatment techniques and tailor them to the individual's needs, circumstances, communication style and cognitive level. Chapter 12 reviews recommendations for medication use for patients with ID. Overall, there is a dearth of literature surrounding diagnosis and treatment of anxiety in the ID population. Randomized controlled studies are needed to improve diagnosis and treatment to this population.

References

Arnold, L.E. (1993). Clinical pharmacological issues in treating psychiatric disorders of patients with mental retardation. *Annals of Clinical Psychiatry* **5**, 189–197.

Bailey, N.M. & Andrews, T.M. (2003). Diagnostic Criteria for Psychiatric Disorders for Use with Adults with Learning Disabilities/Mental Retardation (DC-LD) and the diagnosis of anxiety disorders: a review. *Journal of Intellectual Disability Research* **47**, 50–61.

Barak, Y., Ring, A., Levy, D., Granek, I., Szor, H. & Elizur, A. (1995). Disabling compulsions in 11 mentally retarded adults: an open trial of clomipramine Sr. *Journal of Clinical Psychiatry* **56**, 459–461.

Blankenship, K., Erickson, C.A., Stigler, K.A., Posey, D.J. & McDougle, C.J. (2010). Autism spectrum disorders and mental retardation. In: Stolerman, I. (ed.) *Encyclopedia of Psychopharmacology.* Springer-Verlag, Heidelberg, Germany.

Bodfish, J.W. & Madison, J.T. (1993). Diagnosis of fluoxetine treatment of compulsive behavior disorder of adults with mental retardation. *American Journal of Mental Retardation* **98**, 360–367.

Bodfish, J.W., Crawford, T.W., Powell, S.B., Parker, D.E., Golden, R.N., & Lewis, M.H. (1995). Compulsions in adults with mental retardation: prevalence, phenomenology and comorbidity with stereotypy and self-injury. *American Journal of Mental Retardation* **100**, 183–192.

Branford, D., Bhaumik, S. & Naik, B. (1998). Selective serotonin re-uptake inhibitors for the treatment of preservative and maladaptive behaviors of people with intellectual disability. *Journal of intellectual Disability Research* **42**, 301–306.

Campbell, M. & Malone, R.P. (1991). Mental retardation and psychiatric disorders. *Hospital & Community Psychiatry* **42**, 374–379.

Cook, E.H., Rowlett, R., Jaselskis, C., & Leventhal, B.L. (1992). Fluoxetine treatment of children and adults with autistic disorder and mental retardation. *Journal of The American Academy Of Child and Adolescent Psychiatry* **31**, 739–745.

Cooray, S.E. & Bakala, A. (2005). Anxiety disorders in people with learning disabilities. *Advances in Psychiatric Treatment* **11**, 355–361.

Deb, S., Thomas, M. & Bright, C. (2001). Mental disorder in adults with intellectual disability. I: Prevalence of functional psychiatric illness among a community-based population aged between 16 and 64 years. *Journal of Intellectual Disability Research* **45**, 495–505.

DSM-IV, Work Group (1994). *Diagnostic and Statistical Manual of Mental Disorders: Forth edition.* American Psychiatric Association, Washington, DC.

Fletcher, R. (2007). *Diagnostic Manual-Intellectual Disability: A Textbook of Diagnosis of Mental Disorders in Persons with Intellectual Disability.* National Association for the Dually Diagnosed Press, New York.

Gentile, J.P. & Jackson, C.S. (2008). Supportive psychotherapy with the dual diagnosis patient: co-occurring mental illness/intellectual disabilities. *Psychiatry* **5**(3), 49–57.

Glenn, E., Bihm, E.M. & Lammers, W.J. (2003). Depression, anxiety, and relevant cognitions in persons with mental retardation. *Journal of Autism and Developmental Disorders* **33**, 69–76.

Harper, D.C. & Wadsworth, J.S. (1993). Grief in adults with mental retardation: preliminary findings. *Research in Developmental Disabilities* **14**, 313–330.

Hollins, S. & Esterhuizen, A. (1997). Bereavement and grief in adults with learning disabilities. *The British Journal of Psychiatry* **170**, 497–501.

Hollins, S. & Sinason, V. (2000). Psychotherapy, learning disabilities and trauma: new perspectives. *The British Journal of Psychiatry* **176**, 32–36.

Hurley, A.D., Folstein, M. & Lam, N. (2003). Patients with and without intellectual disability seeking outpatient psychiatric services: diagnoses and prescribing pattern. *Journal of Intellectual Disability Research* **47**, 39–50.

Jackson, C. & Gentile, J. (September 8, 2008). Oral presentation: Medications and psychotherapy for patients with mental illness/developmental disabilities. Dual Diagnosis conference: "Putting the Pieces Together". Wright State University, Dayton, Ohio.

King, B.H., DeAntonia, C., McCracken, J.T., Forness, S.R. & Ackerland, V. (1994). Psychiatric consultation in severe and profound mental retardation. *American Journal of Psychiatry* **151**, 1802–1808.

Khreim, I. & Mikkelsen, E. (1997). Anxiety disorders in adults with mental retardation. *Psychiatric Annals* **98**, 175–181.

Lindsay, W.R., Baty, F.J. & Michie, A.M. (1989). A comparison of anxiety treatments with adults who have moderate and severe mental retardation. *Research in Developmental Disabilities* **10**, 129–140.

Lund, J. (1985). The prevalence of psychiatric morbidity in mentally retarded adults. *Acta Psychiatrica Scandinavica*, **72**, 563–570.

Malloy, E., Zealberg, J.J. & Paolone, T. (1998). A patient with mental retardation and possible panic disorder. *Psychiatric Services* **49**, 105–106.

Masi, G., Favilla, L. & Mucci, M. (2000). Generalized anxiety disorder in adolescents and young adults with mild mental retardation. *Psychiatry: Interpersonal and Biological Processes* **63** (1), 54–64.

Masi, G., Brovedani, P., Mucci, M. & Favilla, L. (2002). Assessment of anxiety and depression in adolescents with mental retardation. *Child Psychiatry and Human Development* **32**(3), 227–237.

Matson, J.L., Smiroldo, B.B., Hamilton, M. & Baglio, C.S. (1997). Do anxiety disorders exist in persons with severe and profound mental retardation? *Research in Developmental Disabilities* **18**, 39–44.

May, M.E., Jackson, J.A., Blodgett, K.A., Huber, H.B., Kishel, E.K., Riediger, A.B. & Kennedy, C.H. (2008). Using functional behavioral assessment to study the effects of citalopram on the obsessive-compulsive verbalizations of a woman with obsessive-compulsive disorder and mental retardation. *Journal of Clinical Psychiatry* **10**, 73–75.

McCarthy, J. (2001). Post-traumatic stress disorder in people with learning disability. *Advances in Psychiatric Treatment* **7**, 163–169.

Mitchell, A. & Clegg, J. (2005). Is post-traumatic stress disorder a helpful concept for adults with intellectual disability? *Journal of Intellectual Disability Research* **49**, 552–559.

Ratey, J.J., Sovner, R., Mikkelsen, E. & Chmielinski, H.E. (1989). Buspirone therapy for maladaptive behavior and anxiety in developmentally disabled persons. *Journal of Clinical Psychiatry* **50**(10), 382–384.

Royal College of Psychiatrists (2001). *DC-LD (Diagnostic Criteria for Psychiatric Disorders for Use with Adults with Learning Disabilities/Mental Retardation)*. Gaskell, London.

Sohanpal, S.K., Deb, S., Thomas, C., Soni, R., Lenôtre, L. & Unwin, G. (2007). The effectiveness of antidepressant medication in the management of behavior problems in adults with intellectual disabilities: a systematic review. *Journal of Intellectual Disability Research* **51**, 750–765.

Sternlicht, M. (1965). Psychotherapeutic techniques useful with the mentally retarded: A review and critique. *Psychiatric Quarterly* **39**(1), 84–90.

Szymanski, L. & King, B.H. (1999). *Practice Parameters for the Assessment and Treatment of Children, Adolescents and Adults with Mental Retardation and Comorbid Mental Disorders.* American Academy of Child and Adolescent Psychiatry, Washington, DC.

Turk, J., Robbins, I. & Woodhead, M. (2005). Post-traumatic stress disorder in young people with intellectual disability. *Journal of Intellectual Disability Research* **49**, 872–875.

Vitiello, B. & Behar, D. (1992). Mental retardation and psychiatric illness. *Hospital and Community Psychiatry* **43**, 494–499.

Vitiello, B., Spreat, S. & Behar, D. (1989) Obsessive–compulsive disorder in mentally retarded patients. *Journal of Nervous and Mental Disease* **177**, 232–236.

Williams, D.T., Hirsch, S. & Coffey, B. (2007). Mood and anxiety symptoms in an adolescent with pervasive developmental disorder not otherwise specified and moderate mental retardation. *Journal of Child and Adolescent Psychopharmacology* **17**, 721–726.

9

Psychotic Disorders

Allison E. Cowan, MD, Assistant Professor, Wright State University, Dayton, Ohio

Historical perspective

The history of individuals with mental illness and intellectual disabilities (ID) is profoundly intertwined. Overlooked by the great ancient physicians of Greece and Rome, thought to be cursed by God or possessed by demonic spirits in prehistory and Medieval times, warehoused together in the asylums of the Enlightenment, and finally returned to the community during the deinstitutionalization of the 1960s and 1970s, individuals with mental illness, ID or both have shared history and treatments.

One of the earliest treatments of mental illness is trephination – drilling into the skull to remove a circle of bone, presumably to let out the demonic spirits possessing the sufferer. The other early treatments were the traditions and herbs of the healers, wise women and shamans. The Greek physician Hippocrates attributed mental illness to an imbalance in the humors – e.g. too much "black bile" would result in the development of melancholia. While Hippocrates' treatments were generally passive, kind, and given with the presumption that the body could restore its own imbalance, treatment of mental illness was not always so. During the Renaissance and the Enlightenment, the humoral theory continued to be used in therapeutic bleedings, purgings and blistering of patients to restore health.

People with ID or mental illness were, for the most part, reliant on family. They were put to work doing simple labor in the fields of agrarian communities. They were used as entertainment as "natural fools" in wealthy families and royal courts, which was viewed as a position of privilege. If unruly, they were kept in dungeons or dark cellars. Treatment in

Psychiatry of Intellectual Disability: A Practical Manual, First Edition.
Edited by Julie P. Gentile and Paulette M. Gillig.
© 2012 John Wiley & Sons, Ltd. Published 2012 by John Wiley & Sons, Ltd.

1542 was for people to be kept in a "chamber where there is little light and with a keeper that the mad man do fear" (Scheerenberger, 1983). In 1997, O'Dwyer wrote of the historical intersections of the mental illness and ID, with Pinel (1802) suggesting that mental illness and ID were different but coexisted, and Kraeplin (1896) reporting that 7% of cases of dementia praecox arose on the basis of then-named idiocy.

When the asylums began to appear, the intention was to provide treatment that was *moral* or humane. Unfortunately, overcrowding and abuse lead to treatment that often was no better. In the asylums, people, both with mental illness and ID, were chained to walls, subjected to cold baths and frequently not given clothing. The upper class was charged admission and toured the facilities for entertainment.

After the discovery of thorazine (chlorpromazine), there was finally an effective treatment for mental illness. This discovery made it possible to deinstitutionalize individuals with ID and severe mental illness.

Prevalence

The psychotic disorders are described by the DSM-IV-TR as Schizophrenia, Schizophreni-form Disorder, Schizoaffective Disorder, Delusional Disorder, Brief Psychotic Disorder, Shared Psychotic Disorder, Psychotic Disorder Due to a General Medical Condition, Substance-Induced Psychotic Disorder, and Psychotic Disorder Not Otherwise Specified.

The prevalence of schizophrenia in the general population is generally thought to be around 1% worldwide (Robins *et al.*, 1984; Kessler *et al.* 1994; Perälä *et al.*, 2007). The prevalence in people with ID, however, has been debated for some time. Historically, there was the misapprehension that people with ID did not have the cognitive ability to develop psychiatric illness, but more recent research has shown that the opposite is likely. Individuals with ID have a three to five-fold increased prevalence of schizophrenia over the general population (Cooper *et al.*, 2007; Lund, 1985), with lower ability levels associated with a higher prevalence of mental ill-health (Perälä *et al.*, 2007; Kessler *et al.*, 1994; Cooper *et al.*, 2007; Melville *et al.*, 2008).

While the ultimate etiology of schizophrenia and the psychotic disorders remains unknown, the link between ID and psychotic disorders remains. A meta-analytic review done by Cannon *et al.* (2002) demonstrated a reportedly small effect size between birth complications, abnormal fetal growth and complications of delivery and the subsequent development of schizophrenia. Birth complications, cerebral palsy and epilepsy are also known to be more prevalent in individuals with ID.

Diagnosis

The diagnosis of psychotic disorders in individuals with ID remains a challenge. Many issues make the definitive psychiatric diagnosis of psychotic disorders more difficult, including diagnostic overshadowing, patient interview and caregiver interview, parsing out problem behaviors and self-stimulation from psychotic symptoms, and the exclusion of individuals with ID from most scientific studies. Another challenge is adaptation of criteria for individuals with ID from individuals without ID, especially when those criteria require a certain amount of cognition and communication.

Diagnostic overshadowing in psychotic disorders

Diagnostic overshadowing (see also Chapter 2) refers to the attribution of psychiatric symptoms to the individual's ID.

Clinical Vignette #1

Diagnostic overshadowing   Marcia, a woman with moderate ID, was brought to the mental health clinic to meet with her psychotherapist for the first time. Her primary caregiver remained in the waiting room to insure Marcia's privacy in therapy. Marcia sat quietly in the session and only answered yes or no to questions.

Marcia's therapist attributed her lack of speech to her ID. Only upon discussing the follow-up appointment with the caregiver did the therapist discover that Marcia was usually chatty and upbeat, even if at times difficult to understand. The therapist quickly re-evaluated Marcia with her caregiver present, and discovered that Marcia had begun suspecting people of poisoning her food at her sheltered workshop.

Matson & Scior (2004) found, via two separate vignette surveys (identical except that one vignette included ID and the other did not), that clinicians were less likely to consider a diagnosis of schizophrenia, less likely to consider psychiatric admission and less likely to recommend medication in individuals with ID. This supports the meta-analysis by White *et al.* (1995) that showed a reliably small to moderate effect size in diagnostic over-shadowing judgmental bias. They posited that overshadowing could be a contributing factor in decreased mental health services to people with ID.

In a meta-analysis of ten overshadowing studies (Jopp *et al.*, 2001), using a multiaxial diagnosis (Axis I-V), lent more correct diagnoses in two of the overshadowing studies. It was postulated that overshadowing was reduced or eliminated because of engaging in a multidimensional, and thus more complex, formulation. Therefore, when seeing individuals with ID, a multiaxial formulation, combined with awareness of diagnostic overshadowing, could lead to more accurate diagnoses and better mental health care delivery.

The patient interview

Depending on the level of communication, adaptive ability and baseline cognition in an individual with ID, reliability of self-reporting symptoms can be a challenge to accurate diagnosis. Compounded by the burden of psychotic symptoms, communication – and therefore diagnosis – can be even more difficult. Individuals with ID in the borderline to mild range are quite likely to be able to discuss their symptoms with the clinician. However, attempting to discuss a timeline or complicated sequence of events (e.g. past medication trials or hospitalizations) can be more difficult for the patient.

Timothy, the patient described in Clinical Vignette #2, is an example of a typical patient with mild ID and a psychotic disorder. He is able to describe his symptoms in detail, but his thinking is not always concrete (his parents brought him in, not the concrete answer of a car). Some clinicians may be surprised at the complexity of positive symptoms that individuals

Clinical Vignette #2

Psychosis   Timothy is a 37 year-old man with mild ID who was brought in by his parents. When asked what brought him in, he said, "My parents thought I should come."

Timothy reported that he thought that an evil Two-Face (a Batman villain) had moved into the house next door, and that Two-Face was planning to hurt Timothy's parents. Timothy said, "I hear him whisper to me at night."

Timothy admitted that he had these problems before and took medicine that helped, but he was not able to remember the names of the medications.

with mild ID can report, but Timothy's are not unusual. The importance of the patient interview had been marginalized in the past, but several studies show that the patient has vital information to aid in diagnosis. Specifically, Moss *et al.* (1996) found that a third of diagnoses were missed if this part of the interview is omitted. Hatton *et al.* (2005) demonstrated that people with mild ID had less complex delusions than people without ID, but that these may have been undiagnosed.

Individuals with a higher degree of communication difficulties and/or more severe cognitive deficits are typically more difficult to elicit symptoms from. Some of these individuals with ID, when confronted with a confusing or unfamiliar situation, might answer questions in a manner to please the interviewer, as in the example in Clinical Vignette #3.

Clinical Vignette #3

Concrete operations   Tony is brought to the mental health clinic because of "bizarre behavior." He sees his psychiatrist regularly for depression.

His psychiatrist asks, "Tony, what brings you in?"
Tony answers, "The van."
His psychiatrist tries a different tack, "How are you?"
Tony, without pause, says "Great, how about you?"
Again the psychiatrist tries, "Are you having any problems?"
Tony, now obviously uncomfortable, says, "No," and looks to his caregiver for help. The caregiver fills in the details: Tony has been staying in his room and pulling all his clothes out of his closet.
The psychiatrist asks, "Tony, do you ever hear people talk to you when no one else is around?"
"Yes."
"What do they sound like?"
Tony responds, "Bad people."

This example demonstrates the difficulty of conducting an interview with someone who is operating at a concrete level of cognition typical of ID, either because of his psychotic illness or because of his baseline ID. The patient is quick to respond in stereotyped and routine answers, much to the befuddlement of the psychiatrist. The need for clear, concise questions is also demonstrated. There also is a tendency for individuals with ID to answer questions in the manner they expect their examiners to want (Scheerenberger, 1983; Cooper *et al.*, 2007) – or, as the DM-ID puts it, "yessing" the examiner.

Another difficulty in the patient interview for diagnosing psychotic disorders is the differentiation of self-talk from psychotic symptoms, such as auditory and/or visual hallucinations, disorganized thoughts and disorganized behavior. While there is scant literature on this topic, self-talk (or inner speech) represent the individual's own thoughts. This can be recognized as "talking to oneself" and sometimes appears as mumbling, both in individuals with and without ID.

Usually, an individual, if prone to self-talk, does so at baseline. Some common presentations are repeating an earlier conversation, talking through a difficult situation (e.g. not being allowed to do an activity) or repeating television, song or movie quotes. These should be carefully considered and monitored for a change for the person's normal routine or behavior. Self-talk might not be self-talk if the individual has a change from his or her normal pattern. The example in Clinical Vignette #4 illustrates a patient's change from baseline behavior.

Clinical Vignette #4

Self-talk versus emergence of psychosis   Normally, Gwen had a brisk and cheerful quality to her self-talk. Her caregivers understood this was how she worked things out in her mind. However, when they noticed that she began spending more time in her room alone, they worried.

Her primary caregiver went to check on her and, from outside the room, overheard Gwen in a heated argument. Thinking that Gwen was on the telephone, the caregiver knocked quietly and opened the door. The caregiver found that Gwen was not on the phone but that she had been yelling at her unplugged radio.

Langdon *et al.* (2009) looked at the inner speech of individuals with schizophrenia (without ID) and compared their inner speech with that of individuals without schizophrenia. Their results showed that the inner speech of both groups had no discernable differences. This study has not been replicated in individuals with ID, but it is not such a stretch of the imagination that the same should remain true in individuals with ID as well. Moss *et al.* (1997) found that the patient report was more likely to elicit hallucinations than caregiver report.

The caregiver interview

Since the caregiver is usually the person to have initiated contact with mental health services, their experiences and knowledge of the patient are important. The caregiver provides perspective to the treatment of individuals with ID – that of an observer.

A careful and thorough interview with both patient and caregiver provides much information that the patient alone cannot. A person with ID can have difficulty answering historical questions, such as medication and medical history, dates and durations of treatment and the types of resources available to the patient.

The Moss *et al.* (1997) report also noted that the caregiver is more likely to be able to report delusions. This is presumably because the individual with ID talks more about delusions, as opposed to hallucinations that are passively experienced. As discussed previously, diagnostic overshadowing is a possibility with caregivers, e.g., a caregiver thinking that responding to internal stimuli (auditory or visual hallucinations) was "normal" or "a behavior."

Clinical Vignette #5

Caregiver interview   Brenda, an individual with ID and schizophrenia, was referred to the mental health clinic from her sheltered workshop. She had started doing paid work since her schizophrenia was controlled with a new medication, and the new job required closer concentration than her previous one.

The workshop reported that Brenda would be working quietly for a time, when her head and neck would flex toward her back. This caused Brenda to lose her place in her work, and she would have to start over. When asked about this, her caregiver reported that Brenda had "been doing it for a while" and that the caregiver did not know that it was something about which to inform anyone.

In Clinical Vignette #5, Brenda's caregiver was also not appropriately educated about symptoms and side effects to watch for with the new medication prescribed, and Brenda was likely having a dystonic reaction to a new antipsychotic medication. See Chapter 12 for more information.

Encountering the push for medication

One difficulty in the caregiver interview is that there are both stated and unstated expectations. The first, and most obvious, expectation is that the clinician will help the identified patient. This is usually the goal on both sides of the desk. Unfortunately, the caregiver's definition of help may differ from the clinician's definition.

One of the most common presentations of individuals with ID to mental health services is problem behaviors. Since there has been a recent shift in mental health away from psychotropics to quell problem behaviors (Unwin & Deb, 2008, Matson *et al.*, 2009), the responses of clinicians are changing. People with ID are much more likely to be prescribed psychotropic medication than the general population, with Unwin citing 20–45% of individuals with ID being prescribed them.

Many studies have investigated whether antipsychotics are effective in treating problem behaviors (See Chapter 14). A caregiver may report that an individual is "psychotic," but it remains the duty of the clinician to determine the meaning of this collateral information. A thorough evaluation for true psychotic symptoms is important in making a definitive diagnosis and treatment with psychotropic medications, but "psychotic" in the common lexicon can mean simply that one is angry, yelling or engaging in property destruction. Problem behaviors alone do not indicate psychotic symptoms.

Table 1 Clinical Pearls: Tips for differentiating problem behavior from psychotic symptoms.

- Problem behaviors have an associated benefit (conscious or unconscious, pleasant or unpleasant), be it:
  - o attention or reaction from caregivers or peers;
  - o avoidance of something unpleasant;
  - o a pattern, even if difficult to determine.
- Psychotic symptoms usually appear more random and are driven from within, rather than seeking something from outside the individual.
- Psychotic symptoms are associated with acute changes from baseline behaviors.

Differentiating problem behaviors from psychotic illnesses

One more challenge for the clinician is the elucidating of psychotic symptoms in individuals with ID from problem behaviors. There still remain all of the previously discussed complications, especially diagnostic overshadowing and limitations of communication. When we add to this mix the idea that people with or without ID, can have difficulty knowing *why* they do what they do (Freud, 1966), the challenge then comes more into focus. See Table 1.

> **Clinical Vignette #6**
>
> *Self-talk*
> 1. Someone without ID: "Why on Earth did I eat that second brownie? I didn't even want it, and I wasn't even hungry any more."
> 2. Someone with ID, who, rather than just dealing with their own thoughts and feelings about eating that extra brownie, usually gets into some amount of trouble for doing it: "Doug! Why on Earth did you eat that second brownie? You already had your brownie, and now you've eaten your roommate's!"

Something to which the clinician often is not privy is the antecedent, or preceding, actions that result in a behavior. Often the clinician is presented with the outcome (e.g. "*He started yelling that he'd eat a brownie if he wanted one.*"). These antecedents, in psychotic illness, can be hallucinations ("*The man was yelling I was stupid. So I threw the chair.*"). However, depression, and not psychosis, has been more strongly linked with problem behaviors (Moss *et al.*, 2000). Therefore individuals presenting with primarily behavioral issues should be considered for depressive or affective disorders before being considered for a psychotic illness, given this link. Another psychotic antecedent would be a delusional belief, e.g. that a staff person was out to harm the patient ("*I hit him because I know he's putting bad things into the food I eat.*"). Again, what is helpful in parsing out these symptoms and behaviors are patterns. People usually have a baseline of problem behaviors, and change from this is what should be examined. The involvement of the entire treatment team – the habilitation staff, behavioral support professionals, therapists, case managers, nurses, primary home care staff and family – is needed to make this determination. While psychotic illnesses can reduce frustration tolerance, a clue that something is a behavior rather than a hallucination or delusion is that the episode happens after the individual does not get what they wanted.

Clinical Vignette #7

Frustration tolerance   Esperanza was brought to the psychiatrist because she was "psychotic." Her mother said, "She refuses to get on the bus to work. She screams and cries and hits herself it if we make her."

This was the only change that her mother and habilitation staff had noticed in Esperanza. When asked, Esperanza said, "I don't want to get on the bus," but would not say more.

Her mother recalled that it had started about a week previously. The habilitation staff remarked that this was when a new person, known to be very disruptive and loud, had started riding the bus as well.

Behavior modifications are difficult and labor-intensive, and they require solidarity of the treatment team (see Chapter 14). Medications can be seen as simpler and less time-consuming on the care staff, but the well-being of the patient can be better served by a behavior plan rather than a psychotropic medication.

Symptoms of psychotic illness can be brought on by interactions with other people or by internal stimuli. Psychotic symptoms usually appear to be more random when carefully tracked on behavior charting.

Clinical Vignette #8

Psychotic symptoms   Elizabeth presented with her mother and father. "We don't know what's gotten into her. She tore the house apart and was screaming. The YMCA, her daytime recreation place, called and said that she was having problems out there, too."

Elizabeth sat in a corner chair, glaring at the psychiatrist. She said, "You can't make me go to a group home." Her parents looked puzzled and said that this was not the plan. Elizabeth said, "The bad people yell at me that you're going to make me go."

Elizabeth said that sometimes she heard people yell at her even when she was alone.

These two examples start with similar presentations, but obviously the etiology of the behavior issues is very different. It is also important in Elizabeth's case to determine whether her thinking is delusional, or if her parents have been discussing group home placement, just as would be determined in an individual without ID.

Some problem behaviors can be shocking and extreme, but an individual with ID should not be diagnosed with a psychotic disorder unless they meet criteria for one.

Clinical Vignette #9

Extreme behavior   Denise was heard screaming from the exam room, "I'm not going to be here. I'm going to kill myself. They can just come to take me away."

Denise was brought into the emergency room by the police after an altercation with her roommate. Denise carried a diagnosis of schizoaffective disorder, and care was taken to evaluate her. She denied auditory and visual hallucinations as well as delusions.

Her caregiver reported that her ex-boyfriend had begun dating her roommate. Denise had punched her roommate, saying, "I'm going to beat her. I'm going to kill her."

Although Denise's presentation in Clinical Vignette #9 is dramatic, she does not meet criteria for a psychotic disorder. She may require emergency medication to ensure her safety and evaluation or detainment until it can be assured that both she and her roommate are safe, which then will be tapered and discontinued.

Differentiating self-stimulation from psychotic illness

Stereotypic behavior, most often called self-stimulation or "self-stim" in the treatment community of individuals with ID, was described by Harris & Wolchick (1979) as "repetitive bodily movement which serves no apparent purpose in the external environment." Some common forms of self-stimulation include rocking the trunk back and forth or side-to-side, hand-flapping, finger-tapping and repetitive vocal sounds. See Table 2.

Self-stimulation is seen in individuals with pervasive developmental disorders, such as autism, Asperger's syndrome, and Pervasive Developmental Disorder Not Otherwise Specified. If the clinician does not know the individual well, differentiating these symptoms is challenging but possible. Because schizophrenia and other psychotic disorders are typically first experienced after childhood, and usually after adolescence, the clinician should look for a change from the baseline of the individual (see Clinical Vignette #2).

Disorganized symptoms appear with the onset of schizophrenia. If an individual has always had the self-stimulating behavior, or a habit of waving his or her arms in the air, this would not be considered a disorganized symptom of emerging schizophrenia.

Additionally, autistic disorder and autism spectrum disorders can be difficult to distinguish from psychotic disorders. Autism, meaning "withdrawing into the self," was even one of Bleuler's "Four As" used to describe Schizophrenia. Autistic disorder is described as a failure in varying degrees since childhood of social relatedness and communication, e.g. poor eye contact, delayed and pedantic speech, and restricted behaviors. Individuals with psychotic disorders can have difficulties with social relatedness but, to qualify as a symptom of a psychotic disorder, a change from the baseline is required. The symptoms of a psychotic disorder also tend to wax and wane more than those of autism.

Exclusion from scientific literature

With the exception for journals devoted to intellectual or developmental disabilities, individuals with ID are usually excluded from major studies (e.g. the NIMH 2005 CATIE

Table 2 Clinical Pearls: Differentiating stereotypies/self-stimulation from psychotic symptoms.

Timeline	Stereotypies/'self-stim' behaviors are present from childhood, while psychotic symptoms of disorganization are not.
Repetition	Stereotypies and self-stim are usually repetitive, while psychotic symptoms of disorganization are much less organized.

study, Lieberman, 2005) that looked at the effectiveness of antipsychotic medications in people with schizophrenia.

People with ID are also excluded from major drug trials and all but completely ignored in the psychotherapy literature. This places more importance on the literature that is published, and Matson *et al.* (2003) argued that the lack of scientific rigor in the published works can be worse at times than none.

Diagnostic manual-intellectual disability (DM-ID)

There are also fewer standardized rating scales for research in individuals with ID, and the DSM-IV-TR criteria are somewhat cumbersome and difficult to use in individuals with ID when diagnosing mental illness.

In 2007, NADD, in association with the American Psychiatric Association, undertook an evidenced-based approach to applying the DSM-IV-TR criteria to individuals with ID, in order to make the diagnoses more applicable to the ID population, publishing the Diagnostic Manual-Intellectual Disability (Fletcher *et al.*, 2007), DM-ID. It is analogous to the DC-LD: Diagnostic Criteria for Psychiatric Disorders for Use with Adults with Learning Disabilities/Mental Retardation, which uses the ICD-10 as a base reference as opposed to the DSM.

Schizophrenia

Historical perspective

In Western medicine, Emile Kraeplin first described what is now known as schizophrenia as *dementia praecox*. Kraeplin noticed that a decline, like that seen in the then-named senile dementia, was occurring in adolescents that resulted in a "mental weakness." Then the term *schizophrenia*, meaning split mind, was coined by Eugen Bleuler in 1911. Bleuler introduced the "four As" of schizophrenia: autism (directing thoughts inward), looseness of associations (words beginning to lose connections or meaning in the context of a thought or sentence), ambivalence (strong and simultaneous conflicting feelings), and affective flattening (loss of the normal range of emotions). When the first DSM was compiled in 1952, the term *schizophrenic reaction* was used. It was described as "a strong tendency to retreat from reality, by emotional disharmony, unpredictable disturbances in stream of thought, regressive behavior, and in some, by a tendency to 'deterioration'." DSM-II (1968) describes schizophrenia as being:

> "...*manifested by characteristic disturbances of thinking, mood and behavior. Disturbances in thinking are marked by alterations of concept formation which may lead to misinterpretation of reality and sometimes to delusions and hallu- cinations, which frequently appear psychologically self-protective. Corollary mood changes include ambivalent, constricted and inappropriate emotional responsiveness and loss of empathy with others. Behavior may be withdrawn, regressive and bizarre.*"

It would only make sense that these vague definitions would have led to inaccurate and imprecise diagnoses in the past. The DSM-III (1980) was the first DSM to include diagnostic criteria (delusions, hallucinations, disorganized behavior) and multi-axial evaluation. The DSM-III included an exhortation diagnosis of individuals with ID:

> *"In Mental Retardation, low level of social functioning, oddities of behavior, and impoverished affect and cognition all may suggest Schizophrenia. Both diagnoses should be made in the same individual only when there is certainty that the symptoms suggesting Schizophrenia, such as delusions or hallucinations, are definitely present and are not the result of difficulties in communication."*

Clinicians today might emphasize the second idea over the first, but these ideas remain applicable.

Current diagnosis

As discussed previously, individuals with ID are thought to have co-occurring schizophrenia in up to 3% of cases, rather than the general population's 1%. This is important to bear in mind when treating individuals with ID.

Hallucinations

Combinations of positive and negative symptoms are specific to each type of schizophrenia: paranoid, catatonic, and disorganized. Auditory hallucinations, considered a positive symptom, are the most commonly occurring hallucinations in schizophrenia. Visual, tactile, gustatory and olfactory hallucinations can be present in varying frequencies, but these are usually more often seen in other conditions, e.g. delirium (visual hallucinations) or substance withdrawal (tactile hallucinations).

Asking the patient about hallucinations is the least difficult way to determine their presence. As discussed above, the clinician needs to differentiate between the patient's own thoughts (inner-speech) and self-talk from true auditory hallucinations. A question such as, "Do you hear people talk to you when you're alone?," followed up by asking for a description of the content, can be helpful.

Caregiver observations are invaluable if the individual with ID is denying hallucinations. Denial of symptoms is, of course, not limited to individuals with ID, but it does appear to happen less frequently than in individuals with schizophrenia but without ID.

Delusions

Delusions, also positive symptoms, are by definition fixed, false beliefs that can take many forms. The most common delusion is paranoia – the idea that someone or something is intending to harm the individual with the delusion.

In order to be considered a delusion, there has to be relative certainty that what the patient fears is not true or not actually happening. For example, if someone is worried about being moved from their group home by the state or county board, it might be just that – a worry. However, if the person is unable to be dissuaded from a false belief, and the state or county board is not considering moving them, or has not considered this, then the belief takes on the proportions of a delusion.

Typically, people with delusions are more likely to want to discuss them (DM-ID: Fletcher *et al.*, 2007) with caregivers and clinicians. Delusions may be nihilistic, erotomanic, jealous, somatic or grandiose. They may seem bizarre, in that the delusion is not possible (e.g. space aliens injecting processing chips into nasal cavities for tracking purposes). Delusions are called "non-bizarre" when they are possible in reality (e.g. thinking the FBI is tracking one's whereabouts). Delusions of control are less frequent in individuals with ID, but it is uncertain whether this is because the level of communication to convey these ideas is not present, or if the symptomatology is not present as often.

Negative symptoms

Affective flattening, impaired cognition, poverty of speech and thought, and avolition are generally considered negative symptoms of schizophrenia and other psychotic disorders. Negative symptoms can be hard to diagnose if the patient is not known well, as some individuals with ID have decreased affective range, idiosyncratic or bizarre-looking behaviors. Interviewing the caregiver then becomes that much more important.

Disorganized symptoms

Disorganized behavior and speech can also be difficult to diagnose, for the same reasons that negative symptoms are hard to diagnose. Disorganized thinking can be observed in the speech pattern of the patient. Loosening of associations, often devolving into "word salad" (a jumbled mix of words with no seeming structure or meaning), can be observed.

Disorganized behavior and catatonic behavior are in the same criteria in the DSM-IV-TR (American Psychiatric Association, 2000) and refer to behavior that is typically nonsensical and done with no apparent connection to reality (e.g. raising arms above the head; standing, then sitting, then standing). Catatonia movement can either be excessive or extremely reduced. A catatonic symptom called catalepsy occurs when a patient becomes "stuck" in a position which can then be held for hours if no intervention is made.

Echolalia (repeating words said by others) or echopraxia (repeating movements done by others) are also symptoms of disorganized behavior and catatonia. In individuals with ID, disorganized behavior must be differentiated from self-stimulating behavior seen in people with ID. Self-stimulation is usually a pattern of behaviors.

Table 3 Clinical Pearls: General recommendations for diagnosis and treatment of psychotic disorder.

Individuals with ID:
- should be diagnosed with much the same rigor and by the same diagnostic criteria as individuals without ID;
- should be offered the same treatment that individuals without ID would be offered: reasonable medications, psychotherapy and case management.

DSM-IV-TR and DM-ID Diagnosis of schizophrenia

The DSM-IV-TR criteria for schizophrenia describe the characteristic symptoms: hallu-cinations; delusions; disorganized speech; disorganized behavior; and negative symptoms. The requirement for social and/or occupational dysfunction is also addressed (see Table 4). The majority of the criteria do not require adaptation for individuals with ID. However, the DM-ID does note:

> "A significant behavior change – for example, an increase in aggressive, self-injurious, or bizarre behavior – should alert the clinician to the possibility of a psychotic process. Assessment of this criterion might be especially difficult in individuals with Severe or Profound ID."
>
> (American Psychiatric Association, 2000)

Criterion A, the characteristic symptoms, also did not require adaptation, but the editors of the DM-ID did note there may be self-talk, which is common and not necessarily interpreted as an extension of Psychotic Disorder. See Tables 3 and 4.

Table 4   DSM-IV-TR and DM-ID criteria for diagnosis of schizophrenia.

			DM-ID adaptation
A	Characteristic symptoms	Two (or more) of the following, each present for a significant portion of time during a one-month period (or less if successfully treated):	None
		1. delusions	
		2. hallucinations	
		3. disorganized speech (e.g., frequent derailment or incoherence)	
		4. grossly disorganized or catatonic behavior	
		5. negative symptoms, i.e., affective flattening, alogia or avolition	
		Note: There may be self-talk, which is common and not necessarily interpreted as an extension of Psychotic Disorder.	
B	Social/ occupational dysfunction	For a significant portion of the time since the onset of the disturbance, on or more major areas of functioning such as work, interpersonal relations, or self-care are markedly below the level achieved prior to the onset (or when the onset is in childhood or adolescence, failure to achieve expected level of interpersonal, academic, or occupational achievement).	None
C	Duration	Continuous signs of the disturbance persist for at least 6 months. This 6-month period must include at least 1 month of symptoms (or less if successfully treated) that meet Criterion A (i.e. active-phase symptoms) and may include periods of prodromal or residual symptoms. During these prodromal or	None

(continued)

Table 4 (*Continued*)

			DM-ID adaptation
		residual periods, the signs of the disturbance may be manifested by only negative symptoms or two or more symptoms listed in Criterion A present in an attenuated form (e.g., odd beliefs, unusual perceptual experiences).	
D	Schizoaffective and mood disorder exclusion	Schizoaffective disorder and mood disorder with psychotic features have been ruled out because either: 1. no major depressive, manic or mixed episodes have occurred concurrently with the active-phase symptoms; or 2. if mood episodes have occurred during active-phase symptoms, their total duration has been brief relative to the duration of the active and residual periods.	None
E	Substance/ general medical condition exclusion	The disturbance is not due to the direct physiological effects of a substance (e.g., a drug of abuse, a medication) or a general medical condition.	None
F	Relationship to a pervasive developmental disorder	If there is a history of autistic disorder or another pervasive developmental disorder, the additional diagnosis of schizophrenia is made only if prominent delusions or hallucinations are also present for at least a month (or less if successfully treated).	None

Source: Reproduced with permission from the Diagnostic and Statistical Manual of Mental Disorders, Fourth Edition, Text Revision (DSM-IV TR), American Psychiatric Association, 2000, page 312; Fletcher, R., Loschen, E., Stavrakaki, C., & First, M. (eds., 2007). *Diagnostic Manual – Intellectual Disability (DM-ID): A Textbook of Diagnosis of Mental Disorders in Persons with Intellectual Disability*. NADD Press, Kingston, NY, pp. 260–261.

Clinical Vignette #10

Schizophrenia, mild ID   Linda was a 29 year old white woman who had been diagnosed with mild ID as a child. She lived in a community group home with three roommates, with 24-hour care providers. Linda was referred by her home manager for "voices."

Linda sat in the chair closest the door upon entering the exam room. She shot a glance to her home manager, Patricia, as she sat in the other chair. When asked what the appointment was for, Linda said, "Because my guts are rotten." Patricia, who had known Linda for ten years, reminded Linda that there were there to discuss her "voices." Linda said, "But my guts are dead. They rotted. There's a snake in there."

Patricia reassured Linda that the gastroenterologist had found nothing out of the ordinary in a thorough workup, but Linda remained unconvinced. She said, "Well, my roommates are all talking about it." Patricia said Linda had always talked to herself, repeating parts of conversations from the day or thinking out loud; however, she had became concerned two or three weeks ago when Linda began accusing people of talking about her when she was alone. Linda had also stopped doing her usual activities of daily living, and she had been hostile to the staff when they had to remind her to take a shower or brush her teeth.

Her psychiatrist asked, "Do you ever hear people talk about you when no one is around?" Linda glared at the psychiatrist and said, "No."

Patricia said that the workshop had reported that she had yelled at her work group to stop talking about her. They had been playing video games, but not talking about Linda. Patricia attempted to reassure Linda that no one had been talking about her, but Linda yelled, "I don't believe you lying snakes." Patricia reported she was especially concerned because she and Linda had always had a good relationship before, but it had become strained due to Linda's belief people were conspiring against her.

Diagnosis

Given the time frame, Linda does not yet meet DM-ID criteria for schizophrenia, but she does have auditory hallucinations in addition to somatic and paranoid delusions. The DM-ID does not make any adaptations in the criteria for mild ID. Individuals with ID have a threefold increased prevalence in schizophrenia over the general population. Attention to changes in baseline function and a good longitudinal understanding of the individual can be very helpful in making an accurate diagnosis.

Self-talk vs. psychosis

In individuals with ID, self-talk may be confused for psychotic symptoms. In Linda's case, the clue that she is having auditory hallucinations rather than just talking to herself is that her baseline behavior has changed. Before her current episode, Linda was observed talking to herself but she had never accused people of talking about her.

Treatment

After a thorough medical evaluation, Linda was started on risperidone and was seen for her routine follow-up. She remained very suspicious of Patricia and her psychiatrist. She was noticed to be attending to internal stimuli during the appointment and spitting into the trashcan. Patricia said her staff suspected that Linda was trying to induce emesis in the bathroom after medication administration.

Linda was started on an orally disintegrating risperidone and monitored medication passes. After two weeks, Linda reported that her roommates were saying fewer things about her. After a month of treatment, she no longer mentioned having snakes inside her guts. She was more productive at work and reported a better relationship with Patricia and with her roommates. She continued to complain that her care providers were talking about her, but the treatment team decided that it was most likely based in reality, due to things like shift-change and check-out procedures in the home.

Clinical Vignette #11

Schizophrenia, severe/moderate: "haze jesus"   "Haze Jesus, haze Jesus, haze Jesus." Elliot, a 24 year old man, was easily heard as he came down the hallway for his initial appointment. When he came into the office, he turned to sit in the chair but did not sit. He crouched above the chair, then stood back up. He did this several times until his father, Mark, firmly guided him to sit.

Mark said, "Elliot just hasn't been himself. About a year ago, he just started having all these problems. He used to be able to answer simple questions. It's so embarrassing, this 'Haze Jesus' thing he says over and over. It's about all he says anymore. And he used to get dressed and brush his hair and teeth. He used to be able to follow directions. Now he does all these weird things – like getting up in the middle of the night pacing, rubbing cooking oil on the doors and windowsills, laughing and crying for no reason. He used to do arts and crafts at workshop, but they say there he stands around repeating the same things. They said one time he even got stuck, like he bent over all weird, and they couldn't get his to stand back up."

Throughout the interview, Elliot responded to all questions by repeating the last word asked, then saying "Haze Jesus." He laughed inappropriately in the interview and he stood up and then sat down again for no reason, several times. He did not appear to be responding or attending to internal stimuli. He was not observed to act in a way that would convey paranoia, and his father concurred that no symptoms had been observed at home or at work. Elliot regularly sees his family doctor.

Diagnosis

Elliot's symptoms appear to be consistent with schizophrenia, catatonic type. According to the DM-ID, there are no adaptations to the DSM-IV-TR criteria. Elliot demonstrated catalepsy, excessive, purposeless motoric activity; peculiarities of voluntary movement and echolalia.

Treatment

In conjunction with a thorough medical work-up, antipsychotics were recommended. Over the course of several months, many antipsychotics were tried, but Mark reported that each one gave Elliot intolerable side effects: vomiting, diarrhea, increased agitation, sedation. Sometimes, the side effects happened after one dose, and then Mark would stop administering the medication.

The psychiatrist met with Mark privately to discuss Elliot's side effects and Mark's concerns. Mark was both worried that the medications would hurt Elliot, and that Elliot would have to take them forever. He said that he would try one more medication if the psychiatrist would agree to start at a low dose and to only increase it very slowly. Low-dose risperidone was started nightly. Elliot tolerated this and, after two weeks, it was increased to twice a day.

The psychiatrist received positive feedback from Elliot's workshop that he had been able to focus on tasks and follow directions. Elliot came back for his follow-up appointment and, when asked how he was doing, he said, "Fine, thank you." He answered a few more questions appropriately before saying "Haze Jesus."

His medication was continued, and his workshop continued to report gains. Soon Elliot was taking care of himself again, and his bizarre behaviors slowed and then stopped over the course of the next two months. Elliot did well at home over the next six months and was participating in arts and crafts at workshop. Unfortunately, he missed his next two appointments despite attempts reschedule, and his workshop reported that the behaviors returned over the next several months.

Discussion

The same issues that plague treatment of individuals without disabilities are present in treatment of individuals with ID. Adherence to medications has been measured at around 55% of the general population with schizophrenia (Fenton *et al.*, 1997). This is likely to be different in individuals with ID because many people live in group homes or have monitored medication administration (staff, family), but concerns of patients and family about the safety and efficacy of medications are still present. Working closely with staff and family is helpful in addressing concerns of diagnoses and treatment.

Schizophrenia subtypes

On the whole, the various types of schizophrenia – paranoid, disorganized, catatonic, undifferentiated and residual – did not require adaptation for individuals with mild to moderate ID in the DM-ID, but caution was advised. The usefulness of utilizing subtypes was also questioned. For individuals with severe to profound ID, the DM-ID lists characteristic symptoms as delusions, hallucinations and a significant change in behavior (increased aggression or self-injurious behavior), and it advises that the subtypes should not be applied to individuals with severe to profound ID.

Schizophreniform disorder

Langfelt (1983) first applied the term "schizophreniform" to individuals with schizophrenic symptoms with good prognosis, to differentiate from those with poor prognosis. The DSM-III incorporated this term and, while Langfelt disagreed with the newer definition, is has come to be applied to individuals who meet DSM-IV-TR Criteria A (characteristic symptoms), D (schizoaffective and mood disorders exclusion) and E (substance and general medical condition exclusion) for at least one month but not more than six months.

The scientific literature is scant on the topic of schizophreniform disorder in general, and particularly in individuals with ID, but it is likely to be more prevalent in individuals with ID as they have higher rates of psychotic illnesses over the general population, thought to be 0.1–0.2% (Myers *et al.*, 1984). The DM-ID makes no adaptations for DSM-IV-TR criteria for individuals with mild to moderate ID or for individuals with severe to profound ID. Individuals diagnosed with schizophreniform disorder may not have a recurrence of psychotic symptoms, but it is estimated that 60–80% of people diagnosed will progress to schizophrenia (Sadock & Sadock, 2003).

The DSM specifies with or without good prognostic features. Good prognostic features are: onset of prominent psychotic symptoms within four weeks of the first noticeable change in usual behavior or functioning; confusion or perplexity at the height of the psychotic episode, good premorbid social and occupational functioning; and absence of blunted or flat affect.

In interviewing an individual with ID who is suspected of having schizophreniform disorder, note should be made of premorbid functioning. Did this person do well at workshop? Did he or she work in the community? Does he or she live independently or at an intermediate care facility? These are factors that influence prognosis.

Chronicity of symptoms is vital in making the schizophreniform disorder diagnosis, so interview of caregivers and habilitation staff should be done meticulously to differentiate between a previously undiagnosed schizophrenia and brief psychotic disorder. As with all patients regardless of IQ, a careful medical history should be taken to exclude underlying medical or substance disorders that could be contributing to symptom presentation. Interviewing techniques described previously in this chapter or in earlier chapters are applicable here as well. Clear, concise questions with minimal jargon are helpful.

Clinical Vignette #12

Medical conditions   Sally has severe ID and was brought to the mental health clinic after her primary caregiver, Linda became concerned.

About two months ago, Sally started acting in an unusual manner. Before going to sleep at night, she would pull Linda to her closet and then to the windows, to have Linda double-check that they were closed. Linda said, "That was pretty strange for her, but we didn't think much of it, until she started to cower in the corner and cover her ears. We took her to the family doctor to get her checked out, but Dr. Jones said her ears were fine. There was nothing else, either."

Sally began having difficulty in her habilitation/supported employment program and was not interested in magazines as she had previously been. She began screaming at people who were not there.

Following up Clinical Vignette #12, after careful evaluation of Sally's medical status (i.e. that she did not have an ear infection, headache or other medical illness), a diagnosis of schizophreniform disorder should be suspected. It should also be determined that nothing was occurring in Sally's bedroom at night, as abuse is, unfortunately, a too-common occurrence in individuals with ID. Continued observation with behavioral monitoring, to rule out antecedent actions to screaming at workshop, should be undertaken as well. Treatment with an antipsychotic medication is indicated. Sally should be monitored closely for side effects as well.

Schizoaffective disorder

Psychiatry and psychology have long struggled with the overlap of the psychotic disorders and the affective disorders. Some clinicians diagnose individuals with schizoaffective disorder as a provisional diagnosis while waiting for more information to make a definitive diagnosis. Other clinicians are more deliberate in their diagnoses. Because this diagnosis has been in flux even in recent history (Levitt & Tsuang, 1988), schizoaffective disorder has been categorized as a "schizophrenic" illness and as an affective one. The DSM-IV-TR categorizes it with the psychotic illnesses such as schizophrenia, but the description is that of a primarily affective disorder (See Table 6), with at least two weeks of a discrete episode of psychotic symptoms.

The prevalence in the general population appears to be less than 1% in lifetime prevalence, and was measured at around 0.3% (Perälä et al., 2007). The scientific literature regarding ID and schizoaffective disorder is also limited, but it is likely that the rate of schizoaffective disorder is higher for individuals with ID, just as it is with other psychotic diagnoses.

In individuals with mild to moderate ID, the DM-ID reports that the criteria can be used successfully without adaptation. The modified criteria for mood disorders should be adhered to (see Chapter 7). In individuals with severe to profound ID, the DM-ID advocates for a longitudinal approach with careful evaluation of corroborative evidence, specialist assessment, and observation. See Clinical Vignette #3 for a discussion of schizoaffective disorder and autistic disorder.

Careful assessment is required in making this diagnosis. The DM-ID exhorts clinicians to remember that a serious change in behavior ("for example, an increase in aggressive, self-injurious, or bizarre behavior") should be a clue to an underlying psychotic disorder. The DM-ID also notes that individuals with severe or profound ID may be more difficult to assess.

As with most psychotic disorders, timeline is important to diagnosis. Because individuals with ID can have difficulty with details and specifics, caregiver input is valuable. Of course, the individual should be carefully assessed for medical and substance disorders that can contribute to psychiatric symptom presentation.

Delusional disorder

Delusional disorder is characterized by the presence of a non-bizarre delusion of at least one month's duration. Non-bizarre delusions must be about phenomena that, although not real, are within the realm of being possible (Patel *et al.*, 2003). The prevalence in the general population is estimated to be around 0.03% and comprising 1–2% of admissions to inpatient mental health units (DSM-IV-TR). Delusions in this disorder may include the famous eponymous syndrome *de Clerambault's Syndrome,* which was historically thought to be caused by unrequited love or excessive physical love (Berrios, 2002).

Persecutory delusions may be one of the more common types of this uncommon illness. The literary-named *Othello Syndrome* describes the jealous delusion that can occur in romantic relationships. Other delusions include somatic (see example below), grandiose, mixed and unspecified.

Prevalence in individuals with ID is unknown. Since individuals with ID tend to have more bizarre delusions, this diagnosis may be difficult to apply. The DM-ID suggests that it is possible to utilize current DSM-IV-TR criteria in people with mild to moderate ID, but that it is likely to be unhelpful and should be removed from the classification system for people with severe or profound ID (see Clinical Vignette #13).

Clinical Vignette #13

Somatic delusional disorder   Howard presented to the mental health clinic after being referred by his primary care doctor. Howard's mother reported that he had been checked over very well, but he continued to believe he was infested with bugs.

His family home had been overrun with bedbugs and had several treatments over the course of months. During this time, Howard became convinced that his clothing, bed, bathroom, and the car had bedbugs. His mother, several exterminators and his brother were not able to convince him otherwise.

Howard continued to go to work, but he had been picking at his skin more and more. He would put stray pieces of fuzz in an old pill bottle and show him to his mother as proof of bedbugs.

In Clinical Vignette #13, while it is likely that Howard and his mother might actually continue to have bedbugs, a few things point to a somatic delusional disorder instead. One is the so-called *matchbox sign* (Lee, 2008), the container that Howard brought in to prove the existence of bedbugs. The other is that he continues to believe the bedbugs are there, despite many otherwise convincing reassurances to the contrary. The DM-ID states that the diagnosis of delusional disorder should not be applied to individuals with severe or profound ID.

Brief psychotic disorder

Formerly called "brief reactive psychosis" and concordant with the ICD-10 diagnosis acute and transient psychotic disorder (Pillmann *et al.*, 2002), brief psychotic disorder is a disturbance of at least one day but not more than one month, usually with abrupt onset. Because of the relatively rare nature of brief psychotic disorder, the literature on it is limited and, in individuals with ID, it is usually lumped in with "other psychotic disorders."

Historically, reactive psychosis required a clear and traumatic stressor and close relationship in time between symptomatology and the stressors. Now, the DSM-IV-TR criteria do not require a stressor. A European study (Jørgensen *et al.*, 1996) found that individuals with acute and transient psychotic disorder were mostly women in early adulthood with good premorbid social functioning and few psychosocial stressors.

Cultural issues in brief psychotic disorder

It is important to remember that different cultures have different norms. This can be easily forgotten in individuals with ID as, unfortunately all too often, families drift apart. For example, the Evangelical Christian tradition of speaking in tongues when moved by the Spirit of the Lord may look unusual to outsiders, just as the Catholic tradition of eating the body and drinking the blood of Christ might also seem unusual.

Clinical Vignette #14

Audrey: schizoaffective disorder and autism   Audrey was a 20 year old woman who had previously been diagnosed with autism. She had also been diagnosed with moderate to severe ID due to her significant limitations in communication. Tony, her primary caregiver at the group home, brought Audrey to the mental health clinic after she returned from vacation with her family. Tony and the other care providers noticed that she was no longer sleeping well at night (1–2 hours), and was smiling and giggling inappropriately.

Tony reported that Audrey normally kept to a very strict routine, including work and her one hobby (watching her favorite movie, *Back to the Future*). Tony said that Audrey had been whispering about vampires. She usually only repeated lines from her movie or a few other stereotyped phrases, but she had begun talking much more frequently about things she had not talked about before. This had only started when Audrey stopped sleeping. In the week before presenting, Audrey had stopped watching movies because she was too occupied with pacing to sit still. Audrey was asked to stay home from her sheltered workshop because of threatening and aggressive behaviors.

Audrey was started on valproic acid, and within a week, she was sleeping and back to watching her favorite movie. She did well for several months but, at a routine check-up, Audrey's mother said, "The look in her eyes isn't right. She seems scared." She mentioned that Audrey seemed less interested in *Back to the Future* and had begun peering out the front window of the group home.

On a weekend visit to his mother's house, Audrey went to the front window every time a car would drive past. Audrey appeared very worried about this, but she was still sleeping relatively well and did not demonstrate any other mood symptoms. During the exam, Audrey had poor eye contact, which was normal for her, but she also appeared to be responding to voices that only she could hear. When the psychiatrist asked about this symptom, Audrey's mother reported that it had only started in the last few days.

Diagnosis
Audrey appears to have schizoaffective disorder, bipolar type. According to the DSM-IV-TR and the DM-ID, schizoaffective disorder is having, at some time during an uninterrupted period of illness, a major depressive, manic, or mixed episode concurrent with symptoms that meet the characteristic symptoms criteria for schizophrenia. In addition, there must be delusions or hallucinations for at least two weeks in the absence of prominent mood symptoms. The mood symptoms are present for a substantial portion of the total duration of the illness.

Initially, it was thought that Audrey had bipolar disorder, until she began developing psychotic symptoms that were separate from her mood symptoms. The DM-ID makes some allowances for the diagnosis of a manic episode in individuals with ID – namely, and applicable in this case, that a person with limited expressive language skills may have two additional symptoms in conjunction with elevated or expansive mood, and three additional symptoms in the presence of an irritable mood, rather than three and four respectively.

Treatment
Audrey was started on aripiprazole after developing psychotic symptoms. Since aripiprazole is indicated in not only schizophrenia but also autism-related irritability and acute bipolar manic episodes, it is the plan of Audrey's treatment team to gradually stop her valproic acid to reduce polypharmacy. Audrey's case is complicated due to her limited communication but, with the observations of her care staff, family, and treatment team, her diagnosis becomes more definitive.

Shared psychotic disorder (Folie à Deux)

Shared psychotic disorder has been documented for centuries. *Folie communiqué*, psychosis of association and double insanity are all terms that have been used to describe the same shared psychotic disorder (Arnone *et al.*, 2006) that remains notorious in popular imagination. The disorder has typically been characterized as one person, designated the "primary," inducing or transferring the delusions to another person or persons, designated as the "secondary" or "secondaries." Lasègue & Falret (1877) posited that the "primary" individual has a psychotic disorder and is in a close relationship with a passive, more suggestible and less intelligent "secondary," who then develops the delusions of the "primary."

More recent data (Arnone *et al.*, 2006) have shown that the idea that the "secondary," who was traditionally described to have a submissive role in the dyad but otherwise mentally sound, could themselves have a significant mental illness. The study also showed that the treatment of separation was inadequate in a number of the cases. Again, there remains little but case reports in the literature on individuals with ID. Wherein the previous descriptions of the "secondary" might fit more with individuals with ID, it remains unknown if individuals with ID are more susceptible to shared psychotic disorder. It could be postulated that they are, given the dependent situations many people with ID are in, e.g. relying on family and community.

A careful interview should be undertaken with both the identified patient and the caregivers. Usually, in individuals with ID, care is sought after the situation has been discovered and the individuals have been separated.

Clinical Vignette #15

Shared delusional disorder vs. brief psychotic disorder   Adam was a 36 year old man who was diagnosed with moderate intellectual disability. His case manager recommended he be seen by a psychiatrist to evaluate grief and loss issues. Adam's mother had died suddenly and his sister, Claudia, had become Adam's guardian.

Claudia discovered that there were many pill bottles in Adam's name for prescription pain pills, anxiolytics and antipsychotics. She reported that she never even knew Adam had been seeing a doctor for any of these issues, and did not give him any of the medications because she did not know what was safe. She suspected that a neighbor had been using Adam to procure drugs.

Around the same time, Adam's father, now his only caregiver, was diagnosed with Alzheimer's Disease. Claudia also discovered that Adam was not receiving the basic care due to his father's dementia. Adam was quickly moved to a group home for health and safety reasons, despite his wish to stay with his frail father.

Upon exam, Adam had extremely poor eye contact and was suspicious of the people and surroundings in the office. Adam reported that he didn't like his roommates because "they're bad guys who want to hurt me." Claudia said, "It's been really hard for him adjusting to his new place. But they're good people there. Mom and Dad would always tell him things like that – that people are bad and will hurt you if you don't watch out. I don't know if that's one of the things somebody told him to say to the doctors, or if it's true." Adam refused to say any more.

Claudia estimated that Adam had been off medications for approximately a month, if he had ever been taking them. The psychiatrist met with Adam privately and he was able to be more open. He said, "I don't like the group home. They don't let you have the window open." He reported that sometimes he heard little boys talking about him outside his window. His caregiver was asked privately about this and reported that there were no boys nearby and that it was unlikely, due to his second floor bedroom, that Adam would be able to hear the conversation of boys on the street. Home staff had not noticed him attending to internal stimuli, but they did mention he was not open or trusting of anyone at his group home. His sleep chart indicated that he was up, pacing and looking out the window, for several hours each night, but Adam did not show any other symptoms of a mood disorder.

Treatment

After a thorough medical evaluation, Adam was started on quetiapine at night and was tapered up to a therapeutic dose. He began sleeping better almost immediately. He was started in the Grief and Loss Group at his daytime habilitation workshop, in addition to his own individual psychotherapy. At first he did not participate, but after a few weeks he started sharing feelings about the loss of his mother. He remained angry at his sister for removing him from his father's house, but he became more open with her as well.

After six months in treatment, the decision was made to slowly taper off Adam's quetiapine. Adam was back to his old self. He was able to enjoy spending time with his roommates, but he always valued his time alone in his room.

Discussion

The diagnosis of brief psychotic disorder is a difficult one to make, especially given that not much was known of Adam's history. Good prognostic indicators in Adam's care are that his psychosis was likely precipitated by an enormous stressor: the loss of his mother; the acute onset of symptoms with no apparent prodrome; and the return to normal functioning after treatment. Another diagnosis to consider in Adam's case is shared psychotic disorder. Little is known about the mental status of his mother or father but, if either one of them were delusional about people being bad or wanting to hurt Adam, the diagnosis could be considered. If that were the diagnosis, separation from the other half of the delusional pair and consideration of an antipsychotic may be indicated.

Psychotic disorder due to a general medical condition

The philosopher René Descartes theorized that the mind and body were distinct and separate entities (Spinoza, 1905), that the body was capable of doing and the mind of thinking. Medicine has long known that the mind and body interact. In Hippocrates' time, cases of hysteria were attributed to the womb periodically traveling to the brain, and they were treated with the urging of marriage. "My prescription is that when virgins experience this trouble, they should cohabit with a man as quickly as possible. If they become pregnant, they will be cured" (Hippocrates, 4th Century BCE). Psychotic disorders due to a general medical condition (GMC) follow along the same idea – that the body influences the mind – albeit with a little more factual evidence than the "wandering uterus."

The prevalence of psychotic disorder due to a GMC is difficult to determine, due to the varied nature of GMCs that can cause mental illness. The vast majority of individuals with psychotic illnesses have a primary psychiatric disorder, such as schizophrenia or schizoaffective disorder. One German study of 4,181 individuals (Jacobi *et al.*, 2004) found that a psychiatric illness due to a GMC was the least common of all mental illnesses, with 1.3% prevalence over a 12-month period. See Table 5.

While an outpatient psychiatric practice sees relatively few cases of psychotic disorder due to a GMC, case reports from hospital consult and liaison services abound. The DSM-IV-TR notes that as many as 20% of individuals presenting with untreated endocrine disorders, 15% of those with systemic lupus erythematosus, and up to 40% or more of individuals with temporal lobe epilepsy, have psychotic symptoms.

Individuals with ID often have higher rates of undiagnosed medical disorders than the general population. Communication difficulties can contribute to a missed diagnosis. When meeting with an individual with psychotic symptoms, it is important to rule out or rule in a general medical condition as a cause of psychosis. The presence of a GMC is often a helpful clue that there is more than a case of schizophrenia, especially if it known to cause psychiatric symptoms. Some common diseases that cause psychotic symptoms are intracranial tumors, systemic lupus erythematosus, neurosyphilis, epilepsy (especially since people with ID also have an increased incidence of seizure disorders), AIDS and Huntington's. "Myxedema Madness," known as psychosis due to hypothyroidism, and hyperthyroidism can both cause psychosis. Remember also that individuals with ID may have different responses to somatic complaints, e.g. head-banging for an earache or headache, self-injurious or aggressive behavior in response to pain, biting fingers for pain of acid reflux, etc.

Table 5 Causes of psychosis due to a general medical condition.

• Epilepsy
• Encephalitis
• Huntington's Disease
• Sydenham's chorea
• Chorea gravidarum
• Manganism
• Creutzfeld-Jakob disease
• Hashimoto's encephalopathy
• Wilson's disease
• AIDS
• Systemic Lupus Erythematosus
• Hyperthyroidism
• Hypothyroidism

Source: Tasman *et al.*, 2003, p. 899.

The coincidental presentation of symptoms of a GMC and of a psychotic disorder should also raise the clinician's level of suspicion. Symptoms atypical of a primary psychotic disorder should also be investigated. For example, a 60 year old woman with no previous mental health history usually does not develop a primary psychotic disorder. Symptoms such as visual or olfactory hallucinations are a sign that there might be a GMC as well.

Psychotic disorder due to a GMC, by definition, is distinctly separate from the diagnosis of delirium, as psychotic disorder due to a GMC occurs in a clear sensorium, while the sensorium in delirium waxes and wanes. In individuals with ID, sensorium can be a difficult thing to determine, due to communication difficulties.

The non-specific and unscientific term "confusion" can describe delirium accurately, e.g. confusion about who caregivers are, where the individual is, talking as if they were in the past, which must be a change from baseline. The entire clinical picture must be examined to make an accurate clinical diagnosis.

Substance-induced psychotic disorder

The discovery of alcohol dates from 9000–4000 BCE (Standage, 2005), with alcohol-induced psychotic disorder probably not following too far behind. Other naturally occurring hallucinogens (e.g. peyote, jimson weed) and other psychoactive substances (e.g. opium, cocaine) have likely been causing substance-induced psychotic disorders for just as long, if not longer. As with psychotic disorder due to a general medical condition, the sensorium must be clear and reality testing must be impaired.

Substance use disorders were once considered rare in individuals with ID but, as individuals with ID are living more in community settings rather than the institutional ones, drugs and alcohol have become more readily available. Recent research (McGillicuddy, 2006) has shown that, while individuals with ID still have lower rates of use than peers, it is a problem for many individuals. Other research indicates that less use than individuals without disabilities may have more of an impact and necessitate more crises (Westermeyer

Table 6   Medications causing substance-induced psychotic disorder.

- Levetiracetam
- Corticosteroids
- Dopaminergic drugs (like those used for Parkinson's)
- Bupropion
- Fluoxetine
- Sympathomimetics

Source: Tasman *et al.*, 2003, p. 902.

et al., 1995). Diagnostic overshadowing is likely present to an extent here, too, so it is always important to remember substance-induced psychotic disorder in the differential diagnosis for psychotic disorders.

In the current iteration of the DSM-IV-TR, if a medication causes psychotic symptoms, it is diagnosed as a substance-induced psychotic disorder. While many medications have many side effects, an incomplete list is provided in Table 6.

Psychotic disorder not otherwise specified

Psychotic disorder not otherwise specified (NOS) remains the catch-all for psychotic disorders that do not fit the criteria for another specific diagnosis. Within this diagnosis are postpartum psychosis, which has been recognized since the time of Hippocrates and Galen, and autoscopic psychosis, the visual hallucination of all or part of the person's own body. More common than these diagnoses, however, is the diagnosis of psychotic disorder NOS when there is not yet enough information to make a complete and definitive diagnosis of one of the other primary psychotic disorders.

Treatment of psychotic disorders

Safety

Of foremost importance is the safety of the individual. The clinician and treatment team should decide whether the patient needs inpatient care, or if his or her illness can safely be managed on an outpatient basis. Risk factors that may require inpatient hospitalization include: command hallucinations; grossly disorganized behavior (in that the person is no longer caring for his or her needs); significant risk of danger to self or others; or having a complicated medical comorbidity that may require monitoring, such as congestive heart failure, diabetes, heart disease or renal failure. The person's past history is helpful in making the determination to hospitalize. If inpatient hospitalization is not warranted, increased staff and caregiver supervision may be necessary until psychotic symptoms abate.

The other factor in ensuring the patient's safety is proper treatment of undiagnosed or untreated medical conditions that could be contributing to ill-health – mental or physical. This is usually accomplished by routine lab work including, but not limited to: complete blood count; thyroid levels; complete metabolic panel; immediate and long-term blood sugar levels; urinalysis; vitamin B12/folate; vitamin D; and levels of psychoactive and psychotropic medications.

Medications (see also Chapter 12)

Antipsychotics for psychotic symptoms (hallucinations, delusions, disorganization)
Psychotic disorders are a diverse group of illnesses, but are often similarly treated. After
careful evaluation and interviewing, psychotic symptoms like auditory and/or visual
hallucination, delusions, and disorganized speech and behavior are usually first treated
with an antipsychotic. There remains healthy debate on whether the effectiveness of atypical
antipsychotics (often called "atypicals" or second generation antipsychotics) is greater than
that of the typical antipsychotics, but the atypicals are usually the first line of treatment for
presenting psychotic symptoms. Just as in individuals without ID, polypharmacy is best
avoided unless symptomatic control cannot be attained with one medication.

Individuals with ID continue to be the group of people most prescribed antipsychotic
medications with some numbers suggesting 22–48% of individuals with ID taking
neuroleptics (Kiernan *et al.*, 1995; Spreat *et al.*, 1997). More recent trends indicate that
physicians are moving toward antidepressants (Santosh & Baird, 1999).

Benzodiazepines for catatonic symptoms (waxy flexibility, catalepsy)   First, the physician
should determine that the catatonia is due to a primary psychotic disorder or mood
disorder, and not because of neuroleptic malignant syndrome, non-convulsive status
epilepticus, metabolic derangement or another medical condition that resembles
catatonia. The care setting for a complicated case such as this would likely be in the
hospital. High-dose benzodiazepines are recommended in catatonia (Rosebush &
Mazurek, 2010). Other treatments include ECT, and dantrolene and carbamazepine
have been cited in case reports.

Mood stabilizers for mood symptoms of schizoaffective disorder   Because schizoaffective
disorder has symptoms that are both affective and psychotic, both affective treatments (mood
stabilizers) and psychotic treatments (antipsychotics) are used. Lithium, carbamazepine, and
valproate are usually first-line treatment of mania and are FDA (Food and Drug
Administration)-indicated as such. The literature remains mixed on bipolar depression,
with lithium being used traditionally but not being FDA-indicated. Quetiapine and
olanzapine plus fluoxetine are FDA-indicated for treatment of bipolar depression.

Psychotherapy

Psychotherapy is a much-overlooked treatment choice in individuals with ID. Some
psychotherapists express trepidation because of the level of difficulty that is assumed to
be needed to treat individuals with ID. Supportive and cognitive behavioral therapies have
been noted to be possible as well as helpful (Oathamshaw & Haddock, 2006; Gentile &
Jackson, 2008; see Chapter 13).

Involvement of treatment team

Bringing in supports and using all available resources is important with severe mental
illnesses like the psychotic disorders. Behavioral support specialists provide invaluable

information which allows tracking of specific behaviors, finding patterns and parsing out behaviors from psychotic symptoms. Caregivers, parents and other family bring important historical information to the proverbial table. Case managers have access to many resources that psychiatrists and other clinicians do not. Nursing staff can also provide valuable information from the workshops or habilitation programs, in addition to more detailed medical observation to supplement the physician's observations.

Summary

Psychotic disorders have had much attention throughout history and can be debilitating and destructive illnesses. However, they need not be. There are effective treatments, including medication, psychotherapy and behavioral strategies, that can help in decreasing suffering and increasing quality of life. Since individuals with ID appear to be more susceptible to psychotic disorders, a thorough, careful assessment of the patient with as many concerned caregivers, family and friends, is paramount in making an accurate diagnosis to begin treatment without delay.

References

American Psychiatric Association (1980). *Diagnostic and Statistical Manual of Mental Disorders*, 3rd Edition (DSM-III). APA, Washington DC.

American Psychiatric Association (2000). *Diagnostic and Statistical Manual of Mental Disorders*, 4th Edition, Text Revision (DSM-IV TR). Arlington, VA.

Arnone, D., Patel, A. & Tan, G.M.Y. (2006). The nosological significance of Folie à Deux: a review of the literature. *Annals of General Psychiatry* **5**, 11.

Berrios, G.E. (2002). Erotomania: a conceptual history. *History of Psychiatry* **13**(52), 381–400.

Bleuler, E. (1911). *Dementia Praecox or the Group of Schizophrenias*. Translated by Zinkin, J. (1950). International Universities Press, Inc., New York.

Cannon, M., Jones, P.B. & Murray, R.M. (2002). Obstetric Complications and Schizophrenia: Historical and Meta-Analytic Review. *American Journal of Psychiatry* **159**, 7.

Chai, S.L. (2008). Delusions of Parasitosis. *Dermatologic Therapy* **21**(1), 2–7.

Cooper, S.A., Smiley, E., Finlayson, J., Jackson, A., Allan, L., Williamson, A., Mantry, D. & Morrison, J. (2007). The prevalence, Incidence, and factors predictive of mental ill-health in adults with profound intellectual disabilities. *Journal of Applied Research in Intellectual Disabilities* **20**, 493–501.

Committee on Nomenclature and Statistics of the American Psychiatric Association (1952). *Diagnostic and Statistical Manual Mental Disorders*. (DSM-I). American Psychiatric Association, Washington, DC.

Committee on Nomenclature and Statistics of the American Psychiatric Association (1968). *Diagnostic and Statistical Manual of Mental Disorders*, 2nd Edition (DSM-II). American Psychiatric Association, Washington DC.

Fenton, W.S., Blyler, C.R. & Heinssen, R.K. (1997). Determinants of medication compliance in schizophrenia: empirical and clinical findings. *Schizophrenia Bulletin* **23**, 637–651.

Fletcher, R., Loschen, E., Stavrakaki, C.& First, M. (Eds.) (2007). *Diagnostic Manual – Intellectual Disability (DM-ID): A Textbook of Diagnosis of Mental Disorders in Persons with Intellectual Disability*. NADD Press, Kingston, NY.

Freud, S. (1966). *Parapraxes from Introductory Lectures on Psycho-Analysis*. W.W. Norton & Co, New York.

Gentile, J.P. & Jackson, C.S. (2008). Dual Diagnosis Patient: Co-Occurring Mental Illness/ Intellectual Disabilities. *Psychiatry* **5**(3), 49–57.

Harris, S.L. & Wolchik, S.A. (1979). Suppression Of Self-Stimulation: Three Alternative Strategies. *Journal of Applied Behavior Analysis* **12**, 185–198.

Hatton, C., Haddock, G., Taylor, J.L., Coldwell, J., Crossley, R. & Peckham, N. (2005). The reliability and validity of general psychotic rating scales with people with mild and moderate intellectual disabilities: an empirical investigation. *Journal of Intellectual Disability Research* **49**(7), 490–500.

Hippocrates: *Writings on Hysteria*. In: Eghigian, G. (Ed.) (2010). *From Madness to Mental Health. Psychiatric Disorder and Its Treatment*. Rutgers University Press, USA.

Jacobi, F., Wittchen, H.U., Holting, C., Hofler, M., Pfister, H., Mufller, N. & Lieb, R. (2004). Prevalence, Co-Morbidity And Correlates Of Mental Disorders In The General Population: Results From The German Health Interview And Examination Survey (GHS). *Psychological Medicine* **34**, 597–611.

Jopp, D.A. & Keys, C.B. (2001). Diagnostic Overshadowing Reviewed and Reconsidered. *American Journal on Mental Retardation* **106**(5), 416–433.

Jørgensen, P., Bennedsen, B., Christensen, J. & Hyllested, A. (1996). Acute and transient psychotic disorder: comorbidity with personality disorder *Acta Psychiatrica Scandinavica* **94** (6), 460–464.

Kessler, R.C., McGonagle, K.A., Zhao, S., Nelson, C.B., Hughes, M., Eshleman, S., Wittchen, H.U. & Kendler, K.S. (1994). Lifetime and 12-Month Prevalence of DSM-III-R: Psychiatric Disorders in the United States. *Archives of General Psychiatry* **51**, 8–19.

Kiernan, C. Reeves, D. & Alborz, A. (1995). The use of anti-psychotic drugs with adults with learning disabilities and challenging behavior. *Journal of Intellectual Disability Research* **39**, 263–274.

Kraeplin, E. (1896) *Psychiatrie. Translated as: Clinical Psychiatry* (1902) by Deferndorf, A.R. MacMillan, New York.

Langdon, R., Jones, S.R., Connaughton, E. & Fernyhough, C. (2009). The phenomenology of inner speech: comparison of schizophrenia patients with auditory verbal hallucinations and healthy controls. *Psychological Medicine* **39**, 655–663.

Langfeld, G. (1982). Definition of "Schizophreniform Psychoses". *American Journal of Psychiatry* **139**, 703.

Lasègue, C. & Falret, J. (1877). La folie à deux. *Ann Med Psychol (Paris)* **18**, 321–355.

Lee, C.S. (2008). Delusions of Parasitosis. *Dermatologic Therapy* **21**(1), 2–7.

Levitt, J.J. & Tsuang, M.T. (1988). The heterogeneity of schizoaffective disorder: implications for treatment. *American Journal of Psychiatry* **145**, 926–936.

Lieberman, J.A., Stroup, T.S., McEvoy, J.P., Swartz, M.S., Rosenheck, R.A., Perkins, D.O., Keefe, R.S., Davis, S.M., Davis, C.E., Lebowitz, B.D., Severe, J. & Hsiao, J.K. (2005). Effectiveness of antipsychotic drugs in patients with chronic schizophrenia. *New England Journal Of Medicine* **353**, 1209–1223.

Lund, J. (1985). The prevalence of psychiatric morbidity in mentally retarded adults. *Acta Psychiatrica Scandinavica* **72**, 563–570.

Matson, J. & Scior, K. (2004). 'Diagnostic overshadowing' amongst clinicians working with people with intellectual disabilities in the UK. *Journal of Applied Research in Intellectual Disabilities* **17**, 85–90.

Matson, J.L. & Neal, D. (2009). Psychotropic medication use for challenging behaviors in persons with intellectual disabilities: An overview. *Research in Developmental Disabilities* **30**, 572–586.

Matson, J.L., Bielecki, J., Mayville, S.B. & Matson, M.L. (2003). Psychopharmacology research for individuals with mental retardation: methodological issues and suggestions. *Research in Developmental Disabilities* **24**, 149–157.

McGillicuddy, N.B. (2006). A Review Of Substance Use Research Among Those With Mental Retardation. *Mental Retardation and Developmental Disabilities Research Reviews* **12**, 41–47.

Melville, C., Cooper, S.A., Morrison, J., Smiley, E., Allan, L., Jackson, A., Finlayson, J. & Mantry, D. (2008). The prevalence and incidence of mental ill-health in adults with autism and intellectual disabilities. *Journal of Autism and Developmental Disorders* **38**, 1676–1688.

Moss, S., Prosser, H., Ibbotson, B. & Goldberg, D. (1996). Respondent and informant accounts of psychiatric symptoms in a sample of patients with learning disability. *Journal of Intellectual Disability Research* **40**(5), 457–465.

Moss, S., Ibbotson, B., Prosser, H., Goldberg, D. & Simpson N. (1997). Validity of the PAS-ADD for detecting psychiatric symptoms in adults with learning disability (mental retardation). *Social Psychiatry and Psychiatric Epidemiology* **32**, 344–354.

Moss, S., Emerson, E., Kiernan, C., Turner, S., Hatton, C. & Alborz, A. (2000). Psychiatric symptoms in adults with learning disability and challenging behavior. *British Journal of Psychiatry* **177**, 452–456.

Myers, J.K., Weissman, M.M., Tischler, G.L., Holzer, C.E. III, Leaf, P.J., Orvaschel, H., Anthony, J.C., Boyd, J.H., Burke, J.D. Jr, Kramer, M. & Stoltzman, R. (1984). Six–Month Prevalence of Psychiatric Disorders in Three Communities 1980 to 1982. *Archives of General Psychiatry* **41**(10), 959–967.

O'Dwyer, J.M. (1997). Schizophrenia in people with intellectual disability: the role of pregnancy and birth complications. *Journal of Intellectual Disability Research* **41**(3), 238–251.

Oathamshaw, S. & Haddock, G. (2006). Do people with intellectual disabilities and psychosis have the cognitive skills required to undertake cognitive behavioural therapy? *Journal of Applied Research in Intellectual Disabilities* **19**, 35–46.

Patel, J., Pinals, D. & Brier, A. (2003). Schizophrenia and other psychoses. In: Tasman, A., Kay, J., Leiberman, J., First, M.B. & Maj, M. (eds) *Psychiatry*, 3rd ed. John Wiley and Sons, Chichester, UK.

Perälä, J., Suvisaari, J., Saarni, S.I., Kuoppasalmi, K., Isometsä, K., Pirkola, S., Partonen, T., Tuulio-Henriksson, A., Hintikka, J., Kieseppä, T., Härkänen, T., Koskinen, S. & Lönnqvist, J. (2007). Lifetime Prevalence of Psychotic and Bipolar I Disorders in a General Population. *Archives of General Psychiatry* **64**(1), 19–28.

Pillmann, F., Haring, A., Balzuweit, S., Bloink, R. & Marneros, A. (2002). The concordance of ICD-10 acute and transient psychosis and DSM-IV brief psychotic disorder. *Psychological Medicine* **32**, 525–533.

Pinel, P.H. (1802) *A Treatise on Insanity*. Translated by Davies, D. (1962). Haffiier, New York.

Robins, L.N., Hlezer, J.E., Weissman, M.M., Orvaschel, H., Gruenberg, E., Burke, J.D. & Regier, D.A. (1984). Lifetime Prevalence of Specific Psychiatric Disorders in Three Sites. *Archives of General Psychiatry* **41**, 949–958.

Rosebush, P.I. & Mazurek, M.F. (2010). Catatonia and Its Treatment. *Schizophrenia Bulletin* **36**(2) 239–242.

Sadock, B.J. & Sadock, V.A. (2003). *Kaplan and Saddock's Synopsis of Psychiatry Behavioral Science/Clinical Psychiatry*. Lippincott, Williams and Wilkins, Philadelphia, PA.

Santosh, P.J. & Baird G. (1999). Psychopharmacotherapy in children and adults with intellectual disability. *The Lancet* **354**(9174), 233–242.

Scheerenberger, R.C. (1983). *A History of Mental Retardation*. Brookes, Baltimore, MD.

Smiley, E., Morrison, J., Williamson, A. & Allan, L. (2007). Mental ill-health in adults with intellectual disabilities: prevalence and associated factors. *British Journal of Psychiatry* **190**, 27–35.

Spinoza, B. (1905). *The principles of Descartes' philosophy*. Open Court Publishing Company, Chicago, IL.

Spreat, S., Conroy, J.W. & Jones, J.C. (1997). Use of psychotropic medication in Oklahoma: a statewide survey. *American Journal of Mental Retardation* **102**, 80–85.

Standage, T.A. (2005). *History of the World in 6 Glasses*. Walker and Company, New York.

Tasman, A., Kay, J. & Lieberman, J. (2003). *Psychiatry*, 2nd Ed. John Wiley and Sons, Chichester, UK.

Unwin, G.L. & Deb, S. (2008). Use of Medication for the management of behavior problems among adults with intellectual disabilities: a clinicians' consensus survey. *American Journal of Mental Retardation* **113**(1), 19–31.

Westermeyer, J., Kemp, K. & Nugent, S. (1995). Substance Disorder Among Persons With Mild Mental Retardation. *American Journal on Addictions* **5**(1), 23–31.

White, M.J., Nichols, C.N., Cook, R.S. & Spengler, PM. (1995). Diagnostic overshadowing and mental retardation: A meta-analysis. *American Journal on Mental Retardation* **100**(3), 293–298.

10

Personality Disorders

Julie P. Gentile, MD, Associate Professor, Wright State University, Dayton, Ohio
Allison E. Cowan, MD, Assistant Professor, Wright State University, Dayton, Ohio

> "...an enduring pattern of inner experience and behavior that deviates markedly from the expectations of the individual's culture, is pervasive and inflexible, has an onset in adolescence or early adulthood, is stable over time, and leads to distress or impairment."
>
> (American Psychiatric Association, DSM-IV, 2000)

Introduction

Personality is a complex compilation of social skills, impulse control, affective modulation, risk assessment and ability to learn from previous experiences (Powers, 2005a). Personality disorders are fundamental and persisting problems related to who people are, how they see themselves, how they cope with problems and how they interface with others (Putnam, 2009). The diagnosis of a personality disorder implies that the individual has, or could have the ability to evaluate interpersonal, social, legal and professional behavior in his- or herself.

The diagnosis of personality disorders in individuals with intellectual disabilities (ID) is complicated and controversial for various reasons. The criteria for personality disorders are all potentially altered in persons with ID, and their behavior may be greatly affected by the severity of cognitive deficits. It is now widely accepted that ID individuals with "severe and profound" disabilities should not be diagnosed with personality disorders (Lindsay *et al.*, 2005).

Psychiatry of Intellectual Disability: A Practical Manual, First Edition.
Edited by Julie P. Gentile and Paulette M. Gillig.
© 2012 John Wiley & Sons, Ltd. Published 2012 by John Wiley & Sons, Ltd.

According to the existing diagnostic criteria for the general population, there are three broad categories of personality disorders:

- Cluster A includes schizoid, schizotypal and paranoid personality disorders. There is a general focus on thought processes including peculiar ideas, magical thinking and social isolation. In persons with ID, these features can overlap with symptoms of autism (Alexander *et al.*, 2010).

- Cluster B includes borderline, antisocial and narcissistic personality disorders, with a general theme of poor impulse control and emotional instability.

- Cluster C includes avoidant, passive and dependent personality disorders, with a general theme of social or professional withdrawal. In persons with ID, dependent personality is especially complicated and can overlap with realistic dependency needs.

The Diagnostic Criteria-Learning Disability (DC-LD: Royal College of Psychiatrists, 2001) attempts to delineate maladaptive behaviors often present in individuals with ID and to diagnosable personality disorders by utilizing a dividing line between "disorder" versus accepted normality, based on the intensity and severity of the traits/characteristics. The DC-LD adds that this delineation may be "arbitrary" in the ID population.

The Diagnostic Manual – Intellectual Disability (DM-ID) notes that persons with ID are "not exempt" from development of personality disorders (Fletcher *et al.*, 2007). The DM-ID cautions that all evaluations of persons with ID must take into account the developmental and cultural framework of the individual. There is also discussion in the DM-ID regarding the distinction between an individual's real need for support and their fear of abandonment. These are realistic concerns in individuals who have inconsistent support systems, and who have experienced multiple losses.

Prevalence

The prevalence of personality disorders in the general population is approximately 11–22% (Powers, 2005a). The prevalence in individuals with ID has sometimes been estimated to be as high as 23–31%.

However, Naik *et al.* (2002), reported a prevalence rate of only 7% in the ID population. In their sample of 29 subjects, 55% of those diagnosed with personality disorders were female and 45% male. Seven percent had borderline intellectual functioning, 79% had mild ID and 14% had moderate ID (Naik *et al.*, 2003). In this sample, 59% had "dissocial" (antisocial) personality disorder, 28% had "emotionally unstable" (borderline) personality, 10% had both disorders and the remaining 3% were diagnosed with "anxious" personality disorder. Fifty-nine percent had been admitted to a hospital in the previous five years and psychotropic medication was prescribed to the vast majority, although only 34% were diagnosed with co-occurring mental disorders.

In Alexander *et al.* (2010), the prevalence of personality disorders was 55.8% in the sample of 138 subjects. Women were more likely to be in the personality disorder group. Depression and substance use was correlated to subjects with personality disorders, while epilepsy and pervasive developmental disorders (autism spectrum) were more common in the subjects without personality disorders (Alexander *et al.*, 2010). For comparison, see Table 1 for the relative frequency of specific personality disorders in a sample of 101 subjects as found by Khan *et al.* (1997).

There is certainly no consistent or reliable data in this area. This is demonstrated by Alexander & Cooray's (2003) review of the prevalence data, which shows rate variance of more than 90-fold. Tyrer *et al.* (2003) summarize this variance as, "one that would make any epidemiologist blanch in horror" and they also note that there is inconsistency in the training of clinicians making the diagnosis of "personality disorder" in the available historical information of the person with ID, and in the knowledge and reliability of collateral data sources.

Assessment

Assessment tools may be difficult or impossible to utilize in individuals with ID, and tests such as the Minnesota Multiphasic Personality Inventory (MMPI) have not been standardized for use in individuals with cognitive deficits. Many personality tests and inventories require that the individual not only answer hundreds of questions, but also that they utilize various recall and memory skills. Most, if not all, of the assessment instruments created for persons with ID have construct validity problems, and there is a lack of conceptual clarity (Torr, 2003). As with other categories of psychiatric conditions, interplay among behavior, personality and psychiatric disorders in individuals with ID is complex.

When treating individuals with ID, it is vital to be knowledgeable of their baseline functioning and to access reliable data from collateral data sources. Behavior must be evaluated with the caveat that it is a form of communication, while keeping at the forefront the individual's developmental framework (Alexander & Cooray, 2003). A detailed history of the person's behaviors, attitudes and interpersonal interactions are core elements of a thorough assessment for personality disorder; medical or other psychiatric causes of the patient's presentation must also be considered and excluded (Powers, 2005a).

Because individuals with ID have realistic dependency needs, there are certain to be complicating factors in applying the diagnostic criteria for dependent personality disorder to this specialized population. The use of this specific disorder in the ID population would be debatable (Alexander & Cooray, 2003). Studies on both schizoid and obsessive compulsive (anankastic) personality disorders suggest that the criteria for these conditions overlap with symptoms of autism (Deb & Hunter, 1991) and so these should be avoided or utilized with caution.

Table 1 Distribution of personality disorders in persons with intellectual disabilities.

Cluster	Type	Percentage
A	Paranoid	5
	Schizoid	10
B	Antisocial	3
	Histrionic	1
	Impulsive	7
C	Dependent	3

Source: Adapted from Khan *et al.* (1997), p. 327.

Khan *et al.* (1997) found that stereotyped behaviors such as "aimless pacing, repeated self-injury, rocking, hoarding and following routines" were significantly increased in those persons with ID with personality traits. Severe behavior problems were significantly more prevalent in those with personality disorders and co-occurring ID (Khan *et al.*, 1997).

The structured assessment of personality (SAP)

The structured assessment of personality (SAP: Mann *et al.*, 1981) utilizes informant account of behavior to establish the diagnosis of personality disorders (Alexander & Cooray, 2003). The SAP is a semi-structured interview found to have satisfactory inter-rater reliability when used in persons with ID in an institutional setting (Flynn *et al.*, 2002). A personality "trait" is established by the presence of three or more criteria. If there is significant personal distress, or occupational or social impairment, the diagnosis of a personality disorder is made. The scale utilizes ICD-10 (World Health Organization, 1992) diagnoses of personality disorders (Flynn *et al.*, 2002).

Despite good inter-rater reliability, when Wink *et al.* (2010) reviewed several studies which used the SAP, they found that this tool has generated a wide range of results in the ID population. One study reported prevalence of personality disorders in the ID population as high as 90% using the SAP (Wink *et al.*, 2010); this contrasts with Naik *et al.*'s (2002) prevalence rate of 7%. Flynn *et al.* (2002) reported a prevalence of 39% in a sample of 36 individuals and showed a significant relationship to early traumatic experience. In the Flynn study, 53% had antisocial personality disorder and 50% had borderline personality disorder.

Use of the SAP is further complicated by the necessity of having an informant who has known the individual for at least five years. This is a limiting factor in many instances. Additionally, as Wink *et al.* (2010) note, because it relies on objective data from a secondary data source, the SAP does not have the capacity to assess the inner mood state of the individual being evaluated.

The diagnostic criteria in learning disability

The diagnostic criteria in learning disability (DC-LD: Royal College of Psychiatrists, 2001) is a multi-axial operationalized criteria system for adults with moderate to profound learning disabilities. See Table 2 for the key points in the classification system.

Issues regarding personality disorder diagnosis in persons with ID

Alexander & Cooray (2003) outline the problems in diagnosis of personality disorders in individuals with ID as follows:

1. In persons of typical intelligence, it is typical for lifelong personality traits to be present at the time of adolescence. For individuals with learning disability (LD), the emergence of these traits can be delayed (Royal College of Psychiatrists, 2001).

Table 2 Royal College of Psychiatrists diagnostic criteria in learning disability (DC-LD) key points regarding personality disorders.

1. The ICD-10 category of organic personality disorder should not be used purely on the grounds that a person has a learning disability or has a learning disabilities syndrome with an associated behavioral phenotype or epilepsy.
2. A higher age threshold (over 23 years) for diagnosing personality disorders is advised.
3. The categories of schizoid, dependent and anxious/avoidant personality disorders are not recommended.
4. The system emphasizes that the diagnosis of personality disorders in severe or profound learning disabilities is unlikely.
5. The problem that these diagnostic criteria have not been primarily designed for use with adults with learning disabilities who offend is noted.
6. Initial diagnosis using the criteria for "Personality Disorder – Unspecified" is suggested. If these are met, further sub-classification should be considered.

Source: Royal College of Psychiatrists (2001). *Diagnostic Criteria in Learning Disability (DC-LD)*. London: Gaskell. In Alexander and Cooray 2003, p. s30. Reproduced with permission.

2. Communication difficulties in addition to medical, sensory and behavior disorders make diagnosis of a personality disorder in individuals with LD complicated (Khan *et al.*, 1997). Because subjective data is required, the process is more complicated in individuals in with severe/profound communication difficulties. A 'personality disorder' may be diagnosed in persons with mild/moderate ID whereas a similar behavior pattern in persons with severe/profound ID may be labeled a 'behavior disorder.'

3. Dissocial and paranoid personality disorders (Goldberg *et al.*, 1995), for example, assume a level of cognitive stability which may not be present in persons with LD. These disorders require that the individual establish complicated concepts such 'conspiratorial explanations of events' which may reveal the severity of cognitive limitations and make diagnosis of certain personality disorders difficult.

4. There is a lack of reliable, standardized assessment instruments for individuals with LD (Khan *et al.*, 1997), in addition to differences in diagnostic criterion sets (i.e. DSM-IV and ICD-10). Variations in personality theories (Goldberg *et al.*, 1995) and difficulty distinguishing personality disorders from childhood psychosis further complicate accurate diagnosis (Corbett, 1979).

5. Some characteristics of behaviors exhibited by individuals with LD may be similar to behaviors exhibited by persons with personality disorders.

Borderline personality disorder

Borderline personality disorder (BPD) is characterized by "the presence of a pattern of unstable interpersonal relationships, disturbances of self-image and affect, and marked impulsivity" (Wilson, 2001). In the general population, BPD often exists with co-occurring psychiatric disorders such as substance use disorders, mood disorders, eating disorders, post-traumatic stress disorder, attention deficit hyperactivity disorder and other personality disorders (American Psychiatric Association, 2000; Wilson, 2001).

Some of the features of BPD occur frequently in individuals with ID, including self-injurious behavior, impulsivity, and affective lability (Mavromatis, 2000). Mood disorders are more prevalent in the ID population and may have analogous presentations to personality disorders (mood changes, impulsivity, etc), so collateral data and detailed history-taking are vital to distinguish these conditions. Mavromatis (2000) endorses these similarities and emphasizes that the clinician should look for additional features of BPD in persons with ID, including:

1. patterns of idealization and devaluation;

2. splitting;

3. manipulative behavior;

4. subjective perceptions of victimization;

5. chronic feelings of emptiness;

6. stress related paranoia;

7. impulsive patterns of self destructive behavior other than self-mutilation.

The Diagnostic and Statistical Manual (Fourth Edition, Text Revision) diagnostic criteria (for the general population) and the DM-ID criteria for borderline personality disorder (for the ID population) are similar. The DM-ID recommends that the clinician take into account that the patient with ID is generally more reliant on caregivers, and that cultural variations should be taken into account. Also, it may be difficult for patients with ID to express identity disturbance, due to communication difficulties, and making the diagnosis of BPD in this population requires sensitive and sophisticated judgment. The DM-ID also notes that self-injury is a frequent issue, and a thorough evaluation is necessary to rule out numerous etiologies. See Chapter 11 for more details on self-injurious behavior.

Clinical Vignette #1 illustrates an individual with mild ID and borderline personality disorder, which is a high utilizer of both ID and mental health community resources. There are layers of complications, including the chaotic relationships which result in recurrent emotional turmoil for the patient and subsequent emergency department evaluations. The chronic suicidal threats of the patient create urgency in the direct care staff, whose goal is to ensure the safety of the patient – the unfortunate consequence being that the patient may consciously or unconsciously seek the attention of medical providers as part of the character pathology.

Hurley & Sovner (1988) emphasize that staff cohesiveness is essential; if direct caregivers are untrained and/or inconsistent, the outcome will likely include disruptive emotional reaction (negative transference) among the staff, which will impede the successful creation of a therapeutic environment. The goals of treatment must include staff training and

Clinical Vignette #1

"I just want to die! Just leave me alone so I can kill myself!" Jolene, a 27 year old white woman with mild ID, was initially seen by the psychiatry resident in the emergency department. Jolene was well known to the resident because of her frequent trips to the hospital.

Dr. W asked, "What's going on, Jolene?" Jolene grudgingly admitted that she got into a fist fight with her home staff, Sue-Ellen, when Sue-Ellen would not drive her over to visit her boyfriend. When Dr W said, "But I thought she was your favorite staff?," Jolene yelled, "Well, not any more!"

Before the fight, Jolene had tried to break into her locked medication box, and this was discovered by staff who heard her yelling about taking all her medications. Jolene said, "I was so mad, I blacked out. I don't remember what I said. I'm depressed because my boyfriend didn't answer his phone when I called."

Jolene has many different boyfriends and does not stay with one for long. She does not have female friends because she says, "I just can't trust them not to steal my boyfriend." She often unceremoniously dumps her boyfriends when she suspects them of cheating on her, whether this is founded or unfounded. She also believes that people talk behind her back and are trying to hurt her. She has been hospitalized 14 times, usually for suicidal ideation and "auditory hallucinations" of "the wind calling my name."

Jolene was typically admitted, stabilized and discharged within two days. At her check-up with her outpatient psychiatrist, Jolene reported that she didn't even know why she "made a fuss," but stated that she was terrified her boyfriend was cheating on her. She was tearful and sobbing throughout much of the exam. Her case manager, who was sitting in on the appointment, asked if getting a Coke after the appointment would help. Jolene stopped crying and beamed, "That would be great!"

Jolene had a difficult childhood. Raised by her mother, she never knew her father but allegedly suffered through her mother's abusive boyfriends. She carries a diagnosis of post-traumatic stress disorder and major depressive disorder. She is treated with sertraline for her comorbid diagnosis of PTSD, buspirone for anxiety, and hydroxyzine for as needed anxiety relief.

Care was taken by Jolene's psychiatrist to rule out bipolar disorder, which can easily be confused for borderline personality disorder. Some hallmarks of borderline personality are Jolene's affective instability, which is associated with external stimuli (e.g. intense anxiety and sadness due to thinking her boyfriend is cheating, or her happiness for a Coke with her case manager). Jolene also sleeps well. She has an involved treatment team, comprising case management, therapist, a behavioral support specialist and habilitation specialists. She attends weekly group therapy for anger management, and another women's group therapy for relationship issues. She is slowly making progress and does well at her sheltered workshop when in attendance.

development of existing resources, to provide consistent and effective interventions which promote positive therapeutic outcome.

As illustrated in Clinical Vignette #1, individuals with ID display a characteristic pattern of BPD symptoms:

1. Unstable and potentially volatile interpersonal relationships, which are often characterized by overreaction toward, and verbal abuse of, caretakers.

2. Impulsivity, as marked by global efforts at environmental disruption rather than the goal-directed patterns seen in the non-disabled population.

3. Labile affect, characterized by sudden shifts in feeling and expression of feeling.

4. Difficulties in controlling anger, along with overblown reactions to stimuli.

5. Self-injurious behavior which is probably geared to gain attention rather than to commit suicide.

Hurley & Sovner (1988) caution that the above signs in persons with ID are sometimes misunderstood by clinicians and "often interpreted as cognitive deficits, emotional immaturity and neurodysregulation" (Hurley & Sovner, 1988, in Wilson, 2001).

In general, BPD may be associated in any person with neurocognitive dysfunction (Wink *et al.*, 2010); it is present in approximately 5.9% of the general population and commonly co-occurs with mood and anxiety disorders, substance use disorders and additional personality disorders (Grant *et al.*, 2008; Wink *et al.*, 2010). The incidence of self-injurious behavior associated with BPD in the general population is thought to be between 69–75% (Wink *et al.*, 2010).

Many individuals in the general population with BPD are shown to have cognitive impairments related to speed of processing, memory and visuo-spatial learning (Judd, 2005). These processes are likely to be impaired at baseline in persons with ID, thereby potentially making them vulnerable to development of BPD. Fertuck *et al.* (2006) studied neurocognitive abnormalities that contribute to negative outcomes when vulnerable individuals are exposed to abuse or a "poor affective fit between parent and child." This results in insecure and disorganized relationships, as well as an impaired ability to process situations and to form secure attachments (Fertuck *et al.*, 2006).

Clinical Vignette #2

Sam is a 34 year old white man who has been diagnosed with major depressive disorder and mild to moderate ID. He lives in a group home with three other roommates. Sam presented to the clinic for continued management of care. "I'm so sad always," he said.

His caregiver, Lucy, said, "But Sam, you have all your friends at work."

Sam said, "But I don't like them."

Lucy became frustrated, stating "You always do this! You're happy and doing well at work until Sara ignores you." Lucy clarified that Sam and Sara, Sam's girlfriend, have an on-off relationship. She told the psychiatrist that she just wished Sam would end the relationship once and for all.

"But I love her," Sam explained. Sam and Sara would get along well for a few days, usually after Sam received his workshop paycheck, and then she would call him names and break up with him. Sam would pine after her for days, groveling for her to come back to him. Sara would relent and the process would happen again.

After an argument with Sara, Sam would attempt to provoke his much larger, intimidating roommate and would occasionally be on the receiving end of physical aggression. More often, however, he would slap his own face or scratch at his skin. Before presenting to the psychiatrist, Sam had started taking the house knives out of the drawer and threatening to kill himself unless Sara took him back.

Lucy was concerned that Sara was taking advantage of Sam, but Sam was not interested in anyone's opinion of Sara. "I just want her to love me. Sometimes Sara wants us to have alone time and I don't really like to but I do it anyway."

Sam's family of origin was dysfunctional at best. The youngest of four siblings, he does not know who his biological father is. Sam and his siblings were removed from his mother's home when Sam was 11 months old. He was placed with his aunt, then his grandmother, and finally he was placed in foster care from the age of 5 through to adolescence. Sam has reported alleged emotional and sexual abuse at his relatives' homes but understandably does not like to discuss the details.

Sam reached out to his treatment team much more frequently when he and Sara were not together, calling upwards of 10–15 times a day if his therapist were unavailable. Unfortunately, despite being in treatment for some time, Sam tried to drown the cat which lived at his group home. When asked why, he said that he was only trying to give it a bath. After talking with his therapist, he was able to admit that he was enraged at Sara for kissing another peer and he wanted to hurt something. He was remorseful after the fact and filled with shame at the thought of hurting an animal.

The goal for Sam's treatment is for Sam to talk about his feelings rather than act on them. To accomplish this, his therapist meets with him weekly to practice anger management techniques and to work on recognizing feeling states. A longer-term goal for Sam is to improve on his self-image and to explore why he feels compelled to stay in a romantic relationship with someone who does not treat him well.

Sam is slowly improving, albeit with frequent setbacks. He is able to work better and is able to go to his room rather than pick a fight with his roommate if he is angry. He continues to date Sara when they're not broken up.

Stable and enduring relationships which offer acceptance and love are difficult for anyone to achieve and sustain. It can be especially difficult for someone with a dysfunctional background and a difficult current situation to find or navigate a healthy relationship. Fear of abandonment is one of the most pronounced symptoms of an underlying personality disorder, but learning to manage intense anger, unstable moods and self-harming behavior are the highest priority in terms of attaining treatment goals and increasing the quality of life for the individual.

Linehan (1993) stated that children with disabilities enter the world with barriers that may correlate to the "poorness of fit" implicated in the vulnerability to development of BPD. Their parents may be unable to validate the child's experiences adequately or appropriately, making them vulnerable to psychopathology. Hollins & Sinason (2000) add that parents of children with ID frequently struggle with their own grief and loss issues, making attachments complicated and potentially dysfunctional. These factors all play roles in the development of a personality disorder in an individual with ID.

Histrionic personality disorder

The diagnostic criteria for histrionic personality disorder (HPD) in the general population, from the DSM-IV Text Revision (American Psychiatric Association, 2000), and in the ID population from the DM-ID (Fletcher *et al.*, 2007) are similar, but the DM-ID highlights some important points. For example, it notes that individuals with ID might show discomfort by being agitated, intrusive or self-abusive, or by engaging in other problematic behaviors. It is also important to establish that the individual with ID understands appropriate sexual behavior and the normal expression of emotion, and to take into account that the individual may have communication difficulties. Although there is a scarcity of literature on HPD in this specialized population, it should be considered as a diagnosis when the patient presents with attention-seeking behavior, is overly theatrical or dramatic, or exhibits sexually inappropriate or sexually offending behavior, as illustrated in Clinical Vignette #3.

Clinical Vignette #3

José is a 45 year old Hispanic man with a history of schizophrenia (paranoid type) and mild intellectual disability. José likes to wear loud Hawaiian shirts and a feather boa. He also flirts outrageously with anyone in hearing distance.

When his therapist asked José why he was coming to the mental health clinic, José smiled charmingly and said, "But the unicorns tell me to." He explained that ever since he was a boy, a troupe of three unicorns had kept him company. He reported that they often talked to him, but that they were more friends than scary things, and they told him encouraging things, such as he was an attractive person.

The therapist was confused and asked for further clarification. José became irritated and said, "Why are you asking me all these stupid questions? Don't you believe me?" The therapist noted that José did not appear to be responding to internal stimuli and had a full affect.

His caregiver, who until then had been quiet, mentioned that José had always had a very active imagination. José interrupted to say, "My unicorns are telling me that they like watching cartoons and that we'll go get a Coke after we leave here." His caregiver pointed out that José's unicorns were more likely to act up when José was not the center of attention, and would behave when staff asked them nicely to go away. José would often make sexually suggestive statements to people in the hope of getting a reaction, but he did not follow through with any sexual acts.

José's therapist asked, "José, why are you here today?"

José replied, "Oh, I don't know. I guess I just wanted to come see you and everybody else here. I think I'm depressed." He flipped his feather boa dramatically and sighed. He perked up immediately when his service coordinator came in the room, and was cheerful for the remainder of the interview.

The therapist was able to discuss José's history with the service coordinator, his mother and his current caregiver. The "hallucinations" that had been the basis for José's diagnosis of schizophrenia were the three unicorns who kept José company. He had never displayed any paranoia and had never appeared to have been disturbed by his "hallucinations." There was no loss of functioning, no social impairments and no impairments in his work. He slept well.

In the case of "José," described in Vignette #3, care is necessary to make sure that José does not have a psychotic disorder, because this spectrum of disorders is more common in individuals with ID. Despite this fact, psychosis is unlikely and it appears most likely that José has HPD. While this is more common in women, men also can develop HPD.

José's need for attention and sexualized behavior are hallmarks of this disorder. He uses dramatic words and actions to keep attention focused on him. His "unicorns" are likely the result of his active imagination, and differ from true hallucinations in that they are mainly visual, not threatening or upsetting, and have been with him since he was a boy. Hallucinations from psychotic disorders are more likely to be auditory, degrading or demeaning, and scary.

José appears to enjoy the attention brought to him by his unicorns. Gentle boundary-setting and psychotherapy would facilitate José in finding other ways to seek attention, although one would expect that he would sometimes talk about his original symptoms (i.e. unicorns) but do so much less frequently and be able to get along without them most of the time.

Antisocial personality disorder

Aggression is quite common in individuals with ID, although the diagnosis of antisocial personality disorder (APD) is not frequently used. Nevertheless, some factors that make an individual vulnerable to development of APD occur commonly in persons with ID (e.g. presence of attention deficit hyperactivity disorder; abuse history; impoverished developmental upbringing; emotional and behavioral problems; minority race; poor family management and child-rearing practices; and family conflict due to antisocial parents) (Hurley & Sovner, 1995; Douma *et al.*, 2007).

In addition, other characteristics related to ID (impulsivity, acquiescence and social desirability, among others) may further put these individuals at risk (Douma *et al.*, 2007). Dekker & Coot (2003) and Emerson (2003) also report that predictors of conduct problems and disruptive disorders in youths with ID include:

- physical problems

- inadequate socialization

- life events of the child

- low parental educational level

- single parenthood

- parental psychopathology

- frequent use of punitive strategies

- family dysfunction.

There is little research on APD in the ID population. Hurley & Sovner (1995) reported on six patients whom they diagnosed as having co-occurring ID and APD. The authors noted that there was no valid research on the delineation of frequency of aggression as a result of APD in the ID population. In their report on these six patients, only one had received the diagnosis of APD prior to the study, despite the fact that there was documentation of the predatory nature and lack of remorse related to the actions of all six of the individuals. It appears that clinicians hesitated to use this diagnosis, possibly due to concern about the limited cognitive abilities of the patients or what were interpreted by staff as "transparent defense mechanisms" (Hurley & Sovner, 1995).

Douma *et al.* (2007) studied antisocial and delinquent behaviors in youths who had either borderline intellectual dysfunction or mild ID. In a sample of 1,556 subjects, 10–20% of individuals with ID exhibited antisocial or delinquent behavior and this behavior had persisted for over five years. The prevalence was higher in younger males, who likely had a conduct disorder, and this appears to be a consistent risk factor (Douma *et al.*, 2007).

Several studies have shown that individuals with mild ID have a higher prevalence of offending behaviors relative to those with more severe ID and those with typical cognitive functioning (Douma *et al.*, 2007). In addition, inmates of penal institutions tend to have lower intelligence quotients as compared to the general population.

Clinical Vignette #4

Becca is a 25 year old Russian-American woman with mild ID. She presented to the mental health clinic with her adoptive mother, Sandy, for continuation of mental health care when they moved to the area. Sandy said, "Becca has problems with stealing and anger. The tighter you try to regulate her, the more she acts up." During the examination, Becca smiled easily, "Yeah, my mom is right. But I'm not doing that anymore, so you don't have to worry about me."

Becca had been prescribed risperidone 4 mg by her previous psychiatrist, but both Becca and her mother agreed that this had not been effective in helping deal with Becca's presenting symptoms. When left to her own devices, Becca would hang out with "shady characters" in her apartment complex and in the community, which concerned her mother. Becca again smiled easily and said, "It's okay. They won't hurt me."

Becca does not live with her mother, but rather lives in her own apartment with ten hours a week of staffed time. Her parents adopted her from a large orphanage in Russia when she was five years old. Upon taking custody of her, they noticed that Becca had bruises and some unusual scars. After returning to the U.S.A., they took her to a pediatrician, who confirmed their suspicions that Becca had been abused in her orphanage.

Sandy said that Becca was always a very friendly child who was very affectionate with everyone. She especially had taken to her dad, who had died four years ago. Sandy said, "She just seemed to do better with him. She and I have always been a little more distant than she was with him."

Becca was diagnosed with ID in school and she was well-liked but always struggled with following rules. Since her father's death, her mother has remarried. Becca had been arrested for fighting several times. Her mother said Becca was involved with the "wrong crowd." However, Becca was also working as part of a janitorial crew that was contracted out to local businesses through the sheltered workshop.

Becca was given a provisional diagnosis of impulse control disorder NOS. Plans were made to begin decreasing the dose of her risperidone, because of the side effect of weight gain. Becca also started weekly therapy to address the stress of relocating to another area, since her mother had remarried and the family has moved.

Becca's mother had a long-standing reward/punishment plan that allowed Becca DVDs for good behavior and restricted her allowed carbohydrate intake for bad behavior. Weight control had been an issue, because risperidone had likely been contributing to a weight increase. Now risperidone had been discontinued, and Sandy had Becca on a strict 1,500 calorie diet as recommended by her family doctor. Despite this diet, Becca continued to gain weight – 20 pounds over three months.

Becca was caught stealing several times. She was caught taking money and soda from peers at her workshop. Things also were discovered missing from the local businesses when Becca was out on her janitorial jobs, and Sandy found these things in Becca's house. When asked, Becca said that she took the items because people let her get away with it "because I have a disability." She said her peers were "too stupid to have money, anyway."

Becca stole a credit card and used it to buy items from McDonald's and the local grocery store. She also had several different "boyfriends" and, when asked, she laughed and proudly explained, "They all give me the things that I want, but they don't know I don't give a crap about any of them."

As Clinical Vignette #4 illustrates, while "Becca's" disorder may be rooted in a childhood diagnosis of attachment disorder, she now meets the criteria for APD. The DSM-IV Text Revision (American Psychiatric Association, 2000) and the DM-ID (Fletcher *et al.*, 2007) criteria for APD in the general population and in the ID population, respectively, are similar. The DM-ID does note that the individual with ID must have the ability to develop an understanding of the laws and mores of society, and so using APD in moderate, severe or profound ID may not be possible. The DM-ID also notes that clinicians should ensure that individuals with ID comprehend present and future for the purposes of planning ahead.

Becca's criminal behavior and her lack of empathy for her victims are the most striking symptoms. While there remain mixed views on the effectiveness of treating APD, Becca's psychotherapist continued working with Becca and her team to reduce the harm that could come to her and to limit the harm she could bring to others. Medication may be helpful on a symptomatic basis for depression, irritability or anxiety, but it is likely not able to bring about a significant change.

Principles of treatment for personality disorders

The gold standard of treatment for personality disorders is psychotherapy, and the success of the therapy is dependent on the patient's diagnoses, motivation, insight, cognitive functioning and willingness to change interpersonal patterns and interactions (Powers, 2005a). The studies reviewed are all in agreement that the need for support and the utilization of resources for individuals with ID and personality disorders distinguishes them from persons with ID who do not have personality disorders (Naik *et al.*, 2002; Tyrer *et al.*, 2003; Lidher *et al.*, 2005).

Overall, psychological and behavioral interventions are preferable to medications, unless there are co-occurring symptoms or conditions which could benefit from pharmacologic management. Any pharmacologic intervention should focus on the target symptoms of mood lability, depression and psychosis, and must be used in combination with psycho-therapeutic and behavioral strategies. Patients presenting with Cluster A pathology may benefit from antipsychotic medications; those with Cluster B conditions, including emotional lability and impulse control, may benefit from mood stabilization (Powers, 2005a). In the general population, individuals with personality disorders often have co-occurring substance use, depressive and anxiety disorders. It is important that the clinician screen for these and treat appropriately.

Dialectical behavior therapy (DBT) is discussed in detail in Chapter 13. It was originally developed by Linehan (1993) for treatment of borderline personality disorder (BPD) in the outpatient treatment setting (Lew *et al.*, 2006). DBT has been found to be effective in reducing self-injurious behavior and the number of days hospitalized in patients with BPD.

There is evidence that this form of treatment may be very fitting for individuals with ID. First, DBT is a skills-based model consistent with the habilitative approach so frequently utilized with other interventions for patients with ID (Lew *et al.*, 2006). It is also positive in its aspirations and does not blame the victim. In addition, the promotion of self-advocacy of the individual is a great fit for persons with ID. This is consistent with assertiveness, independence and empowerment (Lew *et al.*, 2006). DBT recognizes that the individual being treated likely has experienced, or is currently experiencing, an "invalidating" environment, where thoughts, feelings and needs may not have been adequately recognized for a number of reasons.

See Table 3 for characteristics of the invalidating environment and related common invalidating experiences of those with ID. Wilson (2001) describes a four-stage model designed for the management of borderline personality disorder for persons with ID. In the Wilson model, behavioral fluctuations are seen often to occur in four predictable stages. Each stage has identifiable behavioral manifestations of affective states, with specific goals and with treatment guidelines to achieve these goals. Individuals with ID and BPD may fluctuate among the stages outlined in Table 4, and treatment can be modified to include goals and interventions for each stage.

Wink *et al.* (2010) has outlines of clinical pearls for management and treatment of personality disorders in the ID populations:

(a)   Focus on reducing risk of damage to self and others.

(b)   Establish a safe environment.

(c)   Educate staff.

(d)   Conceptualize the personality disorder in a therapeutic framework.

(e)   Debrief staff.

(f)   Encourage consistent cohesiveness and reliability.

Table 3 Characteristics of the invalidating environment.

Standard DBT	Common invalidating experiences of those with ID	Example
Others reject communication of private experience.	Many decisions are made on the individual's behalf despite his/her verbal protests and complaints.	Mother of an individual becomes the guardian for her adult child "for his own good", despite his ability to assert and make choices she does not agree with.
Others punish emotional displays and intermittently reinforce emotional escalation.	Caretakers may not attend to (or hear) individuals' needs until they display a certain crescendo of behavior.	Staff at a group home insist on an individual going on a non-preferred outing despite his verbal protests. When he has a significant tantrum at the ball game, he requires physical restraint in public and ruins the outing for everyone. Ultimately they leave the game early.
Others oversimplify the case of problem-solving and of meeting goals.	Caretakers wonder why individuals haven't already resolved a problem or wonder when they will turn themselves around.	Foster parent is shocked and dismayed after her charge loses her third consecutive job due to interpersonal problems. The parent states, "She does so well when she is home."
Estimates of childhood sexual abuse history for people with BPD is between 65–85%.	A high percentage of ID individuals (25–83%) have been victimized by sexual abuse.	After a recent series of risky incidents and following a stable period, the individual is accused of "going back to old behaviors" in a dismissive "blame the victim" manner.

Source: Adapted from Lew *et al.* (2006), p. 3.

(g) Remain consistent in all aspects of treatment.

(h) Consistent daily schedule and clear behavioral goals.

(i) Reducing staff turnover, providing consistent care of physicians and therapists.

(j) Patient should be given concrete and easily understood rules of behavior, with the goal of eliminating specific negative behaviors.

(k) Rules must make clear consequences of behavior and must be followed consistently across staff and across environments.

(l) Give the patient a means of self-control (relaxation techniques, etc.).

Table 4 General overview of the four-stage format.

Stage 1 Optimal function	Stage 2 Antecedents/precursors	Stage 3 Crisis	Stage 4 Resolution
Behavior: individual is engaged in typical daily activities	Behavior: individual engages in behavior signaling impending instability	Behavior: individual is acting out	Behavior: individual is calm/exhausted
Goal: maintain function at this stage	Goal: return to Stage 1	Goal: maintain physical safety of all involved and move to Stage 4	Goal: gradual return to Stage 1
Interventions: teach and reinforce appropriate behavior; maintain structure; teach and practice skills for coping, soothing and distracting	Interventions: initiate procedures for coping, soothing and distracting; maintain structure	Interventions: initiate safety procedures; observe for signs of resolution	Interventions: reinstate structure; validate feelings; initiate procedures for coping, distracting and soothing

Source: Wilson (2001), p. 71.

Similarly, Nugent (in Wilson, 2001) recommends:

(a) maximizing consistency and structure

(b) appropriate social interactions

(c) supporting the individual to trust others

(d) providing opportunities for closely supervised choices

(e) teaching acceptable ways to communicate emotions.

Conclusion

Morbidity and mortality are greatly increased in individuals with personality disorders. There are many potential consequences of personality disorders, not the least of which is abandonment by family members. Lidher *et al.* (2005) found that a greater number of individuals with ID and no personality disorder (PD) lived with family than did persons diagnosed with PD and co-occurring ID. Deb & Hunter (1991) commented that PDs have a significant effect on the rehabilitation and integration of persons with ID from hospitals to community settings, so the presence of a PD may result in a more restrictive environment.

Diagnosing PDs in individuals with ID is clinically significant for the many reasons stated in this chapter, but many clinicians find a lack of diagnostic clarity and difficulty applying standardized diagnostic instruments to individuals with ID. Alexander & Cooray (2003) noted the need for consensus diagnostic criteria which use objective measures and are specific to developmental framework of the individuals. Accurate diagnosis can have significant implications for reducing stigma, improving treatment options, acceptance into community resources, residential and community placements, reducing psychiatric co-morbidity, improving outcomes and identifying and meeting specific care needs of individuals with ID (Alexander *et al.*, 2010).

Ultimately, the presence or absence of a PD will directly and significantly impact an individual's quality of life.

References

Alexander, R. & Cooray, S. (2003). Diagnosis of personality disorders in learning disability. *British Journal of Psychiatry* **182** (Suppl. 44), a28–a31.

Alexander, R.T., Green, F.N., O'Mahony, B., Gunaratna, I.J., Gangadharan, S.K. & Hoare, S. (2010). Personality disorders in offenders with intellectual disability: a comparison of clinical, forensic and outcome variables and implications for service provision. *Journal of Intellectual Disability Research* **54**(7), 650–658.

American Psychiatric Association (2000). *Diagnostic and Statistical Manual of Mental Disorders*, 4th ed. (DSM-IV). APA, Washington, DC.

Corbett, J.A. (1979). Psychiatric morbidity and mental retardation. In: Games, F.E. & Snaith, R.P. (eds.) *Psychiatric Illness and Mental Handicap*, pp. 11–25. Gaskill Press, London.

Deb, S. & Hunter, D. (1991). Psychopathology of people with mental handicap and epilepsy, III: Personality disorder. *British Journal of Psychiatry* **159**, 830–834.

Dekker, M.C. & Koot, H.M. (2003). DSM-IV disorders in children with borderline to moderate intellectual disability. II: Child and family predictors. *Journal of the American Academy of Child and Adolescent Psychiatry* **42**, 923–931.

Douma, J.C.H., Dekker, M.C., de Ruiter, K.P., Tick, N.T. & Koot, H.M. (2007). Antisocial and Delinquent Behaviors in Youths with Mild or Borderline Disabilities. *American Journal on Mental Retardation* **112**(3), 207–220. May.

Emerson, E. (2003). Prevalence of psychiatric disorders in children and adolescents with and without intellectual disability. *Journal of Intellectual Disability Research* **47**, 51–58.

Fertuck, E.A., Lenzenweger, M.E., Clarkin, J.F., Hoermann, S. & Stanley, B. (2006). Executive neurocognition, memory systems, and Borderline Personality Disorder. *Clinical Psychology Review* **26**, 346–375.

Fletcher, R., Loschen, E., Stavrakaki, C. & First, M. (Eds.). (2007). *Diagnostic Manual – Intellectual Disability (DM-ID): A Textbook of Diagnosis of Mental Disorders in Persons with Intellectual Disability.* NADD Press, Kingston, NY.

Flynn, A., Matthews, H. & Hollins, S. (2002). Validity of the diagnosis of personality disorder in adults with learning disability and severe behavioral problems. *British Journal of Psychiatry* **180**, 543–546.

Goldberg, B., Gitta, M.Z. & Puddephatt, A. (1995). Personality and trait disturbances in an adult mental retardation population: significance for psychiatric management. *Journal of Intellectual Disability Research* **39**, 284–294.

Grant, B.F., Chou, S.P., Goldstein, R.B., Huang, B., Stinson, F.S., Saha, T.D., Smith, S.M., Dawson, D.A., Pulay, A.J., Pickering, R.P. & Ruan, W.J. (2008). Prevalence, Correlates, Disability, and Comorbidity of DSM-IV Borderline Personality Disorder: Results from the Wave 2 National Epidemiologic Survey on Alcohol and Related Conditions. *Journal of Clinical Psychiatry* **69**, 533–545.

Hollins, S. & Sinason, V. (2000). Psychotherapy, learning disabilities and trauma: New perspectives. *British Journal of Psychiatry* **176**, 32–36.

Hurley, A.D. & Sovner, R. (1988). The clinical characteristics and management of borderline personality disorder in mentally retarded persons. *Psychiatric Aspects of Mental Retardation Reviews* **7**, 42–48.

Hurley, A.D. & Sovner, R. (1995). Six Cases of Patients with Mental Retardation who have Antisocial Personality Disorder. *Psychiatric Services* **46**(8), 828–831.

Judd, P.H. (2005). Neurocognitive impairment as a modulator in the development of borderline personality disorder. *Development and Psychopathology* **17**, 1173–1196.

Khan, A., Cowan, C. & Roy, A. (1997). Personality disorders in people with learning disabilities: a community survey. *Journal of Intellectual Disability Research* **41**(4), 324–330.

Lew, M., Matta, C., Tripp-Tebo, C. & Watts, D. (2006). Dialectical Behavior Therapy (DBT) for Individuals with Intellectual Disabilities: A Program Description. *Mental Health Aspects of Developmental Disabilities* **9**(1), 1–13.

Lidher, J., Martin, D.M., Jayaprakash, M.S. & Roy, A. (2005). Personality disorders in people with learning disabilities: follow-up of a community survey. *Journal of Intellectual Disability Research* **49**(11), 845–851 November.

Lindsay, W.R., Gabriel, S., Dana, L., Young, S. & Dosen, A. (2005). Personality Disorders. In: Fletcher, R., Loschen, E. & Sturmey, P. (eds.) *Diagnostic Manual of Psychotic Disorders for Individuals with Mental Retardation.* NADD Press, Kingston, NY.

Linehan, M.M. (1993). *Cognitive-Behavioral Treatment of Borderline Personality Disorder.* Guilford, New York.

Mann, A. H., Jenkins, R., Cutting, J. C. & Cowen, PJ. (1981). The development and use of a standardized assessment of abnormal personality. *Psychological Medicine*, **11**, 839–847.

Mavromatis, M. (2000). The diagnosis and treatment of borderline personality disorder in persons with developmental disability – three case reports. *Mental Health Aspects of Developmental Disabilities* **3**, 89–97.

Naik, B.I., Gangadharan, S. & Alexander, R.T. (2002). Personality Disorders in Learning Disability – The Clinical Experience. *British Journal of Developmental Disabilities* **48** (2), (95), 95–100.

Powers, R.E. (2005a). *Clinical Guide to Assessment and Management of Personality Disorders in the Adult Person with Mental Retardation and Developmental Disabilities (MR/DD)*. http://www.ddmed.org./pdfs/33.pdf

Powers, R.E. (2005b). *Physician Fact Sheet on Therapy for Personality Disorders in Persons with Mental Retardation and Developmental Disabilities(MR/DD)*. http://www.ddmed.org./pdfs/81.pdf

Putnam, C.(Ed.) (2009) *Guidelines for Understanding and Serving People with Intellectual Disabilities and Mental, Emotional, and Behavioral Disorders*, pp. 1–30. Florida Developmental Disabilities Council, Inc. Contract Number 732HC08B. Prepared by Human Systems and Outcomes, Inc.

Royal College of Psychiatrists (2001). *Diagnostic Criteria in Learning Disability (DC-LD)*. Gaskell, London.

Torr, J., (2003). Personality disorder in intellectual disability. *Current Opinion in Psychiatry* **16** (5), 517–521.

Tyrer, P., Conor, D., & Coid, J., (2003). Ramifications of personality disorder in clinical practice. *British Journal of Psychiatry* **182**, s1–s2.

Wilson, S.R., (2001). A Four-Stage Model for Management of Borderline Personality Disorder in People With Mental Retardation. *Mental Health Aspects of Developmental Disabilities* **4**(2), 68–76.

Wink, L.K., Erickson, C.A., Chambers, J.E. & McDougle, C.J. (2010). Co-morbid intellectual disability and borderline personality disorder: a case series. *Psychiatry* **73**(3), 277–287.

World Health Organization (1992). *Tenth Revision of the International Classification of Diseases and Related Health Problems (ICD-10)*. WHO, Geneva.

11

Aggression

Julie P. Gentile, MD, Associate Professor, Wright State University, Dayton, Ohio
Paulette Marie Gillig, MD, PhD, Professor, Wright State University, Dayton, Ohio

Introduction

Aggression in its various forms (verbal, physical, property destruction and auto-aggression or self-injurious behavior) is the most frequent cause for mental health appointments and assessments in patients with intellectual disabilities (ID) (Tenneij *et al.*, 2009; Hurley *et al.*, 2007; Rueve & Welton, 2008; Silka & Hauser, 1997). Patients with ID experience psychiatric and behavioral problems at three to six times the frequency of the general population (Hardan & Sahl, 1997; Larson *et al.*, 2001). "Problem behavior" occurs in approximately 50–60% of individuals with ID, and reported prevalence rates for aggression range widely from 2–40%, according to various reports (Clark *et al.*, 1990; Deb & Fraser, 1994).

The impact of aggression is significant. For the patient exhibiting the aggression, it can result in a decrease or termination of family involvement, in social isolation, or in a placement in more restrictive environments. For the caregiver, it can result in negative transference toward the individual with ID, caregiver anxiety, burnout or injury. For society, it often results in frequent hospitalization or incarceration of the person.

Aggression is a multi-determined problem and it is influenced by biological, psychological, social, spiritual and cultural factors. Psychiatric and behavioral interventions must be tailored to meet the specific needs of the particular individual with ID and aggression. There is rarely an easy answer to the etiology of aggression; however, use of the

Psychiatry of Intellectual Disability: A Practical Manual, First Edition.
Edited by Julie P. Gentile and Paulette M. Gillig.

biopsychosocial formulation can act as a template upon which to build, and with which to perform the detective work necessary.

Rueve & Welton (2008) have posed the question: "Are aggression and mental illness co-occurring conditions, inter-related, or merely coincidental?" We could ask the same of aggression and ID. Aggression in the ID population is often studied in the context of the entire spectrum of challenging behaviors that can be seen, including stereotyped behavior, pica, rumination, noncompliance and nonspecific behavior problems (Antonacci *et al.*, 2008).

Recent empirical findings about neuroanatomical and neuroreceptor correlates of aggression can help guide the clinician in selecting appropriate treatments for impulsivity and aggression. Because aggression cannot be understood outside of its situational context, the use of the "biopsychosocial formulation" when evaluating aggression is important (Campbell & Rohrbaugh, 2006). A biopsychosocial formulation includes "predisposing," "perpetuating" and "protective" factors, and is essential in determining the etiology of

Clinical Vignette #1

Christopher   Christopher is a 19 year old male with history of severe intellectual disability and no mental health history. He was assessed in the emergency department (ED) of a children's hospital near his home for agitation, paranoia and aggression toward his uncle.

The staff in the ED consulted psychiatry to assess the paranoia and aggression. The patient's uncle explained that the aggression had begun approximately 48 hours earlier, when Christopher had started refusing to eat and drink. He would examine the food as if he was suspicious of it, and became agitated and physically aggressive with his uncle if he was encouraged to eat or drink. This was new onset behavior that had never been seen before. The aggression did not occur at other times – only in combination with presentation of food or drink.

After the initial mental health assessment in the emergency department, Christopher was scheduled for follow-up with a local mental health clinic to rule out psychotic disorder due to the aggression, paranoia and agitation. Upon returning home, his caregiver became concerned when he tried to encourage Christopher to drink fluids and eat dinner. He called the clinic and asked for an emergency appointment, but the mental health clinic felt that the acuity of the situation deemed another ED assessment necessary.

Christopher's uncle returned to the ED, again requesting assessment and treatment. Because the patient was refusing food and fluids, mental health team requested that the emergency department physician perform a thorough physical exam to rule out organic causes of the aggression. Routine lab work was obtained and a physical exam was performed. The patient became agitated and aggressive when the physician attempted an exam of the oral cavity.

Upon further investigation, the patient was diagnosed with esophageal ulcers which had likely presented 48 hours earlier. Because of the extent of the pain, Christopher had refused food and fluids from that point forward. He was admitted to the hospital and placed on a medical unit, where his esophageal ulcers were treated appropriately and his nutritional status was stabilized. He followed up with the mental health clinic one month later, but no acute mental health symptoms were found; Christopher did not meet criteria for a mental health condition and was stable at that time.

aggression and in facilitating a proper diagnosis prior to prescribing psychotropic medication. For example, medical conditions should be ruled out through screening laboratory values, a physical examination should be performed, and interdisciplinary referrals and consultations should be obtained when needed.

For patients with ID, "aggression" might be viewed as an *externalizing behavior symptom* – a clue – and really should be an impetus for detective work. It is important for the ID or mental health clinician to be aware of the most commonly missed, untreated or under-treated medical conditions in persons with ID, as these may present as "behavior problems." See Chapter 3 for more information on medical assessment.

The psychiatrist may be the first physician to evaluate a patient with ID because the patient often presents first with "problem behavior," due to an inability to communicate real physical complaints and other medical symptoms. For example, a patient could present with repetitive jamming of his fist into his mouth, viewed as "aggression." However, this patient should be evaluated for possible medical conditions of the upper gastrointestinal tract, the upper respiratory tract and the mouth and teeth, as well as conditions affecting the hands. These could include, for example, gastro-esophageal reflux disease, eruption of third molars, asthma, nausea, gout, or other conditions.

In addition to possible medical causes, there appear to be time periods when patients with mental health diagnoses exhibit a higher incidence of aggression, including at the time of admission to the hospital, as well as the first weeks after discharge from the hospital (Rueve & Welton, 2008). After discharge, it is likely that patients continue to experience active symptoms during this critical period of stabilization.

Prevalence rates: review of the available evidence

Both behavioral problems and mental illness occur more frequently in individuals with ID. Einfeld & Tonge (1999) reported a 3- to 4-fold increase in emotional problems and behavior issues compared to the general population (Hollander *et al.*, 2006). Deb *et al.* (2007, 2008) reported behavior problems in the range of 50–60% in individuals with ID. Nearly one-third of individuals with ID show aggression, self-injurious behavior (SIB), overactivity, screaming, shouting, or similar behaviors (Hollander *et al.*, 2006). Table 1 presents a summary of research findings concerning the frequency of behavioral symptoms in individuals with ID, adapted from Hollander, 2005.

Cooper *et al.* (2009) specifically studied the prevalence and incidence of self-injurious behavior (SIB). In this study, the operationalized definition of "problem behavior" was taken from the DC-LD as described in Table 2.

By way of comparison, in the general population, aggression is most frequent in persons with dementia, those who have experienced loss of independence and/or physical functioning, persons suffering from grief and loss, persons who are trying to escape or avoid unwanted demands or situations, and persons who are seeking attention or who are bored (Rueve & Welton, 2006).

Tenneij *et al.* (2009) studied aggression in longer-term inpatient treatment centers created for individuals with both mild ID and severely challenging behavior. The vast majority of aggressive incidents were toward direct care staff and were precipitated by denial of requests (Tenneij *et al.*, 2009). Approximately 50% of the reported incidents consisted of verbal aggression alone, and in only 4% of the incidents were there severe consequences for the

Table 1 Incidence of behavioral symptoms in individuals with intellectual disability.

Sexual delinquency	4.9%
Wandering	7.9%
Scatter objects	10.9%
Antisocial behavior	10.9%
Destructiveness	11.9%
Nighttime disturbance	17.8%
Objectionable habits	19.8%
Aggression	22.7%
Self-injury	23.7%
Overactivity	25.7%
Screaming/shouting	28.7%
Temper tantrum	35.6%
Seeks attention	37.6%
TOTAL	60.4%

Source: Deb *et al*. (2001).

victims. Among the subjects in Tenneij's study, higher rates of aggression were associated with more severe ID and, in particular, self-injurious behavior (SIB) was associated with more severe or profound ID. The two age groups most likely to exhibit aggression were late adolescence and early adulthood; those at highest risk were men aged 20–35 years (Tenneij *et al*., 2009).

Table 2 Diagnostic criteria for problem behavior and self-injurious behavior (diagnostic criteria for psychiatric disorders for use with adults with learning disabilities/mental retardation).

General diagnostic criteria for problem behavior
   A The problem behavior is of significant frequency, severity or chronicity as to require clinical assessment and special interventions/support.
   B The problem behavior must not be a direct consequence of other psychiatric disorders, drugs, or physical disorders.
   C One of the following must be present:
   1 The problem behavior results in a significant negative impact on the person's quality of life or quality of life of others. This may be owing to restriction of his or her lifestyle, social opportunities, independence, community integration, service access or choices, or adaptive functioning.
   2 The problem behavior presents significant risks to the health and/or safety of the person.
   D The problem behavior is pervasive. It is across a range of personal and social situations, although it may be more severe in certain identified settings.
Self-injurious behavior
   A The general diagnostic criteria for problem behavior are met.
   B Self-injury sufficient to cause tissue damage, such as bruising, scarring, tissue loss and dysfunction, must have occurred during most weeks of the preceding six-month period, e.g. ranging from skin-picking/scratching, hair-pulling, face slapping, to biting hands, lips and other body parts, rectal/genital poking, eye-poking and head-banging.
   C The self-injurious behavior is not a deliberate suicide attempt.

Source: Cooper *et al*. (2009), p. 210.

Correlates of aggression in persons with ID

Deb *et al.* (2007, 2008) found that higher rates of SIB were associated with more severe ID, poorer communication abilities and autism. McClintock *et al.* (2003) found aggression most closely related to visual impairment, hearing impairment, inability to express needs and inability to ambulate, all of which presumably resulted in unfilled needs (Deb *et al.*, 2007, 2008). Sensory impairments are much more common in people with ID, and Carvill & Marston (2002) found that these physical handicaps were closely related both to aggression and SIB.

Rates of psychiatric disorders appeared to be closely associated with aggression in patients with comorbid ID; prevalence rates for mental illness co-existing with ID are reported to range from 10% to more than 80% (Antonacci *et al.*, 2008). The interaction between symptoms of mental illness and a person's developmental framework is complex, and these factors mutually influence each other.

In one study, psychiatric consultations for persons with severe and profound ID who showed aggression or SIB found an association with mental illness in 23% of patients (King *et al.*, 1994). The reported prevalence rates of various mental health conditions in this study were: impulse control disorders (29%); stereotyped/habit disorders (26%); anxiety disorders (12%); and mood disorders (13%). In patients with ID who also were diagnosed with anxiety disorder, 25% presented with agitation. Patients diagnosed with impulse control disorder were likely to be referred for: aggression (36%); self-injury (30%); or evaluation of psychotropic medications (30%).The group who displayed stereotypic behavior was most likely to exhibit SIB (41%). In the mood disorder group, patients with bipolar disorder exhibited: aggression (12%); hyperactivity (12%); and maladaptive behavior (10%). In the unipolar depressed group, the most common referral problem was maladaptive behavior (10%), followed closely by hyperactivity (8%).

Rojahn *et al.* (2004) studied SIB and aggression and their relationship to impulse control and conduct disorders. Stereotyped behavior was linked to pervasive developmental disorders and somewhat less to schizophrenia. Several other studies have produced consistent findings to support a potential link between SIB/aggressive behavior and affective disorders, and this association has also been suggested by previous authors (Rojahn *et al.*, 2004).

Many researchers have studied risk factors for aggression in inpatient treatment facilities for persons with ID (Tenneij *et al.*, 2009; McClintock *et al.*, 2003; Sigafoos *et al.*, 1994; Tyrer *et al.*, 2006; Davidson *et al.*, 1994; Hogue *et al.*, 2006). Behaviors and risk factors which predicted aggression have included: history of violence; male gender; ages 20–35 years; more severe levels of ID; and the presence of personality disorders. The factors more loosely related but thought to play a role included: psychiatric pathology; presence of SIB; and antisocial behavior (Tenneij *et al.*, 2009).

Aggressive incidents in the Tenneij *et al.* study were assessed using the Staff Observation Assessment Scale-Revised or SOAS-R (Nijman & Palmstierna, 2002). Previously, Nijman and Palmstierna had found that at least four types of behaviors were associated with and may be predictive of, severe aggression on inpatient units for individuals with ID:

1 antisocial behaviors

2 impulse control problems

3 psychotic symptoms

4 mood related symptoms (i.e. mood swings, sudden mood changes, and easily upset) (Tenneij *et al.*, 2009).

Auto-aggression (self-injurious behavior)

Tenneij *et al.* (2009) also observed that auto-aggression (SIB) may be a unique feature to the ID population over and above the aforementioned factors, which is indicative of severity of aggression overall. This has been corroborated by other studies (Davidson *et al.*, 1994; Hillbrand, 1995; Tenneij *et al.*, 2009). Tenneij recommends use of assessment instruments to evaluate known risk factors, and also recommends monitoring for auto-aggression, in particular suggesting that careful assessment should include any acute changes in behavior or emotional reactivity.

Earlier studies have reported widely ranging prevalence rates for SIB in persons with ID, ranging from 1.7–41% (Cooper *et al.*, 2009). SIB is a very serious condition for a patient, and a clearer estimate of prevalence rate is necessary. More recent research by Cooper *et al.* (2009) found the point prevalence of SIB to be approximately 4.9%, and a two-year remission rate of 38.2% (point prevalence being the proportion of people in a population who have a disease or condition at a particular time or date).

Cooper *et al.*'s study identified three risk factors in adult patients with ID and SIB that may make SIB more likely to occur: lower cognitive ability; diagnosis of autism; and more serious communication impairments. Other factors which may be associated, but not reaching statistical significance in the study, included: not living with family; not having Down syndrome; diagnosis of attention deficit hyperactivity disorder; visual impairment; and requiring a high level of support in a residential setting. Institutional populations had a higher prevalence of SIB, but this finding was attributed to the increased risk of this subset of the population being admitted to these facilities. No significant association was found between gender and SIB.

Given the unexpectedly high rate of remission of SIB at the two-year mark (38.2%), Cooper *et al.* (2009) concluded that self-injurious behavior may not be as persistent and longstanding as previously thought. The authors also emphasized that the clinician must be cognizant that patients with ID and SIB may have a medical cause and/or suffer medical complications from this behavior, and these must be diagnosed and treated. The most prevalent complications the authors identified were infections and other physical consequences of seclusion and restraint, and the most common medical causes were sensory impairment and side effects of psychotropic medication. Other identified causes and consequences were isolation from supportive persons and other psychological or social consequences resulting from the behavior (Cooper *et al.*, 2009; see Table 3).

Several other studies that included both adults and children with SIB reported an increased prevalence of SIB in individuals with severe and profound ID. Collacott *et al.* (1998) and Emerson *et al.* (2001a, 2001b) found that SIB was associated with younger age, lower cognitive ability, impaired hearing, impaired mobility and severity of autistic disorder (i.e. greater number of symptoms of diagnostic criteria present). No specific association was found between SIB and seizure disorder, gender or visual impairment. Emerson (2001a, 2001b) also found a high (29%) remission rate after eight years.

Table 3 Associations between individual factors and self-injurious behavior.

Personal factors		Whole cohort	Self-injurious behavior
Age	Prevalent cases	Mean (SD)	42.1 years
	Non-prevalent cases		44.0 years
Gender	Male	54.9%	4.8%
	Female	45.1%	5.0%
Ability	Mild ID	38.9%	0.8%
	Moderate ID	24.2%	2.0%
	Severe ID	18.9%	8.3%
	Profound ID	18.0%	14.1%
Lifestyle and supports			
Accommodation/support	Family caregiver	38.1%	2.3%
	Independent of care	10.0%	2.9%
	Paid caregiver	45.7%	7.5%
	Congregate	6.3%	4.7%
No daytime job/occupation	Has job	75.0%	4.8%
	No job	25.0%	5.1%
Health and disabilities			
Autism	No	92.5%	4.2%
	Yes	7.5%	13.0%
ADHD	No	98.5%	4.2%
	Yes	1.5%	52.3%
Down syndrome	No	81.8%	5.7%
	Yes	18.2%	1.1%
Visual impairment	No	53.0%	3.0%
	Yes	47.0%	7.1%
Bowel incontinence	No	75.0%	2.9%
	Yes	25.0%	10.9%
Urinary incontinence	No	64.7%	2.1%
	Yes	35.3%	10.0%

Source: adapted from Cooper *et al.* (2009), p. 207.

Collacott *et al.* (1998) did not investigate several factors which Cooper found to be significantly associated with SIB, including living with a family member, having ADHD or the absence of Down syndrome. They found a higher prevalence of SIB (17.4%) than did Cooper *et al.* (4.9%), but the two studies used differing definitions for SIB, Cooper having used more severe criteria in her study. Although SIB has historically been considered a severe and sustaining condition, both the Cooper and Emerson studies show that it may not be as persistent as originally thought, and that it appears to have a remitting and relapsing course.

Comorbidity

There are several psychiatric diagnoses known to be associated with aggression. These include: substance abuse disorders; psychotic disorders (especially those including paranoia); affective or mood disorders; personality disorders (especially antisocial and borderline); conduct disorder; oppositional defiant disorder; sexual sadism; pervasive developmental disorders;

Table 4 Summary of psychiatric and medical conditions associated with aggression.

Medical conditions	Traumatic brain injury
	Intracranial pathology (trauma, infections, neoplasms, malformations)
	Cerebrovascular accidents
	Degenerative diseases
	Delirium
	Metabolic conditions (thyroid storm, Cushing's disease, hormonal dysregulation, etc)
	Systemic infections/local infections (i.e. otitis media, urinary tract infections, etc)
	Environmental toxins
	Aberrant effects of medications
	Seizures, especially partial complex
	Sleep apnea
	Constipation
	Food and medication allergies
	Fractures
	Pain (acute and chronic, multiple etiologies)
Psychiatric conditions/symptoms	Substance abuse disorders
	Psychotic disorders (especially paranoia)
	Affective disorders (especially mania, depression assoc with irritability)
	Personality disorders (especially antisocial, borderline)
	Conduct disorder
	Oppositional defiant disorder
	Delirium, dementia
	Intellectual disability

Source: adapted from Rueve & Welton (2008), p. 41 and Charlot & Shedlack (2002).

and delirium/dementia (Rueve & Welton, 2008). There are also many medical conditions that are directly associated with aggression. These include: traumatic brain injury (in particular, injuries that are more severe and involve loss of consciousness); intracranial pathology (including tumors, infectious processes and cerebro-vascular conditions); and metabolic disturbances (including thyroid or other hormonal conditions).

Also important to consider are systemic infections, environmental toxins and certain neurological conditions, such as complex partial seizures or temporal lobe foci on abnormal electroencephalograms (Rueve & Welton, 2008; see Table 4).

Cognitive processes

Prefrontal or frontal lobe disorders may play an important role in aggression. The frontal lobe is responsible for executive functioning, which includes such cognitive processes as the ability to recognize consequences resulting from actions. When the patient makes a choice between good and bad, or better and best, this logic and reasoning requires intact frontal lobe functioning (Rueve & Welton, 2008). The frontal cortex is also likely to be the area of the brain associated with the ability to override or suppress unacceptable social responses. Frontal lobe function is associated with planning, organizing and filtering behavioral responses. Because of limitations in frontal lobe functioning, these cognitive processes may be problematic in persons with ID.

Temporal lobe dysfunction also can have a direct effect on the likelihood of aggression. The temporal lobe and its associated structures are involved in fear and response to danger (Rueve & Welton, 2008). Patients with ID are likely to have co-occurring neurologic conditions or dysfunction in the temporal lobes.

Mood and anxiety disorders and aggression

Mood and anxiety disorders are more common in the ID population and are complicated by fragile self-esteem, fear of failing, loss of caregivers, multiple losses and high prevalence of abuse (Ryan, 2003; Silka & Hauser, 1997). The public signs of anxiety include: sweating or diaphoresis; hyperventilation; avoidance behavior; and motor rituals or other stereotyped behavior. The private symptoms of anxiety and depression may include: embarrassment; worry; despair; frustration; and a variety of physical symptoms.

Individuals with ID are more vulnerable to anxiety and mood disorders due to increased rates of social strain and isolation, decreased problem-solving skills and stigmatization (Silka & Hauser, 1997; Matson & LoVullo, 2008; Taylor, 2002). Both spectrums of disorders can present with various forms of aggression and should be considered as an etiology during the assessment. Both mood and anxiety disorders are thought to be under-diagnosed in the ID population (Silka & Hauser, 1997; Aman *et al.*, 2004; Fletcher *et al.*, 2007). Chapters 7 and 8 discuss the evaluation and treatment of these disorders in greater detail.

Psychotic disorders and aggression

Psychotic disorders, especially when accompanied by paranoia, are associated with aggression in persons with ID. Factors that elevate risk of aggression in recently discharged psychiatric patients in the general population are use of substances and non-adherence to antipsychotic medications (Volavka *et al.*, 2006). Patients with both alcohol and drug abuse appear to be at particular risk for aggression. The risk for aggression and schizophrenia among persons with ID is elevated even without comorbid substance use.

The evaluation and treatment of psychotic disorders is discussed in greater detail in Chapter 9. Determining whether a patient with ID has delusions or hallucinations can be difficult, and the clinician who is evaluating the patient for aggression should elicit reports of thoughts and perceptions, especially those that may be auditory, visual, somatic or proprioceptive and related to neurologic conditions (Volavka *et al.*, 2006). However, psychotic disorders are thought to be over-diagnosed in the ID population, often leading to the over-prescription of antipsychotic medications.

The assessment and treatment of psychotic disorders, as well as the differentiation between psychotic thought disorders versus expectations of function at differing cognitive levels, are discussed in Chapter 9.

Syndromes associated with SIB

Patients with ID who exhibit aggression and SIB are a heterogeneous group, and their behavior reflects various biologic, psychodynamic, and social factors. There are several extremely rare syndromes known to be associated specifically with SIB in the ID population: Lesch-Nyhan syndrome, Smith-Magenis syndrome, Cornelia deLange Syhndrome and Prader-Willi syndrome (Dykens *et al.*, 2000; Emerson *et al.*, 2001a; Fletcher *et al.*, 2007). These disorders are discussed in greater detail in Chapter 4.

Static and dynamic risk factors for aggression

There are several static and dynamic risk factors which have a direct association with aggression both in the general population as well as in persons with ID. The *static* risk factors include: past violence (well-documented to have a direct correlation and to be the most reliable indicator); male gender; younger adult age; cognitive deficits; brain injury; dissociative states; military service; weapons training; and major mental illness. The *dynamic* risk factors include: persecutory delusions; command hallucinations; noncompliance; impulsivity; low global assessment of functioning; homicidality; depression; hopelessness; suicidality; and access to weapons (Rueve & Welton, 2008).

Patients with ID have some additional risk factors for aggression. Aggression in patients with ID can be a means of expressing frustration, a learned problem behavior, an expression of physical pain, an acute medical issue including side effects of medication, a signal of an acute psychiatric problem, or regression in situations of stress, pain, change in routine, or novelty (Rueve & Welton, 2008; Deb *et al.*, 2007; Silka & Hauser, 1997; Antonacci *et al.*, 2008).

SIB that is associated with severe/profound ID is not uncommon, and other disabilities (especially cerebral palsy and sensory impairment) can further complicate the assessment of SIB in this population (Deb *et al.*, 2007; Silka & Hauser, 1997; Antonacci *et al.*, 2008). There also is an association between sleep problems and daytime challenging behavior (irritability, SIB, hyperactivity, and screaming) (Didden *et al.*, 2002; Joyce *et al.*, 2001; Allen *et al.*, 2007). Aggression in children with ID is associated with co-occurring sleep problems, more severe ID, polypharmacy, seizure disorders and cerebral palsy (Didden *et al.*, 2002; Joyce *et al.*, 2001; Allen *et al.*, 2007).

Aggression toward others is more likely to be exhibited by persons with less severe cognitive deficits with greater verbal communication skills, while SIB is more common in individuals with severe ID, who may have decreased mobility, reduced self-help skills, more severe hearing impairment, increased stereotypic movements, and less well developed communication skills (Emerson *et al.*, 2001a).

Life transitions and aggression

Transitions are notoriously difficult for individuals with ID, and they experience many of them. For example, the change from an educational setting to occupational setting may be associated with a new residential placement as well. Introduction to school means introduction to a wide variety of new experiences, more noise, transitions and other factors that can precipitate SIB or other aggression. This also may be a transition time for peers, siblings, parents and others, which therefore makes this a particularly vulnerable time for resurfacing of grief and loss issues. Family members themselves may experience symptoms of grief and loss as the individual with ID goes through various developmental stages, or when these stages would normally have appeared in a child or sibling without ID (e.g. entering school, graduating high school, attending college, marriage and having children).

Irrespective of the person's communication skill level, if aggression continues to be a more powerful means of gaining attention than other behaviors that have been tried, then treatment is not likely to be effective (Matson & LoVullo, 2008). In this scenario, patients with ID often begin to use violence to respond to or communicate about psychosocial stressors, as their cognitive deficits make it difficult for them to develop more adaptive, nonviolent ways of responding (Rueve & Welton, 2008; Silka & Hauser, 1997, Deb *et al.*, 2007; Aman *et al.*, 2004). In order to change, individuals need to learn new outlets and to experience less reinforcement (reward) for using aggression.

The biopsychosocial model

In proposing the biopsychosocial model of disease in 1977, George Engel said: "[in order] *to provide a basis for understanding the determinants of disease and arriving at rational treatments and patterns of health care, a medical model must take into account the patient, the social context in which he lives, and the complementary system devised by society to deal with the disruptive effects of the illness.*" (Campbell & Rohrbaugh, 2006).

The biopsychosocial model is useful when attempting to determine the etiology of aggression in a person with ID. The model or formulation involves gathering information through a variety of sources: patient interview; discussion with family members and/or caretakers; review of clinical records; and contact with collaborating agencies. This leads to a formulation of the problem(s), diagnosis and treatment plan (Campbell & Rohrbaugh, 2006).

The biopsychosocial model allows for an assessment that evolves over time and which should be updated serially, even for patients well known to the physician. Some of its components can vary from assessment to assessment, or even from day to day, depending on the disorder and the "supporting, predisposing, perpetuating, perpetual, and protective factors" related to the disorder.

Biological component of biopsychosocial formulation

The *biological* aspects of the formulation include such information as: demographic data; past and current medical illnesses; genetic predisposition and important family history; medications both past and present; and substance use data. The biologic aspects are especially important to consider, since patients with ID who have behavior problems may be communicating information about an undiagnosed or undertreated medical condition. These biological problems can be worsened by restrictions on care, including restrictions on payment for laboratory work, decreased length and frequency of office visits and other managed care restrictions.

In patients with ID, one may find that medications are being used in ways they were never intended for, in an unsafe manner and with abbreviated monitoring protocols (Ryan, 2003). Especially vital is a detailed medication time line (medications, associated transitions/ stressors/hospitalizations, doses, reasons for discontinuing), if available. For example, if a patient's medication history is studied and it is found that historically he/she has experienced increase in agitation with benzodiazepines, and significant improvement in mood symptoms with norepinephrine reuptake inhibitors, this should guide the clinician in decision making to expedite stabilization of acute symptoms.

If a patient was doing well six months prior to assessment, identify:

(a) the medication regimen at the time;

(b) the residential and occupational settings, support system; and

(c) any significant losses or other psychosocial stressors subsequent to that period of stability.

Quantitative and qualitative information on vegetative symptoms is important and can assist in the determination of etiology of aggression. Assessment of sleep, appetite and internal energy help to identify vegetative symptoms that might be associated with a mood disorder or might be contributing to irritability. The use of sleep charts, mood charts and charts that monitor behaviors/symptoms of interest provided by work/school/residential settings can help in identifying physiologic and psychological changes. Assessment of toilet habits and changes, changes in urination and bowel movements, intake and output of food and fluids, any physical complaints, seizures, sensory deficits or changes (visual, auditory, tactile, olfactory and gustatory) should be completed to help identify medical causes of aggression.

Psychological component of biopsychosocial formulation

A family history of violence is an important factor differentiating persons who exhibit violence from those who do not (Rueve & Welton, 2008), but the task of determining whether aggression is a learned behavior or genetically influenced is a complicated one in

Table 5 Laboratory evaluation of the patient with aggression.

- Complete blood count
- Electrolytes
- Liver function
- Renal function
- Calcium level
- Creatinine phosphokinase
- Toxicology screen
- Blood glucose level
- CT or MRI (brain)
- Optional tests: any pertinent medication levels, ammonia level, antinuclear antibody, rheumatoid factor, sedimentation rate, thyroid function, chest radiograph, lipoprotein levels, B12 level, arterial blood gases, additional medical or neurologic assessment (EEG, etc.) if indicated.

Source: Rueve & Welton (2008), p. 31.

any given patient. It is not known whether there is a specific gene locus or if violence is more likely to be a learned behavior (Rueve & Welton, 2008). It is known that patients who are exposed to violence on a regular basis during developmental years are more likely to exhibit aggression in subsequent relationships.

Past abuse history, including physical, emotional and/or sexual abuse will also play an important role in whether or not any person, including persons with ID, exhibits aggression. This history also will affect a patient's understanding of interpersonal boundaries and their ability to navigate relationships. The incidence of abuse is very high for individuals with ID (Campbell & Rohrbaugh, 2006).

Psychological data that is obtained when assessing aggression in a person with ID should include information about the person's developmental years, institutionalizations (if any), and trauma history. A patient who has a history of institutionalization may feel the need to defend him or herself, may collect or hoard items and may steal or lie. These behaviors or responses may have been developed as survival methods, so they will be difficult to alter or replace. It is also important to be aware of any significant losses the patient has endured, as well as any information about the individual's most significant relationships, both past and present.

Especially in cases where patients do not have family members or other loved ones involved in their lives, the clinician should explore whether there are feelings of abandonment and should utilize direct care staff and/or primary caregivers as vital collateral data sources. These are likely to be the closest relationships that exist under these circumstances. This information should be well documented; if the direct care staff are the only ones aware of such important life events, important pieces of the patient's life history could be lost if that caregiver leaves. Unfortunately, there often is a high turnover rate in direct care staff for individuals with ID. Often, these significant changes take place with no warning to the individual, contributing further to feelings of abandonment and complicated grief processes.

The clinician should also determine whether the patient has ever experienced a counseling relationship in the past, or if one is indicated at the time of assessment. Information on the patient's baseline and current coping skills is important because, in a crisis situation, one may need to try to shore up defenses that exist and to assess deviations from baseline. It is also important to explore thoroughly any precipitants that may exist currently, such as life transitions, job changes, stress in residential placement, recent losses or anniversary reactions.

Social component of biopsychosocial formulation

The *social* component of the biopsychosocial model or formulation is equally important. This includes features of residential placement and entitlements, social activities, and work/school/educational environments and feelings of safety in these environments. The patient's hobbies or interests should be taken into account, as well as their spirituality. Does the aggressive individual have social outlets, spending money, access to exercise and physical activity? It can be useful to ask the patient about such things, using questions such as: "Do you feel safe?"; "Do you like your home?" and "Do you feel the need to defend or protect yourself?"

If the patient is nonverbal, it is important to make this assessment through observation and the use of reliable collateral data sources.

Multimodal model of assessment

Gardner and Moffat (in Antonacci *et al.*, 2008) developed a multimodal model for assessment which consists of:

(a) "individual setting conditions"

(b) "environmental setting conditions"

(c) "maintaining variables."

Individual setting conditions include physiologic elements such as factors related to neurological damage – for example, poor attention span, impulsivity and memory impairment. Patients with ID who are exhibiting aggression should be evaluated for individual medical and neurological conditions, including (but not limited to) seizures, pain conditions, food and environmental allergies, endocrine disorders, hormonal disorders and mental health conditions.

Environmental setting conditions include such things as: high staff turnover; untrained or inconsistent staff; excessive noise or heat; limited interpersonal space; exposure to abrupt or provocative interaction styles; exposure to aggressive behavior; a lack of structure and/or predictability; and intermittent reinforcement of aggression.

The Multimodal Model assumes that aggression is instigated by either individual or environmental factors, and has *maintaining variables* that cause it to recur or diminish, which are reinforcers, either negative or positive. Gardner and Moffat specifically identified level of ID, the presence of sensory or motor disabilities and side effects of anti-seizure medications as common precipitants of problem behaviors.

Emergency assessment of aggression in the person with ID

Clinicians and staff should be aware that there exists the notion of the so-called "vanishing" syndrome or problem in the emergency department (ED). An agitated patient in his or her residential or occupational setting may exhibit aggression but, upon arrival at an ED, this behavior may diminish or "vanish" because of the new and unfamiliar environment. This clearly presents a diagnostic dilemma, since it is impossible for the ED physician to treat a behavior that is not now present. Nevertheless, despite the possibility that the symptom will temporarily subside upon arrival, the emergency department is still an appropriate and necessary setting for acute stabilization, emergency sedation if needed, acute medical and acute psychiatric evaluation on the basis of the history, and referral for further treatment.

Van Silka & Hauser (1997) recommend that, ideally, the ED evaluation should occur in a safe, private, quiet environment, and waiting time should be eliminated if at all possible. The patient with ID will usually be more comfortable if a familiar person remains present throughout the assessment. Patients should be informed what to expect; a clear and detailed explanation prior to any procedures or examination is recommended.

The most common categories of acute ED presentation of patients with ID (Silka & Hauser, 1997) include:

1 new onset or escalation of aggression, self injurious behavior, or both;

2 changes in mental status, including: hyperactivity, irritability, confusion/disorientation, lethargy/withdrawal, psychotic symptoms, and other changes in mood, energy, or sleep pattern;

3 medication side effects, especially extrapyramidal side effects;

4 physical complaints or behavior manifestations that might signify physical illness.

When patients present with aggression, the four functions of problem behavior that should be considered in any ED evaluation are presented in Table 6.

Organizing the emergency assessment of aggression

Because there are multiple potential etiologies of aggression, one may simultaneously develop one or more hypotheses about its possible cause(s). When the comprehensive assessment suggests that a medical/biological problem may be present, this hypothesis should be placed at the top and treated first (see Table 7).

Obtaining a history in the emergency department

There are environmental modifications in the ED and elsewhere that are likely to de-escalate the aggressive patient with ID and to increase the likelihood of obtaining accurate and complete information. These include: employing a calm, soothing tone of voice; positive friendly helpfulness; expressing concern for the patient's well-being; offering food or drink; allowing a phone call to trusted support person; decreased waiting times; distraction with a more positive activity; removal of potentially dangerous items from area; and verbal redirection.

Avoid: overcrowding patients; loud and irritating noises; addressing only caregivers while ignoring the patient; intimidating direct eye contact; unnecessary invasion of personal space; direct confrontational stance; provocative comments; and hands concealed in pockets.

Table 6 Potential functions of problem behavior.

1 Socio-environmental control	Aggression and SIB can be reinforced if the function of the behavior is to exit a situation.
2 Medication	Problem behavior can be a nonverbal means of communication of a variety of messages (attention, discomfort, needs).
3 Modulation of physical discomfort	Medical conditions including medication side effects can cause physical discomfort leading to aggression or SIB.
4 Modulation of emotional discomfort	Problem behavior can occur as a state dependent function of such disorders as Bipolar Disorder, Manic episode, or Major Depressive Disorder.

Source: Lowry & Sovner (1991).

Table 7 Strategy for management of aggression in an emergency.

1	Conduct a comprehensive functional assessment of problem behavior.
2	Develop one or more working hypotheses.
3	Select treatments that address the hypothesized function of the behavior.
4	When a behavior serves multiple functions, target/prioritize those derived from biological dysfunction first.

Source: Lowry & Sovner (1991).

Ostensibly modest interventions can have a remarkable impact on violent outcomes. For example, one might ask "How can I help you?" or "Do you want to talk?" or "What do you need right now?" Do not underestimate the significance of education, effective planning, skilled staff and debriefing after the fact for the purpose of helping staff improve skills. Other treatment options and available staff, in addition to pharmacologic management, should always be considered and used in combination with medication when treating aggressive behavior. These include the help of behavior support specialists, psychotherapists and advocates, and an ongoing and continual collection of collateral data from all important parties to update the formulation.

Even where there are communication deficits, it is important to talk directly to the patient as well as obtaining collateral data from other interested parties. There is an art to "managing the triangle," given that the patient will frequently be accompanied by a caregiver or other interested parties to appointments. A caregiver can hold enormous power in the data provided to the prescriber (for example, the externalizing behaviors are typically the first thing that comes to mind in a follow-up appointment, even if it has been 30 or 60 days since the last episode of aggression). The caregiver also may have unresolved anger or negative transference issues if appropriate debriefing was not conducted, or if the aggressive behavior was taken personally or the staff member was physically injured (see Table 8).

Involve the patient in the history-taking, keeping in mind that a patient with ID will commonly have better developed receptive language skills than expressive language skills, so the clinician should assume that the individual can understand the conversation in the room, even if nonverbal or possessing severely limited communication skills.

As always, it is important to set the stage when the appointment begins by making introductions, while balancing collection of collateral data from others present and direct interface with the patient. Collection of information directly from the patient should be accomplished whenever possible. If the patient is nonverbal or has no usable verbal skills, the clinician can still obtain a great deal of data through observation, relatedness, expression of affect, closed or open posture, personal space, impulse control, attention span, activity level and any unusual or repetitive behavior, along with other nonverbal forms of communication. For individuals who cannot communicate adequately or verbally, the clinician must first evaluate self-report and behavior within the appropriate developmental framework. Despite mild to borderline level of ID, this patient subset may retain some prominent features of early development throughout their adult lives (e.g. self-talk or imaginary friends, with whom they may "discuss" issues of anger and frustration), allowing the clinician to gain greater insight into their feelings. See Chapter 6 for additional information on this topic.

Table 8 Comprehensive assessment of individuals with intellectual disability and aggression.

- Evaluate in a safe, private, quiet place. Decrease stimulation and distractions.
- Conduct the evaluation promptly to avoid further deterioration.
- If possible invite familiar staff, family or career to provide collateral data. The individual will benefit from predictable, reassuring stimuli.
- Calm the patient and the caregivers.
- Explain any procedures simply and clearly.
- *Primum non nocere* (first, do no harm). Do everything possible to avoid seclusion and restraint which will likely increase the individual's distress.
- Determine the reason for requesting the assessment at that point in time. Why now?
- Beware of "vanishing" syndrome. An agitated individual who de-escalates upon arrival to the ER is a diagnostic dilemma. Evaluate the underlying problem, assess likelihood of recurrence, and intervene appropriately.
- Do not attempt a definitive diagnosis during an aggressive episode.
- Use caution in how the emergency department is perceived; it should not be a solution for behavior control, nor used as a form of punishment or to tranquilize the individual.
- It is not necessary to resolve in 30 to 60 minutes a problem which has likely existed for a much longer period of time. Propose both acute and long-term interventions as appropriate by utilizing community resources.
- Rule out medical/organic causes of acute aggression by performing physical and laboratory evaluation.
- Collect careful history on acute psychosocial stressors, changes and losses that the individual may have endured.

Source: Silka & Hauser (1997), p. 165.

Comprehensive ongoing assessment and management of aggression in community and residential settings

When evaluating a patient with ID who has shown aggression periodically over time, the clinician must ask about onset and chronology of the aggression and all other associated symptoms. It is important not only to elicit the presenting problem, but also to determine who has defined the problem, how long it has been observed, in what environments it is observed and, if long-standing in nature, why evaluation is being sought at this point in time. It is crucial that the person making the referral for evaluation is present to explain particular concerns.

The patient's premorbid functioning must be understood and described in detail. If a symptom waxes and wanes in intensity, or varies with level of stress or in different environments, then any pertinent details regarding these circumstances must be documented. If a behavior symptom only occurs at home or only in the occupational setting, this is important information. If the behavior increases in frequency or intensity at certain times, or only exists at a certain time of day, a specific environment, before or after certain events (i.e. family visits) or when a certain staff member or family member is present, this can narrow down the differential diagnoses. The behavior may signal a problem for the person that is interpersonal, physical, or environmental.

The clinician must also take into consideration various mental health issues as a possible etiology of the behavior. When was this individual last doing well? What did that look like (i.e. what is their baseline)? Is the care that is provided consistent across shifts

Table 9 Comprehensive assessment of people with intellectual disabilities and aggressive behavior.

- Identify genetic syndromes with known behavioral or psychiatric phenotypes
- Establish any psychiatric diagnoses, based on most recent standardized evidence based diagnostic manual
- Determine if there are undetected or untreated medical problems
- Determine if there is a correlation between drug changes and changes in behavior
- Consider possible role of drug effects including toxicity/delirium, side effects (akathisia, disinhibition), withdrawal effects, interaction effects
- Identify objective measures of symptoms or behaviors: use screening tools as appropriate, measurement of behaviors, assessment of vegetative functions, mood, memory and other mental status information
- Look for any correlation with stressful life events and changes
- Assess all environments including structure/supports to meet cognitive developmental needs
- Collect detailed data on baseline functioning of the individual
- Consider likely developmental effects on the problems described
- Assess the individual's abilities to describe internal states and other communicative abilities
- Determine behavioral repertoire, including areas of strength and weaknesses
- Assess probable functions of the aggressive behavior, including escape, attention, communication, expression of pain or frustration, modulation of stimulation levels, secure tangibles. Triggers? Factors that maintain behavior? Quantify of frequency and severity. Identify variables contributing to a lowering of the threshold for aggression
- Identify changes in behavioral or other psychosocial treatments correlated with increased problems
- Clarify past treatment trials (What helped? What did not help? Was trial adequate? Were there possible confounding variables? Were successful interventions prematurely terminated?

Source: Reproduced with permission from Charlot, L. & Shedlack, K. (2002). Masquerade: Uncovering and treating the many causes of aggression in individuals with developmental disabilities. *NADD Bulletin* 5, 59–64.

and environments? Is there a conflicted relationship with family or other important people? Is there consistent medication administration? Extract every detail about the time period(s) surrounding the incident(s) of aggression, as these can paint a picture that will help in assessing whether treatment is effective. The functional analysis of aggression and the role of various behavior interventions are described in detail in Chapter 14.

The development of a differential diagnosis of aggression can lead to possible treatments that identify target behaviors which may be responsive to medication, such as a mood disorder that is manifesting itself by aggressive behavior associated with a sleep disturbance. Once this is done, it is important to establish the baseline rate of target behaviors in order to monitor response to treatment. A behavioral psychologist or a behavior support specialist can help design, monitor, and educate staff/direct caregivers regarding data collection.

Pary *et al.* (1995) devised a differential diagnosis of aggression and possible treatments (see Table 11). Taylor (2002) identified four levels of intervention strategies for various presentations of aggressive behavior, summarized in Table 12.

Non-pharmacological intervention strategies for aggression

Taylor (2002) concluded that the most effective non-pharmacological interventions for individuals with co-occurring ID and aggression were the non-cognitive components of

Table 10 Conditions to be considered as etiologies of aggression.

- Means of expressing frustration, fear, injustice or anger
- Learned problem behavior
- Relief from boredom
- Modulation of stimulating environments
- Expression of physical pain or acute medical condition
- Means of communication
- Signal of acute psychiatric problem
- Regression in situations of stress, pain, change in routine, or novelty
- Dementia
- Loss of independence and/or physical functioning
- Grief and loss issues
- Escape or avoidance of unwanted demands or situations
- Attention seeking
- Dementia
- Loss of independence and/or physical functioning
- Grief and loss issues
- Escape or avoidance of unwanted demands or situations
- Attention seeking
- Self-stimulatory behavior
- Product of past experiences
- Parental hostility, maternal permissiveness, absence of maternal affection
- Poor parental modeling, limited social supports, poor school experience

Source: adapted from Rueve & Welton (2008); Ryan (2003); and Charlot & Shedlack (2002).

Table 11 Differential diagnosis of aggression and possible treatments.

Formulation	Interventions
Aggression reflects medical illness	Medical assessment and treatment
Aggression reflects medication side effect	Discontinue and/or substitute medication
Aggression reflects pre-seizure irritability	Review anticonvulsant regimen
Aggression reflects irritability secondary to mania, depression, or organic mood disorder	Treat with disorder-concordant drug and utilize anger management
Aggression represents rage attacks or anger control problem	Treat with appropriate medication, e.g. centrally acting beta blocker or others
Aggression is associated with task-related anxiety	Teach cognitive behavior skills to decrease anxiety
Aggression is associated with psychosis	Treat psychosis
Aggression is related to decreased communication ability	Teach functional communication skills and train carers as needed
Aggression is a means for obtaining positive reinforcers	Enhance access to positive reinforcers; teach socially acceptable, alternative behaviors
Aggression represents escape or avoidance behavior in the absence of an underlying dysfunction	Adapt environment to minimize aversive stimuli (e.g. overcrowding). Teach appropriate escape behavior

Source: Pary *et al.* (1995); adapted from Silka & Hauser (1997), p. 166.

Table 12 Levels of intervention strategies for aggressive behavior in persons with intellectual disability.

Level I	
Reactive strategies	Aimed at managing, rather than reducing challenging behavior when it occurs, with reference to clear guidelines (e.g. control and restraint, seclusion, emergency medication).
Level II	
Ecological interventions	Those which alter the environment or routine in order to use or change the contingencies supporting the behavior or to control the antecedents to it (e.g. increasing the amount of personal space available in reduction of noise levels).
Level III	
Contingency management	Procedures based on learning theory which aim to establish new behaviors that will displace or replace challenging behavior through introduction of new contingencies of real enforcement and or punishment (e.g. extinction, differential reinforcement of incompatible behavior, non-contingent reinforcement in timeout).
Level IV	
Positive programming	Procedures, including direct treatment interventions, which aim to teach the client new skills, abilities and strategies to cope with their environment without the need to rely on challenging behavior (e.g. skills training, relaxation training and psychoeducational approaches).

Source: Taylor (2002), p.61.

treatment, including relaxation, self-monitoring and skills training through role-play. Since concentration problems and executive functioning (comprehending, assimilating, recalling and utilization of information) are problematic for many patients with ID, these persons will have difficulty with the cognitive components of various anger treatments.

In the general population, interpersonal skills training can be useful in altering the way in which an individual expresses anger. Although cognitive techniques may be more difficult for the individual with ID to learn, if the core problem is maladaptive thoughts, a cognitive approach would likely be the most appropriate and successful (Hurley, 2005; Fletcher *et al.*, 2007).

Psychotherapy in the treatment of aggression

Countertransference Countertransference is an important consideration in the treatment of aggressive patients. It is the therapist's experience of emotions in response to the patient's issues. In the circumstance of aggression, the direct care staff or others exposed often have feelings of anger or fear as a result, and they may also interpret the aggression as a personal insult if there is a lack of education and/or inadequate debriefing.

Negative countertransference may influence the progress of treatment, including under- or overestimating risk and becoming over-involved with or alternatively neglectful of the patient (Rueve & Welton, 2008). The psychotherapist may inappropriately ignore feelings

Table 13 Non-pharmacologic interventions for the treatment of aggression.

- Utilize behavior therapy and behavior support services based on functional analysis
- Decrease environmental stressors, stimulation
- Create an appropriately stimulating, predictable and safe environment
- Control antecedent conditions
- Utilize preventive measures (alter physical environment, reduce noise levels, normalize routines, use behavioral momentum, offer choices, etc.)
- Teach adaptive alternatives or functional equivalents
- Alter antecedent events and/or consequences
- Eliminate reinforcers of the aggression
- Render aggressive response unnecessary by strongly reinforcing functionally equivalent alternatives
- Promote early success, gradually 'raise the bar'
- Distract with a preferred activity
- Strengthen desirable alternative behaviors
- Consider weighted vests, wrist weights, etc.
- Communication training
- Replacement behaviors
- Relaxation training

Source: adapted from Charlot & Shedlack (2002) and Matson & LoVullo (2008).

of fear or anger while focusing on building a therapeutic alliance. The clinician may struggle to relate to, or empathize with, an aggressive patient.

For example, in a case where a patient has exhibited aggression due to limit-setting by staff, psychotherapy may be viewed by the patient as punishment. This can be especially so if the psychotherapist joins in with others (e.g. direct care staff, family members, primary care physician, etc) and spends the time in the room lecturing the patient about the rules, instead of focusing on the patient's affect, how the patient feels about being controlled by others, or having this decision made without his or her input and imposed without consent (by contrast, adults without ID are given recommendations but have the right to follow through with these or not). Without self-monitoring, the psychotherapist may find it difficult to maintain a supportive, non-judgmental stance and avoid inappropriate reactions when treating a patient with aggression (Rueve & Welton, 2008).

These modalities of psychotherapy have been instituted in the treatment of aggression (as outlined by Rueve & Welton, 2008):

1 *Behavioral focus*: concerned with prior triggers, violent behaviors, and consequences for actions. Many institutions employ these behavioral techniques in the form of levels of privileges that the patient can earn.

2 *Social skills training*: promotes more acceptable assertive behaviors and reinforces self-control mechanisms.

3 *Cognitive approaches*: focus is on incorrect automatic thoughts that precede anger reactions in the context of larger faulty belief systems that direct an individual's perception of external events. The patient is thought to be filtering experiences through inaccurate cognitive schema, which results in distortions of situations with subsequent unnecessary feelings of anger and inappropriate responses.

4 *Group therapy*: this approach creates a microcosm of real-world relationships and interpersonal difficulties for patients. Group therapy can be less intense for potentially violent patients, because the group dilutes transference and countertransference reactions. Interactions with other group members through a course of therapy can be a source of modeling. It also consists of supportive confrontations and conflict resolution.

Pharmacologic interventions for the treatment of aggression

Pharmacology overview

It is a challenge to develop broad and all-inclusive treatment recommendations because of the heterogeneity of aggression. Treatment choices, including the use of medication, should be guided by the biopsychosocial model, with ongoing assessment of the total picture. There are multiple variables to consider when using medications in the ID population, and sometimes they are not indicated. For example, to quote La Malfa *et al.* (2006):

> "*Antipsychotics are the most widely prescribed medications in individuals with intellectual disability even if schizophrenia and other psychotic disorders do not affect more than three percent of such population.*"

In the past, antipsychotic medications have sometimes been inappropriately prescribed for patients with aggression, for their tranquilizing effects alone. However, self-reporting of side effects is often compromised in patients with ID, given their communication limitations. It is estimated that approximately 20% of patients with ID experience adverse drug reactions, with some side effects manifesting more severely (Aman *et al.*, 2004; Habler & Reis, 2010). Neuroleptic malignant syndrome is more frequently fatal in patients with ID, at rates twice that of the general population (Habler & Reis, 2010). There is evidence that the ID population likely experiences increased rates of sensitivities and adverse drug reactions with psychotropic medication, probably as a consequence of damage to the central nervous system, and also metabolic, pharmacodynamic and pharmacokinetic differences (Janowsky *et al.*, 2004). Therefore, all psychotropic medications must be used with special caution.

Approximately 12–46% of individuals with ID receive psychopharmacologic drugs for reasons of aggression or other behavior problems. Aggression, disruptive behavior and/or SIB occur in 10–62% of individuals with ID.

Both impulsivity and aggression start at a younger age in individuals with ID, compared to individuals without ID (Santosh & Baird, 1999). At least 20% of children and adolescents with ID exhibit problem behaviors. Approximately 12–46% of individuals with ID receive psychopharmacologic drugs for behavior problems. Adults with ID receive psychotropic medicine more often, and at higher doses, compared to children with the same conditions. Medication treatment trials for patients with ID have lasted over longer periods and often included polypharmacy, often without any documented Axis I psychiatric diagnoses (Santosh & Baird, 1999).

When psychopharmacologic drugs are needed, appropriate management includes smaller starting doses for children and adolescents than their normally developing peers, and these doses should be increased at slower rates. Treatment plans should not be based on pharmacology alone. Skill deficits, unmet sensory needs and frustration because of an absence of meaningful choices should be addressed. Expert consensus guidelines recommend that treatment should be based upon the most specific psychiatric diagnosis possible (Aman *et al.*, 2004; Cooper *et al.*, 2009; Deb & Unwin, 2007a). When only a tentative, nonspecific diagnosis can be made, as in the presence of severe/profound ID, clinicians should focus on one or more behavioral symptoms as targets of treatment. Psychotropic medication may or may not be one component of treatment, but it should not be the only treatment strategy.

The consideration of various other categories of psychotropic medications, rather than just antipsychotic medications, is important in the treatment of aggression. For example, beta blockers decrease norepinephrine availability, which in turn may decrease aggression (Rueve & Welton, 2008; Aman *et al.*, 2004).

Medications affecting gamma-amino butyric acid (GABA) receptors (such as benzodiazepines) have an inhibitory effect on aggression. Medications that increase GABA typically have a relaxing, anti-anxiety and anti-seizure effect on patients (Rueve & Welton, 2008; Aman *et al.*, 2004). However, potential side effects of these drugs include sedation, as well as anterograde and retrograde amnesia. Individuals with ID commonly have memory deficits at baseline, so this is especially relevant. Also, some patients with ID may experience and exhibit a paradoxical stimulation from this medication class. During the assessment, questions should be asked specifically about whether this has occurred with these types of medications. Inquiries regarding medications that may have been given prior to medical or dental procedures and their effects often reveal this information.

Finally, individuals with low cerebrospinal fluid levels of 5-hydroxyindoleacetic acid (5-HIAA, a metabolite of serotonin), are more likely to exhibit aggression (Rueve & Welton, 2008). The use of selective serotonin reuptake inhibitors (SSRIs) to treat aggression by increasing serotonin availability in the central nervous system is discussed later in the chapter.

Antipsychotic medications

Antipsychotic literature specific to adults   This is the most commonly used class of medications for aggressive behavior in adults with ID, although there is little evidence-based research supporting the efficacy of antipsychotic medications for this indication. Rates of prescription of antipsychotic medications to patients with ID vary across studies, with an average of 30–50% (Antonacci *et al.*, 2008; Matson & Monshawi, 2007; Radouco-Thomas, 2004). Rates in hospitalized individuals were found to be between 22–45%, while in community samples they were approximately 20%.

In a review of psychopharmacology from 1990 to 1999, Matson reported on 14 studies (Matson & LoVullo, 2008). Twelve of the 14 cite use of both first generation antipsychotics (FGA) and second generation antipsychotics (SGA) to treat aggression, and most of the studies reported decreases in frequency and severity of aggression with administration of these medication classes. King (2002) reported that the evidence was growing for the use of antipsychotic medications for management of aggression in patients with ID, and suggested that SGAs held promise. Deb *et al.* (2007) reported a systematic review of empirical research on the effectiveness of antipsychotic medications in adults with ID and aggression.

After reviewing eleven studies, the author found that the data from randomized controlled trials showed risperidone was probably effective for managing problem behaviors. Sample sizes were small, however, and could not be statistically analyzed.

There are several published documents regarding expert consensus guidelines for treatment of psychiatric and behavioral problems in individuals with ID; these are summarized in Chapter 12. SGAs were recommended to treat aggressive behavior, with risperidone being the first choice (Deb *et al.*, 2007). First-line ratings were also given to olanzapine, with quetiapine a high second-line option. Clozapine was reported as useful in reducing self-injury and aggression in two individuals who did not respond to risperidone (Matson & LoVullo, 2008).

Janowski *et al.* (2006) studied relapse rates of aggression in adults with ID. Of the patients who could be successfully withdrawn from antipsychotic medication, 66.3% were still psychotropic-drug free several years later. On the other hand, of patients who experienced rapid recurrence of symptoms following antipsychotic drug withdrawal or dose decreases, only 9% were psychotropic free at follow-up. This study concluded that policies and guidelines which recommend attempts to limit and discontinue use of psychotropic medications are appropriate, but this will not be possible in all cases, and particularly in adults with ID who are in institutions and who have failed this intervention in the past.

Ruedrich *et al.* (2008) reported that SGAs (including risperidone, olanzapine, quetiapine, ziprasodone, clozapine, etc.) improved aggression in adults with ID, except in cases of SIB. A retrospective review of 31 adult residents of a state developmental (institutional) center who were treated for aggression and/or SIB with SGAs was performed; incidents of aggression and SIB decreased over a twelve-month period, as compared to one year with FGA treatment. The findings suggested that if SGAs were substituted for first generation antipsychotics (FGAs, such as haloperidol, thorazine, perphenazine, etc.) in individuals with ID, there was a decrease in frequency of aggression (but not SIB). In addition, in this study, four out of ten institutionalized adults with ID who were later withdrawn from antipsychotic drugs continued to remain stable without psychotropic drugs for an average of ten years afterward. With respect to side effects, patients with ID taking olanzapine experienced weight gain, which highlights the importance of metabolic monitoring in this population.

Challenging behaviors such as aggression, SIB, destructive and disruptive behaviors are more prevalent with more severe ID. Janowski *et al.* (2003a) found that olanzapine is effective for treating challenging behaviors in the ID population, and it can be substituted for FGAs in some cases to reduce extrapyramidal symptoms and the risk of tardive dyskinesia. The Janowski *et al.* (2003a) study specifically monitored aggression, SIB and destructive/ disruptive behaviors, and found a significant decrease in all of these, including SIB. The importance of monitoring for both EPS and metabolic problems was highlighted, as some patients experienced weight gain, especially in the first six months, and the incidence of tardive dyskinesia and other forms of extrapyramidal symptoms was higher in the ID population as compared with the general population, even when using SGA drugs.

Rueve & Welton (2008) reported that, in the treatment of acute violent behavior, haloperidol (an FGA) has repeatedly been shown to be safe in patients with ID, even if their medical histories are unknown. Haloperidol has minimal effects on seizure threshold, which is of particular importance in patients with ID. In comparison with the FGAs for the treatment of acute aggression, with SGAs there are concerns about the cardiac side effect of QT prolongation (especially with ziprasidone) and sedation/cardiorespiratory depression, especially when olanzapine is prescribed with benzodiazepines (Rueve & Welton, 2008).

Clozapine and other SGAs have been shown to be effective in decreasing chronic aggression associated with psychosis, even when other pharmacological agents have provided no benefit or residual symptoms exist (Volavka *et al.*, 2006). Some SGAs have shown equal efficacy to FGAs for managing chronic aggression, including risperidone, olanzapine and quetiapine. These medications have also been shown to improve aggression associated with autism or dementia, although there are serious safety concerns when prescribing SGAs in patients with dementia, including heart-related events and sudden death (Aman *et al.*, 2004, Antonacci *et al.*, 2008; Volavka *et al.*, 2006).

Volavka *et al.* (2006) reviewed the literature on the use of FGAs and SGAs for the purposes of violence reduction and the decrease of use of restraint and seclusion. Risperidone was reported to have selective effects on hostility that were superior to haloperidol. In low doses, risperidone showed promise in the management of aggression and was effective in boys with oppositional defiant disorder (ODD) or conduct disorder (CD). Both olanzapine and quetiapine showed some anti-aggressive effects, but more research is needed regarding the use of these medications.

In a recent review of the literature, Habler & Reis (2010) determined that risperidone was the most frequently used SGA in adults to treat aggression. In one report (Gagiano *et al.*, 2005) about 58% of patients improved, relative to 31% in the placebo group. Recommended doses ranged between 0.5 and 4.0 mg daily.

Antipsychotic literature specific to children/adolescents   Clozapine is not approved for the indication of disruptive behavior in children, and there is no specific evidence for its efficacy in children (Habler & Reis, 2010). It does not have a formal indication for adolescents or children, and literature is scarce in the treatment of patients under the age of 18 years. Clozapine was the first SGA approved for treatment-resistant schizophrenia in adults.

Risperidone has an approved indication for the treatment of irritability associated with autistic disorder in 5–16 year olds. There is also evidence of effectiveness in the treatment of hyperactivity, irritability, impulsivity, aggression against self and others, and stereotypic behavior (Habler & Reis, 2010). Olanzapine proved effective for the treatment of hyper-activity and irritability, but side effects and dropout rates were both higher.

In general, antipsychotics and some antidepressants (maprotiline, clomipramine, bupro-pion among antidepressants; chlorpromazine, olanzapine and clozapine among antipsy-chotics) have relatively high potential to lower the seizure threshold in adults, and risperidone has a lower risk in adults. However, data are less available for children, although it is known that olanzapine has a potential for increasing seizure risk in children (Habler & Reis, 2010).

For all of these types of medications, this seizure threshold-lowering effect is dose-dependent and must be carefully monitored in this specialized population. Quetiapine is approved for treatment of schizophrenia in children and adolescents in the general population, and also indicated for acute treatment of manic episodes associated with bipolar I disorder. Ziprasidone requires further research, but there is limited data suggesting it may play a role in reduced irritability and aggression in children and adolescents with PDD.

Mood stabilizers/anticonvulsants

Mood stabilizer literature specific to adults   No randomized controlled studies were found on mood stabilizers specific to adults in the ID population. Anticonvulsants/mood stabilizers are the second most common psychotropic medication class prescribed in patients with ID, in part because they are used to treat seizure disorders, which are particularly prevalent in this population. Expert consensus guidelines (2004) list anticonvulsants/mood stabilizers as a preferred medication for treatment of aggression and SIB as target symptoms. Sodium valproate was overwhelmingly chosen as the preferred agent for this population. Overall it showed a reduction in target behavior (whether aggression alone or in combination with additional behaviors) at a rate of 50%.

Verhoeven & Tuinier (2001) reported 68% of patients showed some improvement in behavior problems with sodium valproate. Sodium valproate was primarily used in conjunction with other agents at serum levels comparable to those used to treat seizures. Two studies showed clinical improvement in approximately 70% of adults with ID who had behavior problems. Verhoeven & Tuinier (2001) and Rueve & Welton (2008) reported that sodium valproate was shown to promote reduction in aggression across multiple diagnostic categories, including organic syndromes, dementia, ID and bipolar disorder. Weight gain and hair loss are among several important potential side effects, and there is a risk of fetal malformation if there is a pregnancy.

Carbamazepine was the second most preferred anticonvulsant/mood stabilizer recommended by most expert consensus guidelines. Carbamazepine is a metabolism inducer and alters blood levels of many medications. There is a lower risk of weight gain, but potential side effects include nausea, vomiting, sedation, anticholinergic side effects and cognitive dulling. Janowski *et al.* (2003b) reported that, with topiramate, 74% of patients with ID who were treated for aggression improved. However, a review of all of the available data on anticonvulsants/ mood stabilizers used for the treatment of aggression finds the evidence lacking in showing overall effectiveness of topiramate. Janowski *et al.* (2003b) described positive responses to topiramate in the treatment of SIB, aggression and other disruptive behavior. Acutely increased intraocular pressure is a rare but very important potential side effect of topiramate.

Deb *et al.* (2008) reported on three lithium studies in the treatment of aggression. Lithium was used as an adjunct therapy for aggression, SIB and hyperactivity, and it was added to an existing regimen of psychotropic medications; 73% of adults improved, while 9% worsened. The placebo group had 30% improvement. In a second study, 56% of participants showed some decrease in aggression with lithium, while 44% were unchanged. "Lithium responders" were defined as those patients who sustained major reduction or resolution of target symptoms, and this group consisted of 47% of all subjects who received lithium.

Rueve & Welton (2008) reported that lithium has been shown to be effective for aggression in the ID population at serum concentrations of 0.6 to 1.4 mEq per liter, which is similar to the blood level needed in bipolar disorder. Rates of violence were reduced by between 50–73%, depending on samples reported. Lithium also reduces irritability related to aggression in patients with ID who also are diagnosed with bipolar disorder, though the vast majority of these patients required additional medications prescribed in conjunction with lithium.

Older adults and those who presented with psychosis were more likely to respond to lithium, although side effects and blood levels need to be carefully monitored, especially in the elderly. Overall, both Deb *et al.* (2008) and Rueve & Welton (2008) concluded that most patients with aggression improved while taking lithium. On the other hand, Habler &

Reis (2010) reported severe side effects with lithium in patients with ID (including weight gain, hypothyroidism, tremor, polydipsia, polyurea, diabetes insipidus, acne, electrocardiogram (EKG) changes, muscle weakness and even intoxication). Therefore, lithium should be used with extra caution in this specialized population.

In summary, anticonvulsants or other mood stabilizers are used in almost 50% of inpatients with ID (Habler & Reis, 2010; Aman *et al.*, 2004; Deb & Unwin, 2007b; Deb *et al.*, 2008). In the treatment of impulsive and aggressive behavior, expert consensus guidelines suggest using them also as adjunctive agents for patients with schizophrenia who are exhibiting agitation, excitement, aggression, or violence. Sodium valproate is the most commonly used mood stabilizer for inpatients and has been shown to reduce hostility, in particular when combined with an antipsychotic for hospitalized patients experiencing acute psychosis (Aman *et al.*, 2004; Deb & Unwin, 2007b; Deb *et al.*, 2008). It is established as more effective than a placebo to reduce aggression and is considered the first-line agent in most published guidelines. Carbamazepine and lithium were both recommended as second-line adjunct treatment options for aggressive behavior in psychotic patients by the Expert Consensus Statement (Aman *et al.*, 2004).

Mood stabilizer literature specific to adolescents/children Habler & Reis (2010) report that mood stabilizers have been utilized in the treatment of impulsivity, bipolar disorder, and aggression against self and others in children and adolescents. Both Antonnaci *et al.* (2008) and Green (2001) (both in Habler & Reis, 2010) state that lithium is not recommended for use in children under the age of 12 years because of the increased risk of severe side effects (the same as stated above for adults), (Habler & Reis, 2010). Sodium valproate appears to be the treatment of choice for aggression and SIB in children. Carbamazepine was shown to decrease agitation in children with brain injuries (Rueve & Welton, 2008).

Antidepressants

Antidepressant literature specific to adults In the general population, selective serotonin reuptake inhibitors (SSRIs) have established efficacy in decreasing aggression for patients with various psychiatric diagnoses. Janowski *et al.* (2005) reported on the effects of SSRIs and clomipramine (a tricyclic which also has a significant effect on serotonin level) on aggression and SIB. In this study, there were statistically significant decreases in maladaptive behavior, including aggression, SIB, destruction/disruption and depression/dysphoria with the use of all of these antidepressants.

Janowski *et al.* (2004) studied 38 institutionalized patients with ID who were taking SSRIs or clomipramine for depression. The study concluded that serotonergic antidepressants produced a statistically significant decrease in depression-related symptoms and signs related to aggression, particularly with respect to SIB. The SSRIs also have a significant effect on anxiety, and Janowski *et al.* (2004) concluded that although patients who were prescribed antidepressants improved less than 50% of the time, those with underlying pathology in the anxiety disorder spectrum (obsessions, compulsions, etc.) were more likely to show significant improvement.

Antidepressant literature specific to adolescents/children Habler & Reis (2010) reported that SSRIs are effective for the treatment of some anxiety spectrum disorders, particularly obsessive compulsive disorder (OCD) associated with stereotypic behavior and SIB. There are no specific guidelines for the use of antidepressants in children for the purpose of treating aggression. Fluoxetine may have a positive effect on SIB, impulsivity and depressive symptoms in children with ID. Some children with autistic disorder exhibited manic-like activation, so extra caution should be used with this subset.

Currently, fluoxetine is approved for use in pediatric patients between ages 7–17 years with diagnoses of major depressive disorder (MDD) and OCD (Habler & Reis, 2010). Escitalopram is approved for MDD in adolescents 12–17 years of age, and clomipramine for ages 10–17 years. For treatment of OCD, fluvoxamine is approved for patients 8–17 years of age and sertraline for those aged 6–17 years. Findings include reduction of stereotyped behavior with the use of antidepressants, while visual contact rates and communicative behaviors were both improved. More recently, black box warnings were added to many antidepressants for individuals age 25 years and younger regarding risks of increased suicidal thinking or behavior. Results of comprehensive reviews indicate that the benefits likely outweigh the risks in most patients.

Opioid antagonists

The theory behind the use of this medication class is that SIB causes release of androgynous opioids which, in turn, stimulate the reward system in the central nervous system (Habler & Reis, 2010). Simultaneously, the endogenous opioids theoretically calm the physical pain incurred by the SIB, precipitating a cycle of behavior. Deb et al. (2008), in Habler & Reis (2010), published a systematic review on opioid antagonists for treatment of impulsivity and aggression in adults. In one study, naltrexone was compared to a placebo in 33 adults and found to be ineffective. However, the literature on opioid antagonists was found to be contradictory and there was considerable variation and inconsistency in the effectiveness of the drugs.

Overall, despite this latter study, Deb et al. (2008) concluded that about 80% of adults improved in the short term, and there was a minimum of 50% reduction of SIB in 47% of subjects. With regard to children and adolescents, Habler & Reis (2010) reported that opioid antagonists may be effective for short-term acute treatment of hyperactive, impulsive, stereotypic and aggressive behavior. Boys experienced more pronounced improvement than girls in the salient studies.

Benzodiazepines

Side effects of benzodiazepines are of particular concern in patients with ID because of the risk of disinhibition, agitation, aggression, anger, depression and euphoria (Kalachnik et al., 2002). Benzodiazepines usually have been prescribed to the ID population in an effort to manage hostility, hyperactivity, irritability, socially inappropriate behavior, psychosis and temper tantrums. Kalachnik et al. (2002) reported that this medication class was also being prescribed for various other conditions, including psychiatric illness, seizure disorders, or myoclonus/cerebral palsy. The rate of reported side effects ranged from 11–25%, which could be considered frequent relative to rates of common side effect prevalence. The authors recommend using lower doses of the shorter-acting agents for shorter treatment periods. Silka & Hauser (1997) cautioned that benzodiazepines increased the risk of ataxia in patients with autism.

Beta blockers

Volavka *et al.* (2006) reported on beta blockers for the treatment of irritability mediated by the noradrenergic system. Propranolol and nadolol have shown some effectiveness and are the most extensively studied beta blockers in the context of managing persistent irritable and aggressive behavior, particularly in patients with brain injuries. Rueve & Welton (2008) reported that beta blockers are sometimes used as adjunct treatments to help control violence in patients with a variety of symptoms and conditions. In patients recently hospitalized for traumatic brain injury, propranolol was found to be more effective than placebo in reducing agitation..

Psychostimulants and atomoxetine

The prevalence rate for attention deficit hyperactivity disorder (ADHD) among children without ID is approximately 5% (Habler & Reis, 2010). In children with ID, it co-occurs at rates between 8.7–16%. Response rates for stimulants in patients with ID were found to be between 45–65% in a review of 20 controlled studies (Habler & Reis, 2010). Response rates were 10–30% less, compared to children without ID.

In a meta-analysis of seven studies, Connor *et al.* (2002) reported that the strongest predictor for a positive outcome in the use of stimulants for aggression and disruptive behavior was an IQ above 50. This study did not recommend the use of psychostimulants for patients with IQs below 50, due to extremely small response rates (less than 20%) and the prevalence of side effects, including (but not limited to) tics, social withdrawal, emotional irritability, anxiety and anorexia, which were reported in 22–50% of subjects. In general, the ID population appears to experience increased risk of side effects (tics, irritability, and dysthymia) from psychostimulant use (Handen & Gilchrist, 2006).

Atomoxetine is not a psychostimulant, but rather a selective norepinephrine reuptake inhibitor. Atomoxetine is also approved for treatment of ADHD. It has been found to be an effective and safe co-medication for treating hyperactivity and attention deficit in children with ID. Nevertheless, at this time, expert consensus recommends psychostimulants for ADHD and for hyperactive behavior in adults with ID (Aman *et al.*, 2004). Relatively speaking, there is more available research on the use of stimulants rather than for other classes of drugs in this patient population.

Clinical Vignette #3

Eve, a 26 year old single female with history of attention deficit hyperactivity disorder (combined type), profound intellectual disability and impulse control disorder, presented for mental health assessment with aggression, irritability and restlessness. These symptoms had been present and had increased in frequency and severity over the previous three months.

The symptoms were present nearly every day and occurred across her work and home environments, as well as with various staff, on various shifts and during home visits with family on the weekends. She was physically aggressive toward others and had targeted both familiar and unfamiliar people, as well as vulnerable individuals and those who were clearly larger and stronger than her. The aggression was random and had no identified precipitating factors or triggers.

Prior to the last three months, Eve had episodic and very minimal irritability and distractibility. Approximately three months ago, her psychiatrist tapered and discontinued her Adderall XR in an attempt to alleviate the side effects she experienced with this medication, including decrease in appetite and initial insomnia. At the same time, Eve was started on atomoxetine (Strattera). The atomoxetine was increased to 40 mg twice daily, which was thought to be a therapeutic dose.

Over the course of the last three months, Eve's appetite had improved minimally, resulting in a weight gain of three pounds. In an attempt to treat the aggression, irritability, and restlessness, Eve was tried on multiple medications including Zoloft (sertraline), Valium (diazepam), lamotrigine (Lamictal), and Tegretol (carbamazepine), as well as two different second generation antipsychotics – ziprasidone (Geodon) and risperidone (Risperdal).

Eve experienced tachycardia and palpitations within 48 hours of starting each second generation antipsychotic and so these were discontinued very quickly. The other medications are now daily (Zoloft, ativan, topamax and depakote), but they have been only minimally helpful in the treatment of the aggression.

Family history is significant for two twin brothers, both with ADHD and both treated successfully with Adderall XR. It is evident that Eve will not tolerate second generation antipsychotics, given the above stated adverse drug reactions. She was restarted on the Adderall XR and the atomoxetine was tapered cautiously and discontinued.

Her attention span increased, as did her concentration. Over the next two months, she was tapered and discontinued from the diazepam, Lamictal and sertraline. She was continued on a regimen of depakote and Adderall XR and the aggression resolved.

Hormonal treatment

An association between androgens and aggression has been well established (Guay, 2008, 2009; Sajith *et al.*, 2008; Habler & Reis, 2010). Sexual and aggressive behaviors are regulated by androgens; there is not a direct relationship but, rather, androgen activity can increase the probability of response to situations or stimuli (Habler & Reis, 2010). Hormonal agents, including estrogens and anti-androgens, have been used to decrease aggression, but there are no controlled studies or expert consensus guidelines, so their use is limited by both this and the risk of serious side effects, which include (but are not limited to) liver abnormalities, increased risk of certain cancer types, feminization and bone abnormalities (Guay, 2008, 2009; Sajith *et al.*, 2008; Habler & Reis, 2010). For further discussion on the use of hormonal agents, see Chapter 12.

Electroconvulsive therapy (ECT)

Electroconvulsive therapy (ECT) is a safe, effective and some would say underutilized treatment option for affective disorders, acute psychosis and treatment-resistant schizophrenia among other conditions. There are case reports on the use of ECT for catatonic regression, self-injurious behavior and aggression related to autism and other ID and/or mental health issues (Wachtel *et al.*, 2009, 2010; Ligas *et al.*, 2009; Aziz *et al.*, 2001). Specific to the ID population, the clinician must be aware of possible complications of ECT because patients with ID have an increased prevalence of seizure disorders, can be more easily misdiagnosed, have a lower rate of subjective side effect reporting and often include a complicated informed consent process (Aziz *et al.*, 2001).

Most case reports are consistent in that there is clinical improvement in behavioral and psychiatric symptoms after a course of ECT in patients with ID and aggression, although no controlled studies have been conducted. Case studies report increased mood stabilization, reduction in SIB and decreased behavioral disturbance, but even these data are quite limited (Wachtel *et al.*, 2009, 2010; Ligas *et al.*, 2009; Aziz *et al.*, 2001).

There also are limited studies on the effectiveness of ECT in patients with autism and catatonic regression (Dhossche & Rout, 2006; Dhossche & Stanfill, 2004). There is speculation that some individuals diagnosed with autism may actually be experiencing early expressions of catatonia, as both conditions are associated with abnormal gamma-amino butyric acid (GABA) function, small cerebellar structures, and may be associated with chromosome 15. Although this is controversial, some have argued that if such individuals were treated with ECT early in the course of illness, it might be possible that this could serve as a preventive measure for further development of autistic symptoms (Dhossche & Rout, 2006; Dhossche & Stanfill, 2004). Further exploration of this potential link is needed, as there are no clinical trials on this hypothesized relationship.

Conclusions about medication use

Volavka *et al.* (2006) outlined a brief overview of various medication categories utilized in the treatment of aggression. With regard to aggression, clozapine as an anti-aggressive agent is well-established, especially in the inpatient setting. Evidence also exists for risperidone, olanzapine, quetiapine and aripiprazole. Mood stabilizers, including lithium, are widely used to control aggression, but efficacy lacks strong support. Benzodiazepines have a role in acute aggression and agitation, but their long-term use is not recommended (Volavka *et al.*, 2006). There is some evidence for anti-aggressive effects of SSRIs and hormonal agents with anti-androgenic properties. Beta blockers and electroconvulsive therapy are more rarely used in clinical practice to control aggression, but they may be effective.

In general, treatment with pharmacologic agents for the patient with ID does not differ much from pharmacotherapy in patients without ID. Risperidone is well documented to be effective in the treatment of children with ID, particularly those with autism. It is the preferred agent in the treatment of disruptive behavior in children and adolescents with ID (Habler & Reis, 2010; Volavka *et al.*, 2006).

The selection of treatment agents for disruptive behavior in patients with ID depends on the severity of symptoms and the extent to which social, biological, or psychological factors cause the symptoms. Disruptive behavior needs to be addressed (whether with pharmacotherapy or alternate interventions), despite the fact that there are neither clear diagnostic criteria nor consistent ways to measure it. Medications have been shown to help decrease impulsivity, aggression and agitation, regardless of their etiology.

Patients with ID in general have a high prevalence of disinhibition, impulsive behavior and a lack of "filtering" in addition to differing degrees of executive function deficits compared to the general population. Pharmacotherapy is one of the basic options for the treatment of challenging behavior after several requirements are met. Informed consent issues must be carefully attended to and special consideration utilized in patients with cognitive deficits who are acting as their own guardians. Physical and psychological conditions must be evaluated, diagnosed and appropriately treated. Any medication decision must involve careful consideration of risks and benefits. Reviews of the many expert consensus guidelines instruct the prescriber to "start low and go slow."

A number of side effects can be more severe or have variant presentations compared to similar treatment in patients without ID, and patients may not be able to verbally report them. Use of standardized and universal rating scales should be used to identify and track target symptoms and extrapyramidal symptoms, and to screen for metabolic side effects. In case of no response to monotherapy, combinations of psychotropic medications may be useful, but attention to and prevention of unnecessary polypharmacy must be avoided.

Summary: a comprehensive approach to the chief complaint of aggression – detective work and problem solving

Diagnosing and treating aggression in a patient with ID requires careful detective work. The mainstay of this lies in utilizing a comprehensive biopsychosocial formulation and taking the time to determine the most appropriate interventions and treatment measures. This includes strategic use of collateral data from all environments and from various instrumental people in the patient's life.

The acuity of the situation obviously must be taken into account. If the patient is harming him/herself or others, or if there is great risk of either, then it may be necessary to institute immediate measures (e.g. hospitalization, one-on-one monitoring, short-term use of acute psychotropic medications, etc.) until the etiology of the aggression can be determined.

If the aggression or SIB can be defined in terms of a target symptom or behavior, a behavior support specialist can suggest ways to collect quantitative and qualitative data, including the frequency, severity and associated environmental variables.

Table 14 Pharmacology Pearls regarding pharmacologic treatment of aggression.

- Side effects occur more commonly, including neuroleptic malignant syndrome, extrapyramidal side effects and other adverse effects
- Benzodiazepines may cause disinhibition or paradoxical stimulation but may be useful in control of acute aggression or agitation in some individuals with ID
- Clozapine is a well-established anti-aggressive agent, especially in the inpatient hospital setting
- There is evidence to support the use of risperidone, olanzapine, quetiapine and aripiprazole
- Mood stabilizers, including lithium, are widely used to control aggression, but efficacy lacks strong support
- Some evidence exists for the use SSRIs, hormonal agents with anti-androgenic properties and beta blockers
- Risperidone has been shown to be effective in children with ID, particularly in autism
- Use standardized and universal rating scales to screen for side effects
- Use caution or avoid bupropion and other agents that lower seizure threshold in patients with history of seizure disorders

---

Source: adapted from Volavka *et al.* (2006).

Table 15 Interpretations of behavior problems.

Most common causes of behavior problems:
- Pain
- Medication side effects
- Sleep disorders
- Psychiatric illnesses

Common presentations of behavior problems and their possible meaning:

Fist jammed in mouth	Consider gastroesophageal reflux disease, eruption of teeth, asthma, rumination, nausea, anxiety, painful hands and gout.
Biting side of hand	Consider sinus problems, Eustachian tubes/other ear problems, eruption of third molars, dental problems, pain or paresthesia of the hands.
Biting object with front teeth	Sinus problems (also the most common reason for thumb sucking and bruxism), Eustachian tube or ear problems, finger pain or paresthesia, and gout.
Refuses to sit evenly, or at all	Hip pain, genital or rectal discomfort, clue to ongoing or past abuse.
Unpleasurable masturbation	Prostatitis, urinary tract or genital infection, rectal injury or infection, parasitic infection, syphilis or other 'old' conditions, repetition phenomenon (past abuse) or never learned pleasurable masturbation.
Waving head side to side	Attempt to supplement visual field, vertigo or hypervigilance.
Walking on toes	Arthritis in the hips, ankles, or knees, sensory integration issues or tight heel cords.
Intense rocking	Visceral pain, headache, depression, anxiety or medication side effects.
Won't sit	Akathisia, anxiety, depression, back pain or other pain, sleep deprivation.
Whipping had forward	Atlantoaxial subluxation (found in 14% of individuals with Down syndrome and others with joint laxity), dental problems or headaches.
Sudden sitting down or "sit-down strikes"	Cardiac problems, syncope, orthostasis, medication side effects, vertigo, otitis, Atlantoaxial subluxation, seizures or panic.
Waving fingers in front of eyes	Migraine, corneal scarring, cataracts, seizures, glaucoma or medication side effects, e.g. diplopia.
Head-banging	Depression, headache, dental problems, seizures, otitis, mastoiditis, sinusitis, tinea capitis.

Source: summarized from Ryan (2003).

With respect to treatment with medication, there are few published controlled studies that establish best practices or evidence-based principles specific to individuals with ID, so those that exist for the general population, along with inclusion of the existing Expert Consensus Guidelines, should be followed (see Chapter 12 for a review of existing consensus guidelines from acknowledged experts in the field of ID).

Polypharmacy still widely exists for patients with ID and contributes to diagnostic difficulties, increased risk of multiple categories of adverse medication side effects, mental clouding and decreased memory abilities, among many others. If patients present with aggression and polypharmacy, it may seem counterintuitive to taper and decrease medications. However, by categorizing the list and conservatively tapering to a reasonable regimen with no more than on one medication in each indicated category, the clinician will more often than not have a clearer picture with which to make an accurate diagnosis, collect information if available about what medication classes were beneficial in the past and optimize those medications.

If a medication has been given a fair trial and has not worked well, it should be discontinued. In terms of medication management, "fair" trials of medications are dependent on the specific medication, but typically they take several weeks. Daily changes are not likely to be useful unless the patient is on an inpatient unit and monitored closely. Too often, in the pursuit of stability, medications have been added one on top of the next, with nothing discontinued. Consequently, in the acuity of an aggressive situation, a suggestion to discontinue a medication may not be received well by caregivers and family members.

It is essential to find out as much information about the patient's baseline as possible, so that all involved have a clear picture of the treatment goals. When was the patient last doing well? Has there been a functional analysis performed on all target behaviors? It is important to task behavior support staff to collect data regarding aggression, including frequency, severity, quantity, quality, environmental details, reinforcers, precipitants, antagonistic factors and the overall function of the behavior. While the physician or other prescriber awaits behavior support data or has direct care staff document details about aggression, sleep pattern, appetite, mood, changes in physical functioning and status, etc., the physical examination and laboratory evaluation can be performed and all medical records reviewed. If there is any suspicion of other medical or neurological conditions, the patient should be assessed by the appropriate professional.

There should not be pressure on the prescriber alone to "solve" the problem. The best results in attaining the highest quality of life and stability for the patient will be accomplished through a team approach and educated and consistent direct care staff, who can institute positive interventions with consistent boundaries, along with providing accurate collateral data to the multidisciplinary team.

If the aggression is chronically severe and disruptive, it may be useful to hospitalize or to use another facility (i.e. a developmental center or another similar facility) to provide a 30- or 60-day stay for the purpose of performing a comprehensive assessment, while the team and, especially, direct care staff can be provided with education in order to transition the patient back to the community or to the least restrictive environment feasible. Keep in mind that the problem behavior did not occur in 45 or 60 minutes, and it will not be eliminated in this amount of time during a mental health assessment.

It may be the case that no specific etiology for the aggressive behavior can be determined, either immediately or in the long term. In the case of a patient with poor impulse control, there may be an abuse history which has not been processed in a psychotherapy relationship. There may also be personality disorder pathology or a multitude of other conditions and experiences.

When a decision is considered regarding augmenting other non-pharmacological treatment interventions with psychotropic medications, this must be tailored to the individual's circumstances and the biopsychosocial formulation at that point in time. This formulation is fluid, as it is a constantly changing set of circumstances. There are a number of scenarios in which psychiatrists may consider utilizing medication – for example: failure of non-medication based interventions; risk of harm/distress to the patient; risk of harm to others/property; acute or chronic aggression that is still being investigated – or else to provide acute relief of symptoms so that non-medication strategies can be adequately tried, or to

Table 16 Clinical Pearls based on expert consensus for treating the patient with ID who has aggression or SIB.

Treatment should be based upon the most specific psychiatric diagnosis possible. When only a tentative non-specific diagnosis can be made, such as in individuals with more severe ID, clinicians should focus on one or more behavioral symptoms as targets of treatment (Adapted from Aman *et al.*, 2004).
- Utilize neuroreceptor correlates of aggression to guide pharmacologic interventions
- Utilize the biopsychosocial formulation to determine etiology
- Identify "predisposing," "perpetuating" and "protective" factors
- Rule out undiagnosed and/or undertreated medical conditions
- Depression and anxiety tend to be under-diagnosed
- Rule out physical pain (acute and chronic)
- Rule out medication side effects
- Shore up supports during transitions
- Ensure thorough physical examination and laboratory work up are conducted
- Identify grief and loss issues and address appropriately
- Manage the triangle during the data collection process
- Perform a functional analysis
- Enlist a behavioral psychologist or behavior support specialist
- Be familiar with the individual's baseline functioning

temporarily recreate a state of stability using previously successful medication regimens (World Psychiatry Association, 2010).

Conclusion

When using axial diagnoses such as in the DSM-IV TR, consider each axis as a separate and important piece of information about the patient, but also keep in mind that the axes are inter-related and that relationships may change at times. Clinical Vignette #4 illustrates the relationship among the several axes.

Clinical Vignette #4

Mary is a 38-year-old individual with medical history including seizure disorder and hypothyroidism (Axis III) and psychological underpinnings significant for alleged sexual abuse by her father (Axis IV). She who has mild intellectual disability (Axis II) and depressive disorder not otherwise specified (Axis I) and is currently presenting with the global assessment of functioning of 50 (Axis V).

The formulation above is the relationship among behavior, environment and neurochemistry and is flexible, constantly evolving and specific to the individual at any given point in time. Quality of life indicators are considered, including living situation, physical health, subjective sense of well-being, vocational functioning, relationships and symptom frequency.

At best, medications, psychotherapy, and behavior treatment may lead to an increase in quality of life. Symptom reduction or behavior changes in and of themselves are insufficient.

Patients such as "Mary" in Clinical Vignette #4 are complex, dynamic individuals. The goal of the treatment team is to integrate all components of the information into a formulation of the "aggression" presentation in order to understand the causes and treat the patient. This is a dynamic process, and the only constant is change. Aggression is a serious problem and can have multiple and varying potential consequences which can be disastrous. Modifiable risk factors must be addressed. The aggression assessment requires utilizing a team approach, and patients with ID will benefit from the input of all members of the treatment team.

References

Allen, D.G., Lowe, K., Moore, K. & Brophy, S. (2007). Predictors, costs and characteristics of out of area placement for people with intellectual disability and challenging behaviour. *Journal of Intellectual Disability Research* **51**(6), 409–416.

Aman, M.G., Crismon, M.L., Frances, A., King, B.H. & Rojahn, J. (eds.) (2004). *Treatment of psychiatric and behavior problems in individuals with mental retardation: an update of the expert consensus guidelines for mental retardation and developmental disability populations.* Postgraduate Institute for Medicine, Englewood, CO.

American Psychiatric Association (2000). *Diagnostic and Statistical Manual of Mental Disorders*, 4th ed. (DSM-IV). APA, Washington, DC.

Antonacci, D.J., Manuel, C. & Davis, E. (2008). Diagnosis and treatment of aggression in individuals with developmental disabilities. *Psychiatric Quarterly* **79**, 225–247.

Aziz, M., Maixner, D.F., DeQuardo, J., Aldridge, A. & Tandon, R. (2001). ECT and mental retardation: A review and case reports. *Journal of ECT* **17**(2), 149–152.

Baumeister, A.A., Sevin, J.A. & King, B.H. (1998). Neuroleptics. In: Reiss, S., Aman, M.G. (eds.) *The International Consensus Handbook.* pp. 133–150. Ohio State University Press, Columbus, OH.

Campbell, W.H. & Rohrbaugh, R.M. (2006). *The Biopsychosocial Formulation Manual: A Guide for Mental Health Professionals.* Routledge, New York.

Carvill, S. & Marston, G. (2002). People with intellectual disability, sensory impairments and behavior disorder; a case series. *Journal of Intellectual Disability Research* **46**(3), 264–272.

Charlot, L. & Shedlack, K. (2002). Masquerade: Uncovering and treating the many causes of aggression in individuals with developmental disabilities. *NADD Bulletin* **5**, 59–64.

Clark, D.J., Kelley, S., Thinn, K. & Corbett, J.A. (1990). Psychotropic drugs and mental retardation: I. Disabilities and the prescription of drugs for behavior and for epilepsy in 3 residential settings. *Journal of Mental Deficiency Research* **28**, 229–233.

Collacott, R.A., Cooper, S-A., Branford, D. & McGrother, C. (1998). Epidemiology of self-injurious behaviour in adults with learning disabilities. *British Journal of Psychiatry* **173**, 428–432.

Connor, D.F., Glatt, S.J., Lopez, I.D., Jackson, D. & Melloni, R.H., Jr., (2002). Psychopharmacology and aggression. I: a meta-analysis of stimulant effects on overt/covert aggression-related behaviors in ADHD. *Journal of The American Academy Of Child and Adolescent Psychiatry* **41**, 263–261.

Cooper, S-A., Smiley, E., Allan, L.M., Jackson, A., Finlayson, J., Mantry, D. & Morrison, J. (2009). Adults with intellectual disabilities: prevalence, incidence and remission of self-injurious behaviour, and related factors. *Journal of Intellectual Disability Research Special Issue* **53**(3), 200–216.

Davidson, P., Cain, N., Sloane-Reeves, J., Van Speybroech, A., Segal, J., Gutkin, J., *et al.* (1994). Characteristics of community-based individuals with mental retardation and aggressive behavioral disorders. *American Journal of Mental Retardation* **98**, 704–716.

Deb, S. & Fraser, W. (1994). The use of psychotropic medication in people with learning disability: Towards rational prescribing. *Human Psychopharmacology* **9**, 259–272.

Deb, S. & Unwin, G.L. (2007a) *Guide to using psychotropic medication for the management of behaviour problems among adults with intellectual disability.* Technical document, Section 3: Systematic reviews. University of Birmingham, Birmingham, UK. Available at www.ld-medication.bham.ac.uk

Deb, S. & Unwin, G. (2007b). Psychotropic medication for behaviour problems in people with intellectual disability: A review of current literature. *Current Opinion in Psychiatry* **20**, 461–466.

Deb, S., Thomas, M. & Bright, C. (2001). Mental disorder in adults with intellectual disability 2: The rate of behavior disorders among a community-based population aged between 16 and 64 years. *Journal of Intellectual Disability Research* **45**(6), 506–514.

Deb, S., Sohanpal, S.K., Soni, R. Unwin, G. & Lenôtre, L. (2007). The effectiveness of antipsychotic medication in the management of behaviour problems in adults with intellectual disabilities. *Journal of Intellectual Disability Research* **51**, 766–777.

Deb, S., Chaplin, S., Sohanpal, G., Unwin, G. Soni, R. & Lenôtre, L. (2008). The effectiveness of mood stabilizers and antiepileptic medication for the management of behavior problems in adults with intellectual disability: a systematic review. *Journal of Intellectual Disability Research* **52**, 107–113.

Dhossche, D.M. & Rout, U. (2006). Are autistic and catatonic regression related? A few working hypotheses involving gaba, Purkinge cell survival, neurogenesis, and ECT. *International Review of Neurobiology* **72**, 55–79.

Dhossche, D.M. & Stanfill, S. (2004). Could ECT be effective in autism? *Medical Hypotheses* **63** (3), 371–376.

Didden, R., Korzilius, H., van Aperlo, B., van Overloop, C. & de Vries, M. (2002). Sleep problems and daytime problem behaviours in children with intellectual disability. *Journal of Intellectual Disability Research* **46**(7), 537–547.

Dykens, E.M., Hodapp, R.M. & Finucane, B.M. (2000). *Genetics and mental retardation syndromes: A new look at behavior and interventions.* Paul H Brookes Publishing, Baltimore, MD.

Einfeld, S.L. & Tonge, B.J. (1999). Observations on the use of the ICD-10 guide for the mental retardation. *Journal of Intellectual Disability Research* **45**, 408–412.

Emerson, E., Kiernan, C., Alborz, A., Reeves, D., Mason, H., Swarbrick, R., Mason, L. & Hatton, C. (2001a). Predicting the persistence of severe self-injurious behavior. *Research in Developmental Disabilities* **22**, 67–75.

Emerson, E., Kiernan, C., Alborz, A., Reeves, D., Mason, H., Swarbrick, R., Mason, L. & Hatton, C. (2001b). The prevalence of challenging behaviors: A total population study. *Research in Developmental Disabilities* **22**, 77–93.

Fletcher, R., Loschen, E., Stavrakaki, C. & First, M. (eds.) (2007). *Diagnostic Manual – Intellectual Disability (DM-ID): A Textbook of Diagnosis of Mental Disorders in Persons with Intellectual Disability.* NADD Press, Kingston, NY.

Gagiano, C., Read, S., Thorpe, L., Eerdekens, M. & Van Hove, I. (2005). Short- and long-term efficacy and safety of risperidone in adults with disruptive behavior disorders. *Psychopharmacology* **179**, 629–636.

Gardner, W.I. (2002). *Aggression and Other Disruptive Behavioral Challenges: Biomedical and Psychosocial Assessment and Treatment.* NADD Press, Kingston, NY.

Green, W.H. (2001). *Child and adolescent clinical psychopharmacology.* Lippincott Williams & Wilkins, Philadelphia.

Guay, D.P. (2008). Inappropriate Sexual Behaviors in Cognitively Impaired Older Individuals. *American Journal of Geriatric Pharmacotherapy* **6**(5). 269–288.

Guay, D.P. (2009). Drug Treatment of Paraphilic and Nonparaphilic Sexual Disorders. *Clinical Therapeutics* **31**(1), 1–31.

Habler, F. & Reis, O. (2010). Pharmacotherapy of Disruptive Behavior in Mentally Retarded Subjects: A Review of the Current Literature. *Developmental Disabilities Research Reviews* **16**, 265–272.

Handen, B.L. & Gilchrist, R. (2006). Practitioner review: psychopharmacology in children and adolescent with mental retardation. *Journal of Child Psychology and Psychiatry And Allied Disciplines* **47**, 871–882.

Handen, B.L. & Hardan, A.Y. (2006). Open-label, prospective trial of olanzapine in adolescents with subaverage intelligence and disruptive behavior disorders. *Journal of The American Academy Of Child and Adolescent Psychiatry* **45**, 928–935.

Hardan, A. & Sahl, R. (1997). Psychopathology in children and adolescents with developmental disorders. *Research in Developmental Disabilities* **18**, 369–382.

Hillbrand, M. (1995). Aggression against self and aggression against others in violent psychiatric patients. *Journal of Consulting and Clinical Psychology* **63**, 668–671.

Hogue, T., Steptoe, L., Taylor, J., Lindsay, W., Mooney, P., Pinkney, L., Johnston, S., Smith, A.H. W. & O'Brien, G. (2006). A comparison of offenders with intellectual disability across three levels of security. *Criminal Behavior and Mental Health* **16**, 13–28.

Hollander, E., Wasserman, S., Swanson, E.N., Chaplin, W., Schapiro, M.L., Zagursky, K. & Novotny, S. (2006). A double-blind placebo-controlled pilot study of olanzapine in childhood/adolescent pervasive developmental disorder. *Journal of Child and Adolescent Psychopharmacology* **16**, 541–548.

Hurley, A. (2005). Psychotherapy in an essential tool in the treatment of psychiatric disorders for people with mental retardation. *Mental Retardation* **43**(6), 445–448.

Hurley, A.D., Levitas, A., Lecavalier, L. & Pary, R.J. (2007). Assessment and diagnostic procedures. Special considerations for the metal health diagnostic interview for individuals with ID. In: Fletcher, R., Loschen, E., Stavrakaki, C. & First, M. (eds.) *Diagnostic Manual-Intellectual Disability: A Clinical Guide for Diagnosis of Mental Disorders in Persons with Intellectual Disability.* Chpt 2: 9–23. NADD Press/National Association for the Dually Diagnosed, Kingston, NY.

Janowsky, D.S., Barnhill, L.J. & Davis, J.M. (2003a). Olanzapine for self-injurious, aggressive, and disruptive behaviors in intellectually disabled adults: A retrospective, open-label, naturalistic trial. *Journal of Clinical Psychiatry* **64**, 1258–1265.

Janowsky, D.S., Kraus, J.E., Barnhill, L.J., Elamir, B. & Davis, J.M. (2003b). Effects of topiramate on aggressive, self-injurious, and disruptive/destructive behaviors in the intellectually disabled: An open-label retrospective study. *Journal of Clinical Psychopharmacology* **23**(5), 500–504.

Janowsky, D.S., Shetty, M. & Barnhill, L.J., (2004). Serotonergic antidepressant effects on aggressive, self-injurious and destructive/disruptive behaviors in intellectually disabled adults: a retrospective, open-label, naturalistic trial. *International Journal of Neuropsychopharmacology* **8**, 37–48.

Janowsky, D.S., Shetty, M., Barnhill, L.J., Elamir, B. & Davis, JM. (2005). Serotonergic antidepressant effects on aggressive, self-injurious and destructive/disruptive behaviours in intellectually disabled adults: a retrospective, open label, naturalistic trial. *International Journal of Neuropsychopharmacology* **8**, 37–48.

Janowsky, D.S., Barnhill, L.J., Khalid, A.S. & Davis, J.M. (2006). Relapse of Aggressive and Disruptive Behavior in Mentally Retarded Adults Following Antipsychotic Drug Withdrawal Predicts Psychotropic Drug Use a Decade Later. *Journal of Clinical Psychiatry* **67**, 1272–1277.

Joyce, T., Ditchfield, H. & Harris, B. (2001). Challenging behavior in community services. *Journal of Intellectual Disability Research* **45**(2), 130–138.

Kalachnik, J.E., Leventhal, B.B., James, D.H., Sovner, R., Kastner, T.A., Walsh, K., Weisblatt, S. A., & Klitzke, M.G. (1998). Guidelines for the use of psychotropic medication. In: Reiss, S. & Aman, M.G. (eds.) *Psychotropic Medications and Developmental Disabilities: The International Consensus Handbook*, pp. 45–72. The Ohio State Nisonger Center, Columbus, OH.

Kalachnik, J.E., Hanzel, T.E., Sevenich, R. & Harder, Sr., (2002). Benzodiazepine behavioral side effects: Review and implications for individuals with mental retardation. *American Journal on Mental Retardation* **107**(5), 376–410.

Kane, J.M., Leucht, S., Capenter, D. & Docherty, J.P. (2003). The expert consensus guideline series. Optimizing pharmacologic treatment of psychotic disorders. *Journal of Clinical Psychiatry* **64** (Suppl. 12), 1–100.

King, B.H. (2002). Psychopharmacology in mental retardation. *Current Opinion in Psychiatry* **15**(5), 497–502.

King, B.H., DeAntonio, C., McCracken, J.T., Forness, S.R. & Ackerland, V. (1994). Psychiatric consultation in severe and profound mental retardation. *American Journal of Psychiatry* **151** (12), 1802–1808.

La Malfa, G., Bertelli, M. & Conte, M. (2001). Fluvoxamine and aggression in mental retardation. *Psychiatric Services* **52**(8), 1105.

La Malfa, G., Lassi, S., Bertelli, M. & Castellani, A. (2006). Reviewing the use of antipsychotic drugs in people with intellectual disability. *Human Psychopharmacology: Clinical and Experimental* **21**, 73–89.

Larson, S.A., Lakin, K.C., Anderson, L., Lee, N.K., Jeoung Hak Lee, J.H. & Anderson, D. (2001). Prevalence of mental retardation and developmental disabilities: estimates from the 1994/ 1995 National Health Interview Survey. *American Journal of Mental Retardation* **106**(3), 231–252.

Ligas, A., Petrides, G., Istafanous, R. & Kellner, C.H. (2009). Successful electroconvulsive therapy in a patient with intellectual disability and bipolar disorder, with catatonic features misdiagnosed as encephalopathy. *Journal of ECT* **25**(3), 202–204.

Lowry, M. & Sovner, R. (1991). The functional existence of problem behavior: a key to effective treatment. *The Habilitative Mental Health Care Newsletter* **10**, 59–63.

Matson, J.L. & LoVullo, S.V. (2008). A Review of Behavioral Treatments for Self-injurious Behaviors of Persons with Autism Spectrum Disorders. *Behavior Modification* **32**, 61.

Matson, J.L. & Minshawi, N.F. (2007). Functional assessment of challenging behavior: Toward a strategy for applied settings. *Research in Developmental Disabilities* **28**, 353–361.

McClintock, K., Hall, S. & Oliver, C. (2003). Risk markers associated with challenging behaviors in people with intellectual disabilities: A meta-analytic study. *Journal of Intellectual Disability Research* **47**, 405–416.

Nijman, H. & Palmstierna, T. (2002). Measuring aggression with the staff observation aggression scale-revised. *Acta Psychiatrica Scandinavica. Supplementum* **412**, 101–102.

Pary, R.J., Silka, V.R. & Blaha, S.J. (1995). Mental retardation. In: Thienhaus, O.J. (ed.) *Manual of Clinical Hospital Psychiatry*, pp. 287–309. American Psychiatric Press, Washington, DC.

Radouco-Thomas, M., Bolduc, M., Brisson, A., Brassard, P., Fortier, L. & Thivierge, J. (2004). Pilot study on the use of psychotropic medication in persons with mental retardation. *Progress in Neuro-Psychopharmacology and Biological Psychiatry* **28**, 879–883.

Rojahn, J., Matson, J.L., Naglieri, J.A. & Mayville, E. (2004). Relationships between psychiatric conditions and behavior problems among adults with mental retardation. *American Journal on Mental Retardation* **109**(1), 21–23.

Ruedrich, S.L., Swales, T.P., Rossvanes, C., Diana, L., Arkadiev, V. & Lim, K. (2008). Atypical antipsychotic medication improves aggression, but not self-injurious behaviour, in adults with intellectual disabilities. *Journal of Intellectual Disability Research* **52**(2), 132–140.

Royal College of Psychiatrists (2001). *DC-LD (Diagnostic Criteria for Psychiatric Disorders for Use with Adults with Learning Disabilities/Mental Retardation)*. Gaskell, London.

Rueve, M. & Welton, R. (2008). Violence in Mental Illness. *Psychiatry (Edgemont)*, **5**(5) 35–48.

Ryan, R. (2003). *Intensive Conference on Dual Diagnosis*. The Community Circle, Denver, CO. CME Event.

Sajith, S.G., Margan, C. & Clarke, D. (2008). Pharmacological management of inappropriate sexual behaviours: a review of its evidence, rationale and scope in relation to men with intellectual disabilities. *Journal of Intellectual Disability Research* **52**(12), 1078–1090.

Santosh, P.J. & Baird, G. (1999). Psychopharmacotherapy in children and adults with intellectual disability. *The Lancet* **354**(9174), 233–242.

Sigafoos, J., Elkins, J., Kerr, M. & Attwood, T. (1994). A survey of aggressive behaviour among a population of persons with intellectual disability in Queensland. *Journal of Geriatric Psychiatry* **38**, 369–381.

Silka, V.R. & Hauser, M.J. (1997). Psychiatric assessment of the person with mental retardation. *Psychiatric Annals* **27**(3), 162–169.

Taylor, J.L. (2002). A Review of the assessment and treatment of anger and Aggression in offenders with intellectual disability. *Journal of Intellectual Disability Research* **46** (Supplement I) 57–73.

Tenneij, N.H., Didden, R., Stolker, J.J. & Koot, H.M. (2009). Markers for aggression in inpatient treatment facilities for adults with mild to borderline intellectual disability. *Research in Developmental Disabilities* **30**, 1248–1257.

Tyrer, F., McGrother, C., Thorp, C., Donaldson, M., Bhaumik, S., Watson, J.M. & Hollin, C. (2006). Physical aggression towards others in adults with learning disabilities: Prevalence and associated factors, *Journal of Intellectual Disability Research* **50**, 295–304.

Verhoeven, W.M.A. & Tuiner, S. (2001). Cyclothymia or unstable mood disorder? A systematic treatment evaluation with valproic acid. *Journal of Applied Research in Intellectual Disabilities* **14**, 147–154.

Volavka, J., Citrome, L. & Huertas D. (2006). Update on the biological treatment of aggression. A Review. *Actas Espanolas de Psiquiatria* **34**(2), 123–135.

Wachtel, L.E., Contrucci-Kuhn, S.A., Griffin, M., Thompson, A., Dhossche, D.M. & Reti, I.M. (2009). ECT for self-injury in an autistic boy. *European Child and Adolescent Psychiatry* **18** (7), 458–63.

Wachtel, L.E., Griffin, M. & Reti, I.M. (2010). Electroconvulsive therapy in a man with autism experiencing severe depression, catatonia, and self-injury. *Journal of ECT* **26**(1): 70–3.

World Psychiatry Association (2010). Clinical Bulletin of the Developmental Disabilities Division. International guide to prescribing psychotropic medication for the management of problem behaviours in adults with intellectual disabilities.

12

Psychotropic Medications

Christopher T. Manetta, DO, Kirtland Air Force Base Medical
Group, Kirtland AFB, New Mexico
Julie P. Gentile, MD, Associate Professor, Wright State
University, Dayton, Ohio

*"It is not our responsibility to identify necessarily the limits in our patients, but rather
for us to identify the limits in the care that we give them. It is then, and only then, when
we can go beyond them."*

(Albert Einstein)

Introduction

Many individual with intellectual disability (ID) can collaborate and communicate opinions
regarding pharmacologic interventions. Like those with typical cognitive ability, they suffer
physical and emotional pain, complicated by varying limitations in communication, and in
their ability to meet basic needs and in navigating social settings. Their communicative
abilities are affected by their degree of ID, ranging from mild to profound, but all individuals
should be afforded the opportunity to communicate their thoughts about treatment in their
own ways and within their developmental frameworks.

Although people with ID experience and suffer from the entire range of psychiatric
problems, empirical evidence has shown that psychiatric and behavioral problems occur in
individuals with ID three to six times the rate that they occur in the general population
(Stark *et al.*, 1988; Reiss, 1994; Aman *et al.*, 2003). Between 20–45% of individuals with ID

Psychiatry of Intellectual Disability: A Practical Manual, First Edition.
Edited by Julie P. Gentile and Paulette M. Gillig.
© 2012 John Wiley & Sons, Ltd. Published 2012 by John Wiley & Sons, Ltd.

are prescribed psychotropic medications for various reasons and, for 14–30% of these persons, psychotropics are intended to manage behavior problems (Clark *et al.*, 1990; Deb & Fraser, 1994). In one community sample, 36% of patients with ID were receiving three or more psychotropics, illustrating the commonality of polypharmacy as well (Lott *et al.*, 2004).

This chapter is intended to serve as a pragmatic resource for reviewing and integrating concepts that are included in expert consensus guidelines and other material by acknowledged prescribing authorities in the field of ID. The purpose is to assist the reader in decision-making regarding the appropriate prescription of psychotropic medications for psychiatric and/or behavioral problems in patients with ID.

A brief review of the historical perspective of over-medication and polypharmacy that is frequently seen in this specialized population is included, as well as a focus on the importance of informed consent. The utility and significance of the biopsychosocial model is also discussed, as well as how to determine whether pharmacologic intervention is justified, and what to do if no specific indication or diagnosis can be determined. Specific problems and disorders likely to be encountered by providers treating this specialized patient population are described, and relevant nuances to prescribers that deserve attention and distinguish individuals with ID from others are noted. A literature review of medication categories utilized in the treatment of mental illness in the patient with ID will be presented, in addition to a suggested clinical, chronological and medical timeline for prescribers and other interested parties.

A review of commonly associated medical conditions found in individuals with ID is highly relevant to a prescriber, and this can be found in Chapter 3.

Historical review of psychotropic medication guidelines

Individuals with ID are the most medicated segment of the population, whether in institutions or in the community (Nøttestad & Linaker, 2003). Dating as far back as 1952 and continuing through the most recent decade, state and federal entities have worked diligently at establishing, implementing and monitoring rational guidelines for the use of psychotropic medications to target mental illness and behavioral change in the ID patient population (Kalachnik *et al.*, 1998). There has been ongoing concern about developing appropriate policies for informed consent and for: "*empirical monitoring for all psychotropic medication whether such medication was used for behavior change or mental illness ... to focus more on quality of life outcomes*" (Kalachnik *et al.*, 1998).

Because of the longstanding history of over-medication and polypharmacy in patients with ID, in 1974 the United States Food and Drug Administration considered eliminating all "off-label" prescribing practices. This discussion resulted in increased patient advocacy and protection, and increased awareness of the problems involved when using medications in patients without an appropriate diagnostic indication, but also the intention to avoid micromanagement of medication-prescribing habits.

Because there is a higher prevalence of mental illness in patients with ID in addition to an increased vulnerability of adverse drug reactions and side effects, it is very important that these patients have their conditions accurately assessed, diagnosed and treated. Ultimately, the purpose of psychotropic medication, as with any other treatment intervention, should be to improve the patient's cognitive functioning and quality of life.

Biopsychosocial model

The biopsychosocial model of treatment (Engel, 1977, 1980) proposes a shift from a bio-medical model of patient care to a systems theory model, where it is acknowledged that biological, psychological and sociological systems are interdependent. In such a model, an event at one level is recognized as potentially affecting systems at other levels. Therefore, it is argued, in order to provide optimal patient care, biological, psychological and socio-logical aspects of care must be acknowledged and addressed (Kalachnik *et al.*, 1998).

The biopsychosocial perspective emphasizes inclusion of family/caretakers/guardians and any additional knowledgeable and interested collateral data sources, in order to collect accurate, unbiased and reliable information. Additionally, this model reinforces the prerequisites necessary to build a foundation for a strong and healthy therapeutic alliance with the patient and his/her care providers. The model also supports facilitating the involvement of the patient in all treatment-related decisions to the greatest extent possible, which further improves the accuracy of the diagnosis, improves compliance and strengthens the therapeutic working relationship. Treatment components intrinsic to this process include, but are not limited to, identifying the target symptoms or behaviors to be treated; recognizing measurement tools to quantify changes; and utilizing continuity monitoring parameters (Arnold, 1993; Bishop, 1992).

Non-pharmacological interventions

Before initiating treatment with psychotropic medications, it may be possible to enhance the well-being and health of an individual with ID solely by providing psychotherapy and addressing social and environmental factors (Woods & Miltenberger, 1995). Often, no single medical or psychiatric disorder can be delineated as the main factor causing disruption in a person's quality of life. When this is the case, it is important to consider non-pharmacological management strategies and continuation of investigative measures (e.g. collecting behavior support data and collateral data across environments/caregivers, performing physical examination, obtaining laboratory values, etc.).

A number of behavioral interventions have been identified and employed effectively to treat a variety of contingencies. Unwin & Deb (2008) reported a strong expert consensus to use non-medication-based management options as a primary intervention for aggression and self-injurious behavior (Unwin & Deb, 2008a). Long & Miltenberger (1998) reviewed behavioral treatment modalities for "habit disorders" in individuals with ID, including nail biting, bruxism, trichotillomania, tics and Tourette's disorder. Behavioral approaches that have shown efficacy for treating such disorders were self-monitoring, covert sensitization, relaxation techniques, cognitive-behavioral therapy, overcorrection, and positive and negative practice.

Clinical Vignette #1 illustrates the implementation and effectiveness of such types of non-pharmacologic treatment. These topics are covered in further detail in Chapters 11 and 14.

Reasons for pharmacological intervention

Over 30% of people with ID have a comorbid psychiatric disorder, which often has its onset in childhood and persists through adolescence and adulthood (Cooper *et al.*, 2007a; Einfeld

Clinical Vignette #1

Walt is a 26 year old man with moderate ID and a recurrent and unremitting history of skin picking. Throughout his life, there have been several occasions where his repeated skin picking has led to infections and has required prolonged medical hospitalizations. A number of medications have been tried to alleviate his habit, but with little benefit.

Following his last hospitalization Walt was discharged to a supported residential setting in the community. He began working with a psychotherapist, and positive practice procedures were employed to prevent further complications of the skin picking and subsequent hospitalization. He was required to practice bringing his hands up to his face 30–40 times without picking, and then to bring his hands to his sides. Each time he brought his hands to his face, he would also be holding a marble in each hand. As he lowered his hands from his face to his sides, he would drop the marbles into a jar. With an increase in quantity of marbles in the jar every time he did so, he would make every effort to pass the assigned level indicated on the jar. After reaching the designated level in the jar, he was positively rewarded.

This marked overcorrection resulted in a significant decrease in his skin picking, and there were subsequently fewer episodes of infection and hospitalization.

et al., 2006). Of this 30%, 20–40% receive some form of psychotropic medication to target the identified problem, e.g. aggression, self-injurious behavior or a diagnosed psychiatric disorder. Among this group of patients, 14–30% are receiving the medication to manage *problem behaviors* (Clark *et al.*, 1990; Deb & Fraser, 1994).

Problem behaviors

Problem behaviors (PB) have been defined as "socially unacceptable behavior that causes distress, harm or disadvantage to the persons, themselves or to other people, and usually requires some intervention" (Deb *et al.*, 2006). PB has been recognized by multiple sources as being the most prevalent and common indication for medication management in patients with ID.

In order to effectively treat PB, it is important to first elicit the underlying cause that may be propagating the behavior for the individual patient. Much like narrowing down the cause for delirium in a medical patient, solidifying the etiology of PB, whenever possible, is a vital requirement in satisfactorily treating a patient with ID. There are many causes for PBs, and these include mental disorders, physical ailments, the environment, or even one's longitudinal developmental history and characterologic makeup. Therefore, a thorough and comprehensive assessment must take place. If a cause cannot be identified, then the treatment goal should be to minimize the disruption that the behavior causes to the patient's relationships and quality of life (Fletcher *et al.*, 2007; Royal College of Psychiatrists, DC-LD, 2001).

Frequently no treatable illness can be determined, in which case a non-pharmacological approach should be considered. However, even when utilizing a non-medication-based treatment option, it may become necessary to augment the treatment with medication. This practice must be tailored to the specificity of each unique case, and cannot be based on a pathognomonic algorithm.

There are a number of scenarios in which a psychiatrist may consider using indicated medications. These include:

- failure of non-medication based interventions;

- risk of harm/distress to the patient;

- risk of harm to others/property;

- high frequency of PB;

- treating target symptoms known to respond to medication (i.e. dangerousness to self or others, hyperactivity, etc);

- treating an underlying psychiatric disorder;

- providing acute relief of symptoms so that non-medication strategies can be adequately tried;

- recreating a state of stability using previously successful medication regimens (World Psychiatry Association, 2010).

As always, the primary objective should be to *first do no harm* and to institute a multidisciplinary treatment plan that is in the best interests of the patient. The treatment plan should always be discussed fully with the patient (regardless of the level of his/her cognitive deficits), as well as with the guardian/care provider (World Psychiatry Association, 2010). For a more detailed explanation of the presentation and assessment of PB, see Chapter 11.

In 2010, the Clinical Bulletin of the Developmental Disabilities Division of the World Psychiatry Association outlined a guide for prescribing psychotropic medication for the management of psychiatric disorders and problem behaviors in adults with ID. In order to ensure first doing no harm, it is imperative to monitor the safety and efficacy of the instituted medication(s) (World Psychiatry Association, 2010; Unwin & Deb, 2008a). This is accomplished through regular encounters with the patient and the family, as well as conducting serial mental status examinations and physical examinations. Additionally, depending on the chosen medication, it is important to obtain routine blood tests and diagnostic studies, according to universally accepted recommendations.

Monitoring protocols should not be overlooked or abbreviated in patients with ID. In fact, it may be crucial to increase the use of standardized, measurable instruments in such instances as in assessing for extrapyramidal side effects in those patients with muscular disorders like cerebral palsy (Unwin & Deb, 2008b).

It is recommended to begin with the lowest starting dose, to titrate slowly, and to remain within the dose range outlined by the Physician Desk Reference, the Food and Drug Administration and/or alternate prescribing authorities. An empiric and standardized measure of target symptoms and behaviors must be instituted, including a format to quantify the benefits and adverse effects of psychotropic medications. Also, putting the treatment plan in writing for the patient and his/her care provider is standard practice.

Once the decision to prescribe a medication is made, it is beneficial to identify a point of contact on the treatment team who will administer the medication if the patient with ID requires assistance. Finally, having a safety plan in place is imperative; the person and/or family/guardian need to be educated on the appropriate steps to take should an adverse reaction occur, or should an emergent situation arise (e.g. evidence of imminent harm to self or others). Careful screening and psychoeducation at each visit is crucial.

If the patient improves to such an extent that medication can be withdrawn, there are certain steps that should be followed (Ahmed *et al.*, 2000). It is not safe, nor is it in the best interest of the patient, for the caregiver to stop a medication abruptly unless it would actually be life-threatening to continue the medication (as in the case of errantly continuing a dopamine blocker with neuroleptic malignant syndrome, for example). Attention should be given to the myriad of factors that may influence the success of withdrawing a medication. The following general recommendations are to be emphasized:

1 Try to stabilize the person's PB with a minimum number of medications prescribed at the lowest possible dosages.

2 Withdraw one medication at a time.

3 Withdraw medication slowly.

4 If necessary, allow time after withdrawing one medication and before starting to withdraw another (Ahmed *et al.*, 2000).

Branford (1996) pointed out that it may not always be optimal to withdraw a patient fully from a medication as other aspects, such as social and environment factors, play a pivotal role in the decision. As such, tapering to a lower effective dose may be the most ideal clinical decision.

Clinical Vignette #2

Florence is a 45 year old woman with a history of severe ID. She has been treated with a first generation antipsychotic (FGA) for years to help manage and control her head-banging behavior. She was also being prescribed another medication to combat the development of any common side effects.

A taper of her first generation antipsychotic was initiated due to a complete resolution of this behavior for several years. A full taper of the medication was completed in a short period of time, and within several weeks Florence's caregiver started to notice her tongue protruding from her mouth in what appeared to be in an involuntary manner. Florence also began walking with an abnormal gait, and she would yell intermittently. During these episodes of yelling, her caregiver noticed that Florence was exhibiting a "wryneck." Her head-banging behavior recurred and quickly increased in frequency, and she cried inconsolably on a daily basis. She also had to change residences and physicians during this time period.

Florence was re-started on a much lower dose of the first generation antipsychotic in order to reduce the risk of side effects, and she continued on other medications that she had been taking. After Florence settled into her new home and had attended regularly scheduled appointments with her new psychiatrist, her crying spells began to diminish, the head-banging subsided, and she appeared to tolerate the medication dose reduction well. It was decided that a complete withdrawal of the medication at this time was not in her best interest.

PBs are the reason why greater than 90% of patients with ID present for a mental health evaluation, even when they have undiagnosed and under-treated medical conditions. PBs are the most frequent reason for psychiatric hospitalization, the biggest cause for morbidity and mortality, and the reason that many prescribers feel the only intervention available is to prescribe antipsychotic medications. This is especially prevalent in mental health delivery systems in which no behavior support services are available, and where managed care restrictions (e.g. short office visits, infrequent follow up) are the standard of care (Smith *et al.*, 1996; Qureshi & Alborz, 1992; Emerson *et al.*, 2001; Lowe *et al.*, 2007).

Comorbid psychiatric disorders and habit disorders

Other common reasons for psychotropic medication intervention in the ID patient population include comorbid psychiatric disorders and habit disorders. Again, diagnosis may be difficult due to the limitation in the patient's expressive language skills. It is important to address these problems as soon as possible and to intervene prior to any worsening behavior, because many psychiatric disorders are chronic once they develop.

In the patient with ID who is nonverbal, it is important in the mental status examination to focus on non-verbal behavior signs, for example responding to internal stimuli or if there are changes in the patient's attention or level of arousal. Changes in baseline attention or sensorium may indicate new onset or worsening of a psychiatric or organic comorbidity. It is important to collect collateral information from third parties regarding the patient's current functioning, including any changes in activities of daily living or medical status. Viewing behavior as a form of communication will serve the patient well (Bongiorno, 1996). This has been discussed in detail in previous chapters.

The ID patient population is probably more at risk for developing disorders such as schizophrenia, bipolar disorder, depression, generalized anxiety disorder, obsessive compulsive disorder and panic disorder. Additionally, common "habit disorders" may occur because of poorer self-regulatory control. These can include behaviors such as biting, trichotillomania, bruxism, motor and vocal tics and Tourette's disorder (Long & Miltenberger, 1998).

Some of the most common psychopathologies that warrant pharmacological intervention in the ID patient population are "aggressive, antisocial, and self-injurious behavior" (Aman, 1991). These types of behaviors have been compared by Aman & Gharabawi (2004) to "disruptive behavior disorders" as defined by the DSM-IV TR (American Psychiatric Association, 2000). They are sub-divided there by symptom specificity into oppositional defiant disorder, conduct disorder and disruptive behavior disorder not otherwise specified.

Sexual aggression

Sexual aggression can be another behavior for which psychotropic medication may be considered in the ID patient population. Although this problem may be of low prevalence, it is also of high acuity and potentially devastating, especially in the case of sexual aggression toward others. In addition, nearly all individuals with ID have some degree of impulsivity, as well as difficulties in executive functioning, and less ability to filter behaviors, so the risk is higher.

One important factor to consider when performing an assessment of the behavior is the patient's knowledge of sexuality. Some sexual offending behaviors may be due to a lack of education and knowledge of how to navigate relationships. It is also prudent to keep the patient's developmental level in mind if the sexually offending behavior involves children. Psychoeducation, interpersonal and social skills training and group therapy can all be helpful in assisting the individual in the development of healthy relationships with appropriate boundaries.

Sexual aggression can be defined and illustrated by many and various aberrant behaviors. For example, disrobing, masturbating, frotteurism, voyeurism, exhibiting hostile or destructive behavior or practicing coercion all can represent examples of sexual aggression, and all can be without limit, restriction or control. When these actions occur and imminent threat or harm is present, immediate intervention is necessary. Aside from guardianship issues in dealing with this dilemma, medication may be helpful.

However, evidence-based studies of pharmacological intervention for this problem in the ID patient population are quite limited. Most of the current literature on sexual aggression is focused on forensic patients or those with dementia. However, Sajith *et al*. (2008) and Guay (2008, 2009) have investigated and reviewed the literature on inappropriate sexual behaviors in older individuals with cognitive impairment/memory loss and men with ID. In general, when evaluating these behaviors, it is recommended that the examiner first discern if the deviant sexual behavior is due to some underlying primary affective or psychotic disorder (e.g. bipolar disorder, type I) or some other reversible/treatable cause. If this can be accomplished, then treatment should be implemented for the specific psychiatric diagnosis.

If no specifically treatable disorder is found, then a first-line pharmacological intervention may involve a selective serotonin reuptake inhibitor (SSRI). However, there is potential for a paradoxical effect with the use of an SSRI, where the patient may become hyper-stimulated, leading to worsening behavior (e.g. agitation, anger, restlessness, etc.).

Antipsychotics such as risperidone may be helpful, and these have been said to have a theoretical advantage due to their tendency to induce hyperprolactinemia, which can decrease libido and sexual impulses.

Oral or long-acting injectable forms of medroxyprogesterone also have been used. However, before instituting this latter category of medications, a clear and comprehensive risk/benefit analysis should be carried out due to the potential for serious side effects, including weight gain and decreased bone density. Alternately, there are some other long-acting injectable progesterones that may be prescribed. It is recommended that progestins should be used before luteinizing hormone releasing hormone (LHRH) agonists or estrogens. Cyproterone acetate and medroxyprogesterone are preferred as oral and intramuscular (IM) progesterones, respectively (Guay, 2009).

Medications with anti-androgenic side effects are used, though no clear evidence currently exists that shows whether these side effects have any significant impact on quelling sexual impulsive behavior.

Finally, in a review of drug treatment for paraphilia and non-paraphilic sexual disorders, Guay (2009) reported that serotonin and prolactin may inhibit sexual arousal. Most of the currently used pharmacologic treatments of paraphilias have serotonin and testosterone/ dihydrotestosterone as their targets.

For offenders in the general population, cognitive behavioral psychotherapy (CBT) is highly recommended, whether alone or in combination with medication, but no studies have been completed with respect to sexually offending behavior in patients with ID regarding the efficacy of CBT. This is discussed in more detail in Chapter 13.

General principles for the use of antipsychotic medications in the ID population

In addition to patient diagnosis, several variables have been found to have significant impact on the type, quantity and likelihood of utilization of antipsychotic medication in the ID population. Treatment setting has played a role and has had influence over the percentage of psychotropics being prescribed.

In a study examining 302 Danish patients with ID, 19% were being treated with psychotropic medications. Of those, 42% of the usage occurred when patients with ID were under long-stay hospitalizations. Those living in halfway houses, group homes or other specialized institutions accounted for 20%, and those living in the general community comprised less than 5% (Lund, 1985). Spreat et al. (2004) found similar results, with 33% of 3,789 patients with ID receiving the highest prescribed usage of psychotropic medication in the intermediate care type facilities, followed by nursing homes. Those living in the general community were prescribed the lowest number of medications.

The majority of the medications utilized in patients with ID are from the antipsychotic medication class, although there has been limited consensus data to support the utilization of first generation antipsychotics (FGAs). Spreat et al. (1997) found that, in the state of Oklahoma, as much as 66% of all medications being prescribed to the ID patient population were antipsychotic medications.

Of late, there has been a shift in prescribing to more second generation antipsychotic (SGA) medications, due to their lower risk of extrapyramidal side effects and the benefit of targeting negative symptoms of schizophrenia. In a review of 21 articles using second generation antipsychotics in patients with ID, five studies (two using clozapine and three using risperidone) found improvement in aggression, self-injury and agitation. Another study of risperidone found that partial or complete substitution of risperidone for a FGA led to resolution of side effects with no change in behavior, and three other studies reported decreases in maladaptive behavior, including self-injury. Generally, the studies showed reductions in repetitive or compulsive behavior and self-injury, with some studies reporting reduced agitation, increased social awareness, and improved sleep hygiene (Aman & Madrid, 1999).

Psychosis is an ailment that afflicts the patient with ID in rates thought to be slightly higher than the general population (Cooper et al., 2007b). The clinical presentation of psychosis in the patient with ID is covered in detail in Chapter 9. Once the psychosis is found to be due to a mental health condition (following an appropriate medical evaluation ruling out of organic causes), then an antipsychotic medication should be considered.

Suffering from a psychotic disorder can involve two major pillars of symptomatology, commonly referred to as positive and negative symptoms. In the general population, positive symptoms are defined as: delusions; disordered thoughts and speech; and tactile, auditory, visual, olfactory and gustatory hallucinations. Negative symptoms include: flat or blunted affect and emotion; poverty of speech; inability to experience pleasure; lack of desire to form relationships; and a lack of motivation (DSM-IV TR: American Psychiatric Association, 2000). For details about presentations of this type of psychopathology in patients with ID, see Chapter 9.

When selecting an antipsychotic medication, one should first have an understanding of the mechanism of action of both the FGA (typical) and SGA (atypical) antipsychotics to target either positive or negative symptoms (or both). There are five dopaminergic pathways in the brain which are affected by antipsychotic medications. All antipsychotics, of both generations, involve post-synaptic blockade of dopamine along these pathways.

The FGAs block dopamine along the mesolimbic pathway, which is effective in reducing positive symptoms of psychosis. However, the typical antipsychotics are also more specific to blocking dopamine along the nigrostriatal pathway, which can predispose a patient to develop extrapyramidal side effects (EPS). Medications that cause torsade de pointes prolong the QTc interval on EKG; cardiac rhythm should be periodically monitored in all patients prescribed antipsychotic medications.

The difference between the first and second generation antipsychotics is that the SGAs work on the mesolimbic pathway but less on the nigrostriatal pathway, leading to a lower prevalence of the development of EPS. Additionally, the second generation antipsychotics affect the mesocortical tract (involved in normal cognition), and therefore have increased efficacy in treating negative symptoms than do the first generation antipsychotics (Stahl, 2008).

The ID patient population is more prone than the general population to develop serious adverse reactions and extrapyramidal side effects to antipsychotic medications (Fodstad et al., 2010; Friedlander et al., 2001; Wszola et al., 2001), and also muscle stiffness, especially in the presence of co-occurring disorders such as cerebral palsy. Prescribers should use extra caution in prescribing FGAs to patients with ID because these medications are also more likely to:

- lower seizure threshold;

- decrease cardiac conduction (leading to a decrease in cardiac contractility);

- induce orthostatic hypotension (dizziness upon standing);

- cause an elevation in serum prolactin (which can cause galactorrhea, amenorrhea, gynecomastia, decreased libido and erectile dysfunction in men); and

- lead to anticholinergic side effects (such as blurry vision, constipation, urinary retention, dry mucosal membranes, and confusion) (Matson, 2010).

In general, when prescribing antipsychotics to patients with ID, it is best to avoid use of long-term "as needed" orders, use of anticholinergics without signs of EPS and use of higher than usual doses of antipsychotic medications, as well as off-label prescribing such as the use of medications such as phenytoin, phenobarbital and cardiac medications for treatment of psychiatric illness.

Patients with ID are more vulnerable to psychotropic side effects, with potential catastrophic results, including fatalities related to such conditions as neuroleptic malignant syndrome (Viejo et al., 2003). Neuroleptic malignant syndrome is more frequently fatal in patients with ID. The antipsychotic medications also place individuals at risk for EPS, including both reversible and irreversible forms.

Acute dystonias are involuntary muscle contractions which usually occur early in the treatment with antipsychotic medications. This condition is more common in young African American males and can be treated with use of an anticholinergic such as benztropine (Cogentin) or a benzodiazepine.

Akathisia is experienced by the patient as internal restlessness and it is physically uncomfortable. Usually, the trunk and legs are involved and most significantly affected. This condition may be misinterpreted as psychotic behavior, as the patient may be pacing or alternately sitting/standing, so the clinician may increase the medication, making the condition worse. Akathisia can be treated with a benzodiazepine, benztropine or a beta blocker, but changing to another medication, administering the medication in smaller and more frequent doses or lowering the total daily dose may also be effective.

Parkinsonism is the third reversible form of extrapyramidal side effect and it may appear to be Parkinson's disease, although the symptoms (such as resting tremor, cogwheel rigidity, bradykinesia and masked facies) are not symmetrical in parkinsonism as they are in Parkinson's disease. Elderly women are more vulnerable to this condition, and it can be treated by lowering or discontinuing the causative agent, or by using benztropine (Cogentin), a benzodiazepine or diphenhydramine (Benadryl). The patient with parkinsonism should *not* be given dopamine replacement as is advised in the patient with Parkinson's Disease.

Finally, tardive dyskinesia is the irreversible form of extrapyramidal side effect. It occurs more frequently with the first generation antipsychotics, although medication in both generations can be causative agents. It normally occurs with higher dosages and with longer use, and elderly patients and female patients are at highest risk. Tardive dyskinesia consists of abnormal, involuntary, irregular choreoathetoid movements of the head, limbs and trunk. The most common presentation is perioral movements, including the tongue, jaw and lips; the face and hands are also commonly affected. The condition may be quieted by decreasing or discontinuing the offending dopamine antagonist agent, or by changing it to either olanzapine (Zyprexa) or clozapine (Clozaril), as these two agents appear to present less risk of worsening this irreversible condition.

Clinical Vignette #3

Juan is a 31 year old male with history of moderate ID, schizophrenia (paranoid type) and hypothyroidism. He was referred for an evaluation for "sleeping at work." His medication regimen consisted of haloperidol (a FGA), benztropine, sertraline, lithium and carbamazepine. No medication changes had been made for approximately eleven years.

His mother reported that the carbamazepine, an anticonvulsant, had been started by a neurologist after an incident in high school when Juan had a "shaking" episode that was thought to be "possible seizure activity." Since that time, the patient's primary care physician had prescribed all of the medications, in addition to synthroid, for the treatment of hypothyroidism.

After the initial interview by the psychiatrist, a neurology consult was arranged to determine if the carbamazepine was, in fact, necessary for the prevention of seizure activity.

The neurologist ruled out seizure disorder and recommended a cautious and conservative taper of this medication over several months, which was accomplished successfully. Subsequently, Juan was seen by the psychiatrist monthly, during which time he was tapered and discontinued from several of his other medications. After his lithium was discontinued, the psychiatrist requested that the primary care physician consider that the lithium may have precipitated the hypothyroidism. The synthroid was successfully tapered and discontinued after lithium was stopped, and thyroid functions returned to normal values.

Juan was started on a second generation antipsychotic medication prior to discontinuation of the haloperidol. He tolerated this cross-taper process well, without a recurrence of psychotic symptoms. His final regimen consisted of ziprasidone, sertraline and trazodone. He no longer napped at work, being less sedated and with normal thyroid function. He remained stable and without acute symptomatology.

Although second generation antipsychotics generally are recommended, there are many metabolic effects that can arise from the use of both FGA and SGA psychotropic medications. Weight gain, for example, is a common problem with both FGAs and SGAs in patients with ID (Hellings *et al.*, 2001; Janowsky *et al.*, 2003). Prescribers should be aware of the potential onset of diabetes and weight gain with the use of both atypical and typical antipsychotics.

Signs and symptoms of diabetes can include an increase in thirst, frequency of urination, appetite, gastrointestinal complaints, dizziness and light-headedness. Because of the elevated risk of developing such an illness from the use of these medications, it is within the standard of care to obtain baseline body weight and vital signs, to monitor body weight at each appointment, to educate patients/caregivers on healthy diet and exercise and to use metabolic monitoring tools including blood work on a regular basis.

Prior to starting treatment with these medications, the physician should order a baseline chemistry panel, including fasting, blood glucose and lipid profile. Also, serial laboratory work should be monitored throughout the treatment period and a comprehensive family medical and psychiatric history should be obtained. Although atypical antipsychotics have a ten-fold lower risk of tardive dyskinesia than FGAs, and have a significantly less likelihood of inducing acute EPS, they have been associated with the development of high blood glucose, hyperinsulinemia, type 2 diabetes, cataract formation, and QT prolongation (Alvarez & Pahissa, 2010).

If patients have residual symptoms when taking therapeutic doses of an antipsychotic, switching from one FGA to another may not provide added benefit, due to similar mechanisms of action. If there is no response to an FGA, switch to a SGA; and, if there is no response to one SGA, switch to another SGA. Each SGA is unique and different with regard to relative receptor systems activity (see Table 1). When changing from one antipsychotic medication to another, the current medication should be continued, if possible, while starting the new medication, in order to avoid an interruption in antipsychotic coverage.

Combining two FGAs is not likely to produce additional benefits, as dopamine (D2) receptor blockade will have already been accomplished with a sufficient dose of a single agent. There is also significant risk for EPS with two FGAs (Reiss & Aman, 1998). Combining a SGA with an FGA, however, may be of some benefit if one medication cannot

Table 1 Relative receptor-binding affinities of atypical antipsychotics.

	Geodon	Risperidone	Olanzapine	Quetiapine	Clozapine	Aripiprazole
D_2	+++++	+++++	+++	++	+	++++
5-HT$_{2A}$	+++++	+++++	+++	++	+++	++++
5-HT$_{2C}$	+++++	+++	+++	-	++	++++
5-HT$_{1A}$	++++	+++	-	+	+	++++
5-HT$_{1D}$	+++++	++++	+++	-	-	N/A
A$_1$-adrenergic	++++	++++	+++	+++	++++	++
M$_1$-muscarinic	-	-	+++	+++	+++++	-
H$_1$-histaminergic	+++	++	+++	++++	+++++	++
5-HT reuptake	+++	-	-	-	-	+
NE reuptake	++	-	-	+	+	N/A

Affinity represented as: +++++ very high, ++++ high, +++ moderate, ++ low, – negligible.
Source: adapted from Zorn *et al.* (1999) and Schmidt *et al.* (1998, 2001).

provide symptom relief. Combining two SGAs is not well-studied and can be cost-prohibitive.

Caution is advised when performing a medication taper, because an abrupt discontinuation can induce short-term effects such as cholinergic rebound, dopamine rebound, withdrawal dyskinesia/dystonia and rebound psychosis.

Clinical Vignette #4

Anne was a 22 year old female with history of Asperger's syndrome, bipolar disorder and post-traumatic stress disorder (PTSD), who presented for psychiatric assessment following hospitalization for acute exacerbation of her PTSD. She had a history of alleged sexual and physical abuse at the hands of her father during her developmental years, and now resided in a supported group home setting with two other females with ID. She had been hospitalized five times in the previous six months, and it was discovered that, despite being assigned an independent guardian who mandated no unsupervised contact with her parents, her father had furnished her with a cellphone and had been calling her several times weekly, creating emotional upheaval, increased ritualistic behavior and panic attacks.

Throughout the previous six months, Anne's medical records contained 13 different Axis I diagnoses and she was taking a regimen that included four antipsychotics, four mood stabilizers, three antidepressants and multiple adjunct agents. There were a total of 18 psychotropic medications on board, and she appeared sedated and had difficulty responding to questions. The psychiatrist asked Anne and her caregivers to identify the last time she had been doing well and to describe everything about that point in time (i.e. medication regimen, social support system, residential and occupational settings, physical health, etc).

Anne had been stable for several years on divalproex and risperidone, but these were discontinued eight months prior to this assessment. Anne revealed that her father (her alleged abuser) had told her during one of his phone calls that these medications would make her "fat" if she continued taking them, and she subsequently told her psychiatrist at the time that she would no longer take them. They were both tapered and discontinued, and she did not regain adequate symptom control with the multiple alternate medications prescribed to her since that time.

The psychiatrist discussed the side effect profiles of both medications with Anne and her guardian, including metabolic changes and strategies to monitor and prevent these. A discussion about healthy eating and exercise was reviewed with Anne's caregivers, and all agreed to support the multidimensional treatment plan. The decision was made to restart the two previously successful medications and, after several months of tapering and discontinuing the existing medications, Anne was stable on a regimen of divalproex, risperidone and citalopram.

The multidisciplinary team met with Anne and her guardian to further discuss supervision and enforcement of the prohibition of Anne's family members from any unsupervised contact with her. They also discussed the importance of a therapeutic alliance with the patient and explored the fact that she felt "too scared" to disclose the phone calls with her caregivers, guardian or mental health professionals.

Table 2 Circumstances for the use of medication.

One study by Unwin and Deb (2008a) compiled responses from 108 clinicians working in the ID field regarding the reasons for prescribing psychotropic medications. The most common justifications included failure of non-drug interventions (61.1%), risk/evidence of harm/distress to self (55.6%), risk/evidence of harm/distress to others or property (52.8%), and high frequency/severity of behavior problem (46.3%).

Source: Unwin & Deb (2008a), p. 27.

See Table 2 for the ten most common stated circumstances under which the expert panel would consider prescribing medication (Unwin & Deb, 2008a).

See Table 3 for potential clinical effects and complications of actions on various receptor sites.

Anticonvulsants and mood stabilizers

Mood disorders are common in patients with ID who suffer from a psychiatric condition. The classes of medications called anticonvulsants and mood stabilizers are also often prescribed because of the common co-occurrence of seizure disorders in the ID population. Due to this fact, interdisciplinary networking and collaboration between psychiatry and neurology is vital regarding the prescription of anticonvulsants/mood stabilizers.

Expert consensus supports the use of mood stabilizers and anticonvulsants for bipolar disorder (manic and depressive phases), self-injurious or aggressive behavior, agitation and psychiatric or behavioral problems that occur in individuals with epilepsy (although the literature is limited on these subjects) (Aman *et al.*, 2004). A review of the literature (Deb *et al.*, 2008) shows some support and promise for the use of anticonvulsants for

Table 3 Potential clinical effects and complications.

D_2 antagonism	Positive symptom efficacy, EPS, endocrine effects
5-HT$_{2A}$ antagonism	Negative symptom efficacy, reduced EPS
High 5-HT$_{2A}$/D$_2$ affinity ratio	Antipsychotic efficacy, reduced EPS (compared with D_2 antagonism alone)
5-HT$_{1A}$ agonism	Antidepressant and anxiolytic activity, improved cognition, reduced EPS
5-HT$_{1D}$ antagonism	Antidepressant activity
5-HT$_{2C}$ antagonism	Antidepressant activity
Mixed 5-HT/NE neuronal reuptake inhibition	Antidepressant and anxiolytic activity
Alpha$_1$ antagonism	Postural hypotension
H$_1$ antagonism	Weight gain, sedation
M$_1$ antagonism	Anticholinergic side effects (i.e. cognitive impairment)

Source: adapted from Zorn *et al.* (1999) and Tandon *et al.*, (1977).

behavior problems in individuals with ID. Deb *et al.* also reviewed three studies with lithium (Craft *et al.*, 1987; Langee *et al.*, 1990; Tyrer *et al.*, 1993), two studies with valproate (Ruedrich *et al.*, 1999, Verhoeven and Tuinier, 2001) and one study with topiramate (Janowsky *et al.*, 2003; Reid *et al.*, 1981). All demonstrated an improvement in target problem behaviors in a high percentage of participants.

Valproate is the mood stabilizer preferred by most clinicians, but it brings with it potential side effects, including sedation, nausea/vomiting, increased appetite and weight gain, cognitive dulling, tremor, brittle hair and alopecia. Multivitamins fortified with zinc and selenium may help with hair loss. Valproate can also cause elevations of liver function tests and serum ammonia, skin rash, hemorrhagic pancreatitis and leucopenia/ thrombocytopenia.

Lithium is an effective agent for classic, euphoric mania, although lithium is one of the most lethal medications in overdose, with a small therapeutic index and a large side effect profile that includes weight gain, fluid retention, nausea/vomiting, diarrhea, sedation, cognitive dulling, acne and skin rashes, and fine hand tremors. Lithium can also cause a metallic taste and hypothyroidism in 5–35% of patients. Renal function must be monitored and testing should include evaluating for renal insufficiency and decreased urine-concentrating ability.

Carbamazepine also has been used as a mood stabilizer. Its potential side effects include nausea, vomiting, diarrhea, dermatitis, anticholinergic side effects (structurally similar to tricyclic antidepressants), sedation, cognitive dulling, dizziness, ataxia, diplopia and acute confusional states. However it is associated with less weight gain compared to other mood stabilizers. Of most importance is the fact that it is a metabolism inducer and it reduces the blood levels of many medications, including numerous psychotropics and oral contraceptives. Patients must be monitored for hepatitis or hepatic failure, as well as for syndrome of inappropriate antidiuretic hormone, causing fluid retention (SIADH).

Topiramate's potential side effects include anorexia and weight loss (especially at higher doses), but weight loss is typically not sustained over time. It can also cause sedation, fatigue, cognitive dulling, confusion, memory problems, dizziness, ataxia, tremor and a reduced ability to sweat (with potential for hyperthermia). Patients should also be monitored for kidney stones, metabolic acidosis and acute myopia and secondary angle-closure glaucoma that is not responsive to available glaucoma medications. Topiramate was found poorly efficacious in bipolar disorder for patients in the general population.

An update of the Expert Consensus Guidelines (2004), the Statement on Mood Stabilizers from the Treatment of Psychiatric and Behavioral Problems in Individuals with Mental Retardation, is as follows:

> *"The experts recommended use of mood stabilizers/anticonvulsants for bipolar disorder (manic and depressive phases), self-injurious or aggressive behavior, and agitation, and to treat psychiatric or behavioral problems that occur in individuals with epilepsy. Among the mood stabilizers, the experts considered divalproex the agent of choice (rated first line by 90% or more), followed by carbamazepine. These recommendations reflect the findings in the literature."*

For additional literature review on mood stabilizers in the treatment of PBs and aggression, see Chapter 11.

Antidepressants and anxiolytics

Individuals with ID are at high risk of developing mood and anxiety disorders. Depression is a common psychiatric disorder, but it is often unrecognized, under-diagnosed and, consequently, under-treated in patients with ID (Lunsky & Palucka, 2004). Antidepressants in general are underutilized in the patient with ID.

Unfortunately, even with medications that seem relatively benign, such as the selective serotonin reuptake inhibitors (SSRIs) and some other antidepressants, it has been estimated that approximately 20% of patients with ID will experience adverse drug reactions. This is further complicated by the decrease in self-reporting of side effects, due to limited communicative capabilities.

To lower the incidence of serious or life-threatening side effects of psychotropic medications in this patient population, it is best to start the dose low and go slow in titrating to therapeutic levels. In comparison to the general patient population, it is recommended to use the same (or lower) maintenance and maximum doses, and periodically to consider a gradual dose reduction based on clinical assessment. If a taper is initiated, the physician should proceed conservatively. It is best to avoid frequent dose or drug changes (Expert Consensus Guideline Series, 2000). A regular and systemic review of treatment outcomes should be done at least every three months and within one month of dose or drug changes. The prescribing physician should see the patient at every appointment, and collateral data should be collected from a reliable source.

It is important to be aware of the receptor systems that the antidepressants affect in the treatment of anxiety and depression. There are five major receptor systems involved in the mechanism of action of antidepressants, which include the histamine, serotonin, dopamine, muscarinic and alpha adrenergic receptors. Each receptor is unique in its modulation of action, and each also has its own unique potential benefits as well as its own side effect profile. Dopamine effects can induce stimulation or positive symptoms, as seen in schizophrenia (e.g. auditory or visual hallucinations), while histamine effects can lead to sedation and/or weight changes. Serotonin plays a role in depression and anxiety, and antidepressants work to block the reuptake of serotonin so there is more serotonin available in the synaptic cleft to modulate one's mood. Norepinephrine works with the alpha adrenergic receptor system to target depression and anxiety as well as pain.

It is always necessary, when deciding on a medication, to conduct a risk/benefit analysis with the patient and/or guardian and caregiver(s) to select the most appropriate agent. Obtaining serial laboratory work when starting an antidepressant is also imperative and within the standard of care. Ordering a comprehensive metabolic panel to evaluate blood glucose, electrolyte equilibrium and liver function at least annually is recommended. Evaluating the functional status of the liver is critical, due to the fact that most medications are competing to be metabolized or broken down, which is typically accomplished in the liver. If the liver is not healthy in its ability to metabolize medications, this may alter the blood levels of medications, making them less effective or producing dangerously high plasma levels. Liver enzymes such as GGT, AST and ALT are markers indicating the level of function. GGT levels often indicate acute or short-term changes to the function of the liver, while AST and ALT indicate potential long-term changes.

Though there is a high probability of comorbid mental health diagnoses in the patient with ID, intra-class polypharmacy (using several drugs within the same class) is rarely justified.

If inter-class polypharmacy (using medications from different classes) is considered, the rationale for such a treatment decision should be clear. For example, there may be present both mood and/or anxiety symptoms and co-occurring psychotic symptoms. In other words, clear symptoms in separate categories should be present to justify the use of psychotropic medications in two categories. In addition, there should have already taken place a medication trial failure or only a partial response to a single medication.

In general, when treating anxiety and depression, medication management should be tailored to the needs of the patient, taking into account other prescribed medications, chronic and acute medical conditions, medication half-life and other pertinent factors. Use the most benign agents to minimize risk while attempting to maximize the effect.

Clinical Vignette #5

Daniel was a 58 year old male with history of mild ID and anxiety disorder, who presented for psychiatric evaluation upon transfer from another psychiatrist due to a change in residence. He was currently stable, with no acute symptoms and had been stable for several years. He had never been hospitalized and was currently taking a medication regimen including quetiapine, benztropine, clonazepam, fluoxetine, divalproex and carbamazepine.

Neither the thorough medical record review nor the comprehensive psychiatric intake revealed any present or past history of psychotic symptoms, nor of any mood cycling component. Because of the increased potential for long-term irreversible movement disorders (e.g. tardive dyskinesia) with antipsychotic use, the psychiatrist recommended discontinuation of the quetiapine, and this was accomplished over the next two-month period.

With no recurrence of any mental health symptoms, the patient was then tapered off from the benztropine, divalproex and carbamazepine, one at a time. He was continued on the fluoxetine and clonazepam regimen and remained stable. After further investigation of his previous anxiety symptoms, Daniel's Axis I diagnosis was changed to panic disorder with agoraphobia.

Serial evaluations of the medication regimen should be performed, whether during periods of stability or instability. A trial of taper and discontinuation of psychotropic medications which have been on board for long periods of time should be carefully considered, in particular with medications which have long-term and potentially irreversible side effects. Withdrawal studies suggest that medication can be successfully withdrawn in approximately one third of cases with no re-emergence of behavior problems. In approximately another one third of cases, a reduction in dose can be achieved. In only one third of cases can no reduction in dose be achieved (Deb *et al.*, 2006).

Patients with ID are more vulnerable to developing anxiety disorders for a variety of reasons. They often have limited internal resources to deal with stress, and therefore have circumscribed problem solving skills. Furthermore, they may be more vulnerable to embarrassment, worry or physical symptoms. Though the SSRIs can target and combat these symptoms, it is all too often the case that large doses of anxiolytics such as benzodiazepines are prescribed to the patient with ID. Benzodiazepines, in particular, are prescribed both long-term and on an as-needed basis, despite this being a practice to avoid or minimize in patients with ID.

There are general principles that all members of the multidisciplinary treatment team should be aware of, including the patient and the caregiver, should a benzodiazepine be prescribed. Often, these medications can negatively impact the patient's memory (both anterograde and retrograde) and cognitive sensorium, and they can also suppress respiratory function.

Benzodiazepines can lead to sedation and can also create a physiologic tolerance and dependence, leading to an addictive potential. It is noteworthy that benzodiazepines may have a paradoxical impact on patients with ID, leading to states of disinhibition or disorientation, and can increase the risk of impulse control problems, agitation or PBs. The benzodiazepines with longer half-lives also can accumulate with long-term use in patients with ID. Overall, it is best to minimize or eliminate long-term use of benzodiazepines whenever possible in this patient aggregate.

Clinical Vignette #6

Eric was a 25 year old male with a history of mild ID and attention deficit hyperactivity disorder, combined type. He had been managed on a long-acting psychostimulant for many years, with adequate symptom control. Eric had recently started working in the community through an enclave (supported vocational program), which afforded him the opportunity to work in a laundromat five days per week with on-site supervision.

After the first week, his caregiver started to notice that Eric was not attending to some of his baseline activities of daily living, and there were reports that he was beginning to exhibit anger outbursts while he was out in the community at his job. His caregiver brought him to his primary care physician, and it was concluded that Eric was becoming more anxious since the change in his daily environment had occurred. He was started on an as-needed, short-acting benzodiazepine to target and treat his increased agitation.

When Eric returned to work the following week, it was noticed that he was more aggressive and anxious in appearance. He was also eating much more, and was pointing to his stomach and yelling. Additionally, he was noted to be more somnolent intermittently on the job. During one anger episode, he was administered the "PRN" or "as-needed" benzodiazepine. Approximately 20 minutes later Eric was found sleeping in the bathroom. When an attempt was made to awaken him, he became startled and attacked the supervisor. He remained agitated, threw clothes on the floor and punched several of the washing machines. He then stumbled outside and fell to the ground, hitting his head on the pavement and losing consciousness.

Eric was taken to the closest emergency department, where he underwent a computerized tomography (CT) scan of his head and was found to have a subdural hematoma from the fall. He was hospitalized, treated and eventually discharged. Once he was back at his residence, a review of his medications was performed before he was released to return to work. It was discovered that, after starting the job, his psychostimulant had not been administered mid-morning as it had been previously. Over time, he had become more distracted and anxious, and he had become unable to focus and concentrate without the therapeutic effect of the stimulant. As a result, his symptoms were misconstrued as anxiety due to an environmental change and he was started on an anxiolytic, which ultimately led to a more disinhibited state.

Once the PRN benzodiazepine was eliminated and he was restarted on his stimulant, Eric became an integral part of the work team at the laundromat. It was clear that the anxiolytic had a paradoxical effect on Eric, which is not atypical in the ID patient population.

In studies investigating the efficacy of medications for the treatment of anxiety disorders and related symptoms, Kolevzon et al. (2006) reported a systematic review of SSRI trials (three random controlled and ten open-label) which revealed improvements in anxiety, repetitive behavior and global functioning. In general, when treating anxiety, SSRIs and other newer antidepressants (except bupropion) are first-line anxiolytics; buspirone is very useful, and prior to treatment with these anxiolytics it is vital to rule out side effects of antipsychotics, especially akathisia (an internal sense of restlessness) which can present as "anxiety."

Buspirone has proven efficacy in the treatment of anxiety in patients with ID (Buitelaar *et al.*, 1998). Adults with ID showed reductions in anxiety and aggression with buspirone in one small study (Ratey *et al.*, 1991), and nine out of 14 individuals with pervasive developmental disorder, anxiety, aggression and self-injurious behavior responded favorably to buspirone (Ratey *et al.*, 1989). Buspirone offers several benefits, including the fact that it is not sedating and has no addictive or tolerance potential or withdrawal risk. It is indicated for generalized anxiety disorder, but it is not effective for panic disorder, obsessive compulsive disorder or alcohol withdrawal. It takes up to several weeks to start working and it requires at least twice-daily dosing.

In summary, expert consensus recommends SSRIs in patients with ID (though the literature support is limited) for major depressive disorder, posttraumatic stress disorder, obsessive compulsive disorder, suicidal ideation/behavior and other anxiety that does not meet criteria for a DSM-IV-TR disorder (Aman *et al.*, 2004). When used for the management of behavior problems in adult individuals with ID, the evidence is scant and mixed. Clomipramine showed favorable results when studied for the treatment of stereotyped and related repetitive movement disorders associated with ID (Lewis *et al.*, 1995). Of the SSRI studies for treatment of self-injurious behavior, aggression and agitation, four were favorable (Markowitz *et al.*, 1992; La Malfa *et al.*, 1997; La Malfa *et al.*, 2001; Janowsky *et al.*, 2005), but there were also three that showed negative results for treatment of perseverative and maladaptive behaviors in patients with ID (Bodfish & Madison, 1993; Branford *et al.*, 1998; Troisi *et al.*, 1995). Finally, there were two studies with mixed results (Cook *et al.*, 1992; Davanzo *et al.*, 1998).

The Sohanpal *et al.* review (2007) stated that: "based on poor quality evidence, it can be concluded that antidepressants, particularly SSRIs, improve aggression, self-injurious behavior and other behavior problems on average in less than 50% of cases, and the rest show either no improvement or deterioration." SSRIs seem to be more helpful in the presence of underlying anxiety and an associated diagnosis of obsessive compulsive disorder. "This review does not suggest that they are ineffective, but that there is not enough good quality evidence for their usefulness" (Sohanpal *et al.*, 2007). Potential benefits of SSRIs, when compared to older antidepressants, include a lower risk of causing seizures, lower cardiovascular side effects, less orthostatic hypotension and a high margin of safety in overdose.

Expert consensus guidelines and other documents by prescribing authorities

Every author in the field of ID, from every part of the globe, describes a need for increased quantity and quality of evidence-based research. Expert consensus recommends utilizing the same medications which are used to treat disorders in the general population for those with ID. Use of general evidence-based conclusions is appropriate and logical until more specialized research is available. Table 4 includes a list of citations for documents written by acknowledged prescribing authorities in the field of ID.

In conclusion, taken as a whole, the parameters laid out above provide a comprehensive framework for prescribers to utilize in adhering to the guidelines of best practices and evidence-based medicine in the care of patients with ID and co-occurring mental illness. Both basic and detailed data points have been illustrated to prioritize use of existing best practices and evidence-based medicine principles for the general population in this specialized patient subset.

In linking medical health and mental health, it is possible to use the biopsychosocial formulation and institute treatment plans that treat symptoms and improve quality of life. It appears that long-held beliefs and assumptions about treating patients with ID require ongoing review and modification, as was illustrated in exploring the past 50–100 years of methodology. The information discussed herein is intended to be applied to the care of all individuals with ID and their families/caregivers. It is a great accomplishment to eliminate unnecessary psychotropic medications, to update regimens and to fully treat mental illnesses with the least number of medications, each at the lowest effective dosage.

Table 4 Evidence-based guidelines for prescribing psychotropics.

- Reiss, S. & Aman, M.G. (1998). Chapter 4. Guidelines for the Use of Psychotropic Medication. Ohio State University Publishing. Columbus, Ohio.
- Reiss, S. & Aman, M.G. (eds) (2000). Psychotropic Medications and Developmental Disabilities: The International Consensus Handbook (AAMR).
- *Treatment of Psychiatric and Behavioral Problems in Individuals with Mental Retardation. An Update of the Expert Consensus Guidelines* (2004).
- Deb, S., Clarke, D. & Unwin, G. (2006). *Using medication to manage behavior problems among adults with a learning disability: Quick Reference Guide* (QRG). University of Birmingham, Royal College of Psychiatrists & Mencap, Birmingham, UK. www.ld-medication.bham.ac.uk.
- Fletcher, R., Loschen, E., Stavrakaki, C. & First, M. (eds.) (2007). *Diagnostic Manual – Intellectual Disability (DM-ID): A Textbook of Diagnosis of Mental Disorders in Persons with Intellectual Disability.* NADD Press, Kingston, NY.
- Problem Behaviour in Adults with Intellectual Disabilities: International Guide for Using Medication. The World Psychiatric Association (WPA): Section on Psychiatry of Intellectual Disability (SPID) September 2008. The Section of Psychiatry of Intellectual Disability (SPID): World Psychiatric Association (WPA): Working group.
- Unwin, G.L. & Deb, S. (2008a). Use of medication for the management of behavior problems among adults with intellectual disabilities: a clinicians' consensus survey. *American Journal of Mental Retardation* **113**(1), 19–31.
- World Psychiatry Association (2010). Clinical Bulletin of the Developmental Disabilities Division. International guide to prescribing psychotropic medication for the management of problem behaviours in adults with intellectual disabilities.

Table 5 Clinical Pearls.

1. *Dosing strategies*: keep medication regimen as simple as possible; consider use of once-a-day dosing and extended-release formulations when possible (Aman *et al.*, 2004).
2. *Start low and go slow*: use lower initial doses and increase more slowly than in individuals without ID (Aman *et al.*, 2004).
3. Use the *same (or lower) maintenance and maximum doses* as patients without ID: periodically consider gradual dose reduction; avoid frequent drug and dose changes unless there is a valid reason for the change (e.g., no response, adverse effects) (Aman *et al.*, 2004).
4. *Evaluate treatment effects*: collect baseline data before beginning medication; evaluate medication efficacy by tracking specific index behaviors using recognized behavioral measurement methods (e. g. frequency counts, rating scales). Evaluate the medication's effect on functional status. (Aman *et al.*, 2004).
5. *Evaluate side effects*: monitor for side effects regularly and systematically; at least once every 3–6 months and after any new medication is begun or the dose is increased; a standardized assessment instrument can be helpful in monitoring for side effects. (Reiss & Aman (1998), pp.45–72.)
6. If an antipsychotic is prescribed, *assess for tardive dyskinesia* at least every 3– 6 months. (Aman *et al.*, 2004).
7. If utilizing an atypical antipsychotic, monitor for changes in *weight and glucose and lipid levels* per guidelines (American Psychiatric Association, American Association of Clinical Endocrinologists & North American Association for the Study of Obesity (2004) and Marder *et al.* (2004)
8. *Polypharmacy: avoid using two medications from the same therapeutic class* at the same time; intraclass polypharmacy (e.g. two SSRIs), defined as using two or more medications from different therapeutic classes at the same time, is rarely justified. Interclass polypharmacy (e.g. two psychotropic medications from different categories) may be appropriate and needed in certain situations (e.g. psychotic or bipolar depression, partial response to one drug, comorbid conditions). This requires a diagnosis to justify both medications (i.e. if antidepressant medication and antipsychotic medication are prescribed together, a diagnosis in both categories of symptoms is required). (Aman *et al.*, 2004).
9. *Medication Practices to Avoid*:
   • Long-term use of benzodiazepine antianxiety agents (e.g., diazepam) or shorter acting sedative hypnotics (e.g., zolpidem)
   • Use of long-acting sedative hypnotics (e.g., chloral hydrate)
   • Use of anticholinergics without extrapyramidal symptoms
   • Higher than usual doses of psychotropic medications
   • Use of phenytoin, phenobarbital, primidone as psychotropics
   • Long-term use of 'PRN' or 'as needed' medication orders
   • Failure to integrate medication with psychosocial interventions (Aman *et al.*, 2004).
10. Expert consensus *recommends the new atypical antipsychotics* (though the literature is limited) for schizophrenia, other psychotic symptoms (e.g. psychotic disorder NOS, psychotic depression), self-injurious or aggressive behavior. (Aman *et al.*, 2004).
11. If patient keeps improving as you judiciously increase one medication, it is better to *maximize that medication* (until the therapeutic benefit levels out) *before considering another.* Include all parameters to accurately assess impact of medication; remember to factor in compliance and life stressors/changes appropriately to most accurately assess medication effectiveness (e.g. if events in life are particularly distressing and overwhelming, concluding that the antidepressant "is not working" during this tumultuous time would likely be misguided).
12. *Change one medication at a time*, if possible, to best assess its effect; often, "cleaning up" a long list of psychotropics by judiciously tapering off unnecessary medications is the most helpful intervention. Withdrawal studies show that approximately one third of patients can be tapered and discontinued from medications with no adverse effects or recurrence of pre-existing symptoms or behavior. (Deb *et al.*, 2008)

(*continued*)

13. Several factors were identified that suggested the need to *include medication in the treatment plan in the absence of the diagnosed psychiatric illness*. These factors included *SIB that posed a risk of lasting harm, aggression to others that posed up at physical risk, very severe symptoms, good response to medication, lack of response to psychosocial interventions, and symptoms that interfere significantly* with the ability to participate in education and rehabilitation. (Unwin & Deb, 2008a).

14. The first choice medication class for the *management of both aggression and SIB was antipsychotics*. There was a strong preference for atypical antipsychotics over typical antipsychotics for the management of both aggression and SIB. Risperidone was the most preferred second generation antipsychotic, followed by olanzapine, and then quetiapine. Citalopram was the most preferred new generation antidepressant, followed by fluoxetine and sertraline. (Unwin & Deb, 2008a).

15. Guide to using psychotropic medication to manage behavior problems among adults with ID: the use of *interdisciplinary working* with effective communication and information sharing can facilitate prescribing with person centered planning; the *input of the individual with ID, their family and caregivers* is essential when prescribing within the premise of person-centered planning. (Deb *et al.*, 2006).

16. Guide to using psychotropic medication to manage behavior problems among adults with ID: *the most pronounced effect of antidepressants on behavioral problems emerged where anxiety or obsessive-compulsive symptoms were prominent*. Some evidence to support the use of mood stabilizers and anticonvulsants in the management of behavior problems was found. There is evidence that indicates sodium valproate, carbamazepine and topiramate as well as lithium may be effective. Evidence currently exists for opioid antagonists, with some studies showing better results on large doses and others on small doses. (Deb *et al.*, 2006).

Patients with ID are more vulnerable to the side effects of antipsychotic medications. Psychotropic medications should improve cognitive function, not worsen it. Medications should treat mental illness fully, and we would expect no less for a patient in the general population. Finally, the medication regimen for a patient with ID should look no different than the regimen for any other patient.

References

Ahmed, Z., Fraser, W., Kerr, M.P., Kiernan, C., Emerson, E., Robertson, J., Felce, D., Allen, D., Baxter, H. & Thomas, J. (2000). Reducing antipsychotic medication in people with a learning disability. *British Journal of Psychiatry* **176**, 42–46.

Alvarez, P.A. & Pahissa, J. (2010). QT alterations in psychopharmacology: proven candidates and suspects. *Current Drug Safety* **5**, 97–104.

Aman, MG. (1991). Assessing psychopathology and behavior problems in persons with mental retardation: A review of available instruments. (DHHS Publication No. [ADM] 91-1712.) US Department of Health and Human Services, Rockville, MD.

Aman, M.G. & Gharabawi, G.M., for the Special Topic Advisory Panel on Transitioning to Risperidone Therapy in Patients with Mental Retardation and Developmental Disabilities. (2004). Treatment of behavior disorders in mental retardation: report on transitioning to atypical antipsychotics, with an emphasis on Risperidone. *Journal of Clinical Psychiatry* **65**, 1197–1210.

Aman, M.G. & Madrid, A. (1999). Atypical antipsychotics in persons with developmental disabilities. *Mental Retardation and Developmental Disabilities Research Reviews* **5**, 253–263.

Aman, M.G., Lindsay, R.L., Nash, P.L. & Arnold, L.E. (2003). Individuals with mental retardation. In: Martin, A., Scahill, L., Charney, D.S. & Leckman, J.L. (eds.) *Psycho-pharmacology: Principles and Practice*, pp. 617–630. Oxford University Press Oxford, UK.

Aman, M.G., Crismon, M.L., Frances, A., King, B.H. & Rojahn, J. (eds.) (2004). *Treatment of psychiatric and behavior problems in individuals with mental retardation: an update of the expert consensus guidelines for mental retardation and developmental disability populations.* Postgraduate Institute for Medicine, Englewood, CO.

American Psychiatric Association (2000). *Diagnostic and Statistical Manual of Mental Disorders*, 4th ed., text revision (DSM-IV). APA, Washington, DC.

American Psychiatric Association, American Association of Clinical Endocrinologists & North American Association for the Study of Obesity (2004). Consensus development conference on antipsychotic drugs and obesity and diabetes. *Diabetes Care* **27**, 596–601 and Journal of Clinical Psychiatry 65, 267–272.

Arnold, L.E. (1993). Clinical pharmacological issues in treating psychiatric disorders of patients with mental retardation. *Annals of Clinical Psychiatry* **5**, 189–197.

Bishop, A.C. (1992). Empirical approach to psychopharmacology for institutionalized individuals with severe or profound mental retardation. *Mental Retardation* **30**, 283–288.

Bodfish, J.W. & Madison, J.T. (1993). Diagnosis of fluoxetine treatment of compulsive behavior disorder of adults with mental retardation. *American Journal of Mental Retardation* **98**, 360–367.

Bongiorno, F.P. (1996). Dual Diagnosis: Developmental Disability Complicated by Mental Illness. *Southern Medical Journal* **89**(12), 1142–1146.

Branford, D. (1996). Factors associated with the successful or unsuccessful withdrawal of antipsychotic drug therapy prescribed for people with learning disabilities. *Journal of Intellectual Disability Research* **40**, 322–329.

Branford, D., Bhaumik, S. & Naik, B. (1998). Selective serotonin re-uptake inhibitors for the treatment of preservative and maladaptive behaviors of people with intellectual disability. *Journal of intellectual Disability Research* **42**, 301–306.

Buitelaar, J.K., van der Gaag, J. & van der Hoeven, J. (1998). Buspirone in the management of anxiety and irritability in children with pervasive developmental disorders: results of an open-label study. *Journal of Clinical Psychiatry* **59**(2), 56–59.

Clark, D.J., Kelley, S., Thinn, K., & Corbett, J.A. (1990). Psychotropic drugs and mental retardation: I. *Disabilities and the prescription of drugs for behavior and for epilepsy in 3 residential settings. Journal of Mental Deficiency Research* **28**, 229–233.

Cook, E.H., Rowlett, R., Jaselskis, C., & Leventhal, B.L. (1992). Fluoxetine treatment of children and adults with autistic disorder and mental retardation. *Journal of The American Academy Of Child and Adolescent Psychiatry* **31**, 739–745.

Cooper, S-A., Smiley, E., Morrison, J., Williamson, A. & Allan, L. (2007a). Mental ill-health in adults with intellectual disabilities: Prevalence and associated factors. *British Journal of Psychiatry* **190**, 27–35.

Cooper S-A., Smiley, E., Morrison, J., Allan, L., Williamson, A., Finlayson, J., Jackson, A. & Mantry, D. (2007b). Psychosis and adults with intellectual disabilities: Prevalence, incidence and related factors. *Social Psychiatry and Psychiatric Epidemiology* **42**(7), 530–536.

Craft, M., Ismail, I.A., Kristnamurti, D., Matthews, J., Regan, A., Seth, V. & North, P.M. (1987). Lithium in the treatment of aggression in mentally handicapped patients: a double blind trial. *British Journal of Psychiatry* **150**, 685–689.

Davanzo, P.A., Belin, T.R., Widawski, M.H. & King, B.H. (1998) Paroxetine treatment of aggression and self-injury in persons with mental retardation. *American Journal on Mental Retardation* **102**, 427–437.

Deb, S. & Fraser, W. (1994). The use of psychotropic medication in people with learning disability: Towards rational prescribing. *Human Psychopharmacology* **9**, 259–272.

Deb, S., Matthews, T., Holt, G. & Bouras, N. (2001). *Practice guidelines for the assessment and diagnosis of mental health problems in adults with intellectual disability*. Pavilion, Brighton, UK.

Deb, S., Clarke, D. & Unwin, G. (2006). *Using medication to manage behavior problems among adults with a learning disability: Quick Reference Guide* (QRG). University of Birmingham, Royal College of Psychiatrists & Mencap, Birmingham, UK. www. ld-medication. bham. ac. uk.

Deb, S., Chaplin, S., Sohanpal, G., Unwin, G. Soni, R. & Lenôtre, L. (2008). The effectiveness of mood stabilizers and antiepileptic medication for the management of behavior problems in adults with intellectual disability: a systematic review. *Journal of Intellectual Disability Research* **52**, 107–113.

Einfeld, S.L., Piccinin, A.M., Mackinnon, A., Hofer, S.M., Taffe, J., Gray, K.M., Bontempo, D. E., Hoffman, L.R., Parmenter, T. & Tonge, B.J. (2006). Psychopathology in young people with intellectual disability. *JAMA* **296**, 1981–1989.

Emerson, E., Kiernan, C., Alborz, A., Reeves, D., Mason, H., Swarbrick, R., Mason, L. & Hatton, C. (2001). Predicting the persistence of severe self-injurious behavior. *Research in Developmental Disabilities* **22**, 67–75.

Engel, G.L. (1977). The need for a new medical model: A challenge for biomedicine. *Science* **196** (4286), 129–136.

Engel, G.L. (1980). The clinical application of the biopsychosocial model. *American Journal of Psychiatry* **137**, 535–544.

Fletcher, R., Loschen, E., Stavrakaki, C. & First, M. (eds.), (2007). *Diagnostic Manual – Intellectual Disability (DM-ID): A Textbook of Diagnosis of Mental Disorders in Persons with Intellectual Disability*. NADD Press, Kingston, NY.

Fodstad, J.C., Bamburg, J.W., Matson, J.L., Mahan, S., Hess, J.A., Neal, D. & Holloway, J. (2010). Tardive Dyskinesia and intellectual disability: an examination of demographics and topography in adults with dual diagnosis and atypical antipsychotic use. *Research in Developmental Disabilities* **31**(3), 750–759.

Friedlander, R., Lazar, S. & Klancnik, J. (2001). Atypical antipsychotic use in treating adolescents and young adults with developmental disabilities. *Canadian Journal of Psychiatry* **46**, 741–745.

Guay, D.P. (2008). Inappropriate Sexual Behaviors in Cognitively Impaired Older Individuals. *American Journal of Geriatric Pharmacotherapy* **6**(5). 269–288.

Guay, D.P. (2009). Drug Treatment of Paraphilic and Nonparaphilic Sexual Disorders. *Clinical Therapeutics* **31**(1), 1–31.

Hellings, J.A., Zarcone, J.R., Crandall, K., Wallace, D. & Schroeder, S.R. (2001). Weight gain in a controlled study of risperidone in children, adolescents and adults with mental retardation and autism. *Journal of Child andAdolescent Psychopharmacology*. **11**, 229–238.

Janowsky, D.S., Barnhill, L.J., Davis, J.M. (2003). Olanzapine for self-injurious, aggressive, and disruptive behaviors in intellectually disabled adults: A retrospective, open-label, naturalistic trial. *Journal of Clinical Psychiatry* **64**, 1258–1265.

Janowsky, D.S., Shetty, M., Barnhill, L.J., Elamir, B. & Davis, JM. (2005). Serotonergic antidepressant effects on aggressive, self-injurious and destructive/disruptive behaviours in intellectually disabled adults: a retrospective, open label, naturalistic trial. *International Journal of Neuropsychopharmacology* **8**, 37–48.

Kalachnik, J.E., Leventhal, B.B., James, D.H., Sovner, R., Kastner, T.A., Walsh, K., Weisblatt, S.A., & Klitzke, M.G. (1998). Guidelines for the use of psychotropic medication. In: Reiss, S. & Aman, M.G. (eds.) *Psychotropic Medications and Developmental Disabilities: The International Consensus Handbook*, pp. 45–72. The Ohio State Nisonger Center, Columbus, OH.

Kaplan, H.I. & Sadock, B.J. (1988). *Synopsis of psychiatry. Behavior sciences. Clinical psychiatry* (5th ed.). Williams & Wilkins, Baltimore, MD.

Kolevzon, A., Mathewson, K.A. & Hollander, E. (2006). Selective serotonin reuptake inhibitors in autism: a review of efficacy and tolerability. *Journal of Clinical Psychiatry* **67**(3), 407–414.

La Malfa, G.P., Bertelli, M., Ricca, V., Mannucci, E. & Cabras, P.L. (1997). Fluvoxamine and mental retardation: clinical use. *Italian Journal of Intellective Impairment* **10**, 3–6.

La Malfa, G., Bertelli, M. & Conte, M. (2001). Fluvoxamine and aggression in mental retardation. *Psychiatric Services* **52**(8), 1105.

Langee, H.R. (1990). Retrospective study of lithium use for institutionalized mentally retarded individuals with behavior disorders. *American Journal on Mental Retardation* **94**, 448–452.

Lewis, M.H., Bodfish, J.W., Powell, S.B. & Golden, R.N. (1995). Clomipramine treatment for stereotype and related repetitive movement disorders associated with mental retardation. *American Journal on Mental Retardation* **100**, 299–312.

Long, E.S. & Miltenberger, R.G. (1998). A review of behavioral and pharmacological treatments for habit disorders in individuals with mental retardation. *Journal of Behavior Therapy and Experimental Psychiatry* **29**, 143–156.

Lott, I.T., McGregor, M., Engleman, L., Touchette, P., Tournay, A., Sandman, C., Fernandez, G., Plon, L. & Walsh, D. (2004). Longitudinal prescribing patterns for psychoactive medications in community-based individuals with developmental disabilities: Utilization of pharmacy records. *Journal of Intellectual Disability Research* **6**, 563–571.

Lowe, K., Allen, D., Jones, E., Brophy, S., Moore, K. & James, W. (2007). Challenging behaviours: prevalence and topographies. *Journal of Intellectual Disability Research* **51**, 625–636.

Lund, J. (1985). The prevalence of psychiatric morbidity in mentally retarded adults. *Acta Psychiatrica Scandinavica* **72**, 563–570.

Lunsky, Y. & Palucka, A.M. (2004). Depression in intellectual disability. *Current Opinion in Psychiatry* **17**(5), 359–363.

Marder, S.R., Essock, S.M., Miller, A.L., Buchanan, R.W., Casey, D.E., Davis, J.M., Kane, J.M., Lieberman, J.A., Schooler, N.R., Covell, N., Stroup, S., Weissman, E.M., Wirshing, D.A., Hall, C.S., Pogach, L., Pi-Sunyer, X., Bigger, J.T., Friedman, A., Kleinberg, D., Yevich, S.J., Davis, B. & Shon, S. (2004). Physical health monitoring of patients with schizophrenia. *American Journal of Psychiatry* **161**, 1334–1349.

Markowitz, P.I. (1992) Effect of fluoxetine on self-injurious behavior in the developmentally disabled: a preliminary study. *Journal of Clinical Psychopharmacology* **12**, 27–31.

Matson, J.L., Fodstad, J.C., Neal, D., Dempsey, T. & Rivet, T.T. (2010). Risk factors for tardive dyskinesia in adults with intellectual disability, comorbid psychopathology, and long-term psychotropic use. *Research in Developmental Disabilities* **31**(1), 108–116.

Nøttestad, J.A. & Linaker, O.M. (2003). Psychotropic drug use among people with intellectual disability before and after deinstitutionalization. *Journal of Intellectual Disability Research* **47**, 464–471.

Qureshi, H. & Alborz, A. (1992). Epidemiology of challenging behaviour. *Mental Handicap Research* **5**, 130–145.

Ratey, J.J., Sovner, R., Mikkelsen, E. & Chmielinski, H.E. (1989). Buspirone therapy for maladaptive behavior and anxiety in developmentally disabled persons. *Journal of Clinical Psychiatry* **50**(10), 382–384.

Ratey, J., Sovner, R., Parks, A. & Rogentine, K. (1991). Buspirone treatment of aggression and anxiety in mentally retarded patients: a multiple-baseline, placebo lead-in study. *Journal of Clinical Psychiatry* **52**(4), 159–162.

Reiss, S. (1994). *Handbook of Challenging Behavior: Mental Health Aspects of Mental Retardation*. IDS, Publishing, Worthington, OH.

Reiss, S. & Aman, M.G. (1998). *Psychotropic medications and developmental disabilities: The international consensus handbook*. The Nisonger Center UAP, Columbus, OH.

Royal College of Psychiatrists (2001). *DC-LD (Diagnostic Criteria for Psychiatric Disorders for Use with Adults with Learning Disabilities/Mental Retardation)*. Gaskell, London.

Ruedrich, S., Swales, T.P., Fossaceca, C., Toliver, J. & Rutkowski, A. (1999) Effect of divalproex sodium on aggression and self-injurious behaviour in adults with intellectual disability: a retrospective review. *Journal of Intellectual Disability Research* **43**, 105–111.

Sajith, S.G., Margan, C. & Clarke, D. (2008). Pharmacological management of inappropriate sexual behaviours: a review of its evidence, rationale and scope in relation to men with intellectual disabilities. *Journal of Intellectual Disability Research* **52**(12), 1078–1090.

Schmidt, A.W., Lebel, L.A., Johnson, C.G., Howard, H.R. Jr., Lowe, J.A. & Zorn, S.H. (1998). The novel antipsychotic ziprasidone has a unique human receptor binding profile compared to other agents. *Society for Neuroscience* **24**, 2177.

Schmidt, A.W., Lebel, L.A., Howard, H.R. Jr. & Zorn, S.H. (2001). Ziprasidone: a novel antipsychotic agent with a unique human receptor binding profile. *European Journal of Pharmacology* **425**, 197–201.

Simon, E.W., Blubaugh, K.M. & Pippidis, M. (1996). Substituting traditional antipsychotics with risperidone for people with mental retardation. *Mental Retardation* **34**, 359–366.

Smith, S., Branford, D., Collacott, R., Cooper, S.A. & McGrother, C. (1996). Prevalence and cluster typology of maladaptive behaviours in a geographically defined population of adults with learning disabilities. *British Journal of Psychiatry* **169**, 219–227.

Sohanpal, S.K., Deb, S., Thomas, C., Soni, R., Lenôtre, L. & Unwin, G. (2007). The effectiveness of antidepressant medication in the management of behavior problems in adults with intellectual disabilities: a systematic review. *Journal of Intellectual Disability Research* **51**, 750–765.

Spreat, S., Conroy, J.W. & Jones, J.C. (1997). Use of Psychotropic Medication in Oklahoma: A Statewide Survey. *American Journal on Mental Retardation* **102**(1), 80–85.

Spreat, S., Conroy, J. & Fullerton, A. (2004). Statewide Longitudinal Survey of Psychotropic Medication Use for Persons With Mental Retardation: 1994 to 2000. *American Journal on Mental Retardation* **109**(4), 322–331.

Stahl, SM. (2008). *Stahl's Essential Psychopharmacology Neuroscientific Basis and Practical Applications*. Cambridge University Press, New York.

Stark, J.A., Menolascino, F.J., Albarelli, M.H. & Gray, V.C. (1988). *Mental Retardation and Mental Health: Classification, Diagnosis, Treatment, Services*. Springer-Verlag, New York.

Tandon, R., Harrigan, E. & Zorn, S.H. (1997). Ziprasidone: a novel antipsychotic with unique pharmacology and therapeutic potential. *Journal of Serotonin Research* **4**, 159–177.

Troisi, A., Vicario, E., Nuccetelli, F., Ciani, N. & Pasini, A. (1995) Effects of fluoxetine on aggressive behavior of adult inpatients with mental retardation and epilepsy. *Pharmacopsychiatry* **28**, 73–76.

Tyrer, S.P., Aronson, M.E. & Lauder, J. (1993) Effect of lithium on behavioural factors in aggressive mentally handicapped subjects. In: Birch, N.J., Padgham, C. & Hughes, M.S. (eds.) *Lithium in Medicine and Biology*, pp. 119–25. Marius Press, Carnforth.

Unwin, G.L. & Deb, S. (2008a). Use of medication for the management of behavior problems among adults with intellectual disabilities: a clinicians' consensus survey. *American Journal of Mental Retardation* **113**(1), 19–31.

Unwin, G. & Deb, S. (2008b). Psychiatric and behavioral assessment scales for adults with learning disabilities. *Advances in Mental Health in Learning Disability* **2**, 37–45.

Viejo, L.F., Morales, V., Puñal, P., Pérez, J.L. & Sancho, R.A. (2003). Risk factors in neuroleptic malignant syndrome. *A case-control study. Acta Psychiatrica Scandinavica* **107**, 45–49.

Verhoeven, W.M.A. & Tuiner, S. (2001). Cyclothymia or unstable mood disorder? *A systematic treatment evaluation with valproic acid. Journal of Applied Research in Intellectual Disabilities* **14**, 147–154.

Woods, D.W. & Miltenberger, R.G. (1995). Habit Reversal: a review of applications and variations. *Journal of Behavior Therapy and Experimental Psychiatry* **26**, 123–131.

World Psychiatry Association (2010). Clinical Bulletin of the Developmental Disabilities Division. International guide to prescribing psychotropic medication for the management of problem behaviours in adults with intellectual disabilities.

Wszola, B.A., Newell, K.M. & Sprague, R.L. (2001). Risk factors for tardive dyskinesia in a large population of youths and adults. *Experimental and Clinical Psychopharmacology* **9**, 285–296.

Zorn, S.H., Lebel, L.A., Schmidt, A.W., Lu, Y., Braselton, J.P., Reynolds, L.S., Sprouse, J.S. & Rollema, H. (1999). Pharmacological and neurochemical studies with the new antipsychotic ziprasidone. In: Palomo, T., Beninger, R.J. & Archer, T. (eds.) *Interactive Monoaminergic Brain Disorders*, pp. 377–393. Editorial Sintesis, Madrid, Spain.

13

Psychotherapy

Carroll S. Jackson, LISW-S, Montgomery County Board of Developmental Disabilities, Dayton, Ohio
Julie P. Gentile, MD, Associate Professor, Wright State University, Dayton, Ohio

Introduction

Historically, there have been significant misperceptions regarding the effectiveness of psychotherapy when working with patients with intellectual disabilities (ID). From the 1950s through the 1980s, despite some limited research in this area, the amount of literature being published was minimal, and the stereotype persisted that this specialized population could not benefit from psychotherapy. In fact, the majority of research on the provision of psychotherapy to individuals with ID during this time span concluded that it had no benefit at all, and indicated that there were no substantial differences in outcomes when treatment was provided (Prout & Browning, 2011). A lack of information and education to clinicians contributed to the absence of appropriate mental health services for persons with ID.

While some clinicians thought that individuals with ID could not benefit from treatment with psychotherapy, others considered them immune from developing mental illnesses, believing that having ID protected individuals from developing a mental disorder. This was, supposedly, because their cognitive disabilities would prevent them from experiencing emotional discord or affect (Davidson & Cain, 2006). It also was a widely held belief that this population did not possess the necessary skills to participate actively in the process of psychotherapy, due to their diminished ability to use abstract reasoning. It was assumed that this meant that the patient did not possess the skills needed to examine their own behaviors

Psychiatry of Intellectual Disability: A Practical Manual, First Edition.
Edited by Julie P. Gentile and Paulette M. Gillig.
© 2012 John Wiley & Sons, Ltd. Published 2012 by John Wiley & Sons, Ltd.

or actions, to explore potential antecedents, or to understand the benefits of making positive changes (Lynch, 2004).

It is now understood that individuals with ID are even more susceptible than other people to the development of mental illness, because they are typically more vulnerable to stress, have fewer coping skills and possess a smaller system of natural supports. Much work has been done in recent years to disprove the myth regarding the lack of efficacy of mental health treatment with this population. Informed clinicians are now cognizant of the fact that psychotherapy is, in fact, a best practice when working with patients with ID.

Patients can grow, change and recover from mental illness. It is increasingly clear that level of intelligence is not the sole indicator for appropriateness of psychotherapy and that mental health services can help to improve quality of life for patients with ID. Fortunately, the amount of research on this subject has grown considerably over the last ten years, and there also has been an increase in the amount of workshop and training opportunities available for clinicians. That said, while we have come a long way in a relatively short period of time, there is much more work to be done, as this remains a significantly underserved population.

Although it is now widely understood that patients with ID can benefit from psychotherapy, research on this topic has demonstrated the need to adjust the mode of therapy provided to fit the developmental level, dependence needs and verbal/cognitive abilities of the patient who is to receive treatment (Hurley *et al.*, 1998). Therefore, in order to provide effective mental health services to this population, clinicians will need to be flexible in their approach and need to adapt interventions to accommodate for differences in intellectual ability. Insistence upon the use of traditional models of treatment will result in poor treatment outcomes and will prevent patients with ID from receiving appropriate care (Whitehouse *et al.*, 2006).

This chapter will focus on common issues of concern that may arise in treatment, barriers that complicate treatment, and modifications in the provision of psychotherapy modalities that can increase the efficacy of the treatment provided.

Issues related to the presence of ID

Impact on the family

The diagnosis of ID often means that individuals and their involved family members will experience seemingly insurmountable stressors. Often the initial diagnosis is slow to arrive, coming after family members or the primary care provider recognize the presence of developmental delays. It can be difficult for family members to adjust to the idea that their child has a disability and to accept the loss of the "perfect" child they had envisioned. Instead, their reality may be a child who looks different compared to other children, who exhibits behavior unlike that of peers of the same age and who requires continual care that disrupts previously established daily routine. This is coupled with the stigma that comes with the diagnosis, which sometimes causes friends and even extended family members to pull away, and which may lead to family members feeling alone and isolated at a time when additional support would be invaluable.

As their children grow, parents may experience emotional pain when watching other children in the family, or even non-disabled peers, achieve anticipated milestones such as graduating from college or having children. These events often trigger a resurfacing of sadness and loss as family members process the grief at each developmental milestone.

This distress increases significantly when the child also suffers from a mental illness. Family members may become overwhelmed or may feel ill-equipped to deal with the onset of behavioral changes that are related to a mental illness. When they attempt to seek treatment, they may be shocked to find an absence of treatment providers who are willing and able to help.

Historically, a diagnosis of mental illness plus ID equated to tremendous difficulty in finding appropriate care, with neither the mental health nor the ID system feeling equipped to provide the necessary services and supports. The diagnosis of mental illness can also cause increased stress, because the family has to accept that their child has not one, but two, conditions which will significantly impact the child's functioning and life course.

Impact on the individual

Individuals with ID will experience many various transition periods in their lives that may trigger feelings of stress or loss. These include graduating from educational programs, transitioning from school programs to occupational settings, and moving from family settings into supported residential environments. It also can be extremely difficult to watch siblings achieve milestones that they, too, dream of, but which are out of their reach, such as driving a car or going away to college. As adults, they may long for a level of independence that is out of their grasp, because they may need support with managing their finances, finding and maintaining employment, accessing reliable transportation and navigating the activities of daily living.

Societal stigmas regarding a diagnosis of ID can have a devastating impact, as internalization of these negative messages can lead to low self-esteem, feelings of inadequacy and depression. Individuals with mild ID may be particularly susceptible to this, because they tend to have an increased awareness and understanding of the fact that they have a disability, and of the societal prejudices associated with it. Jahoda *et al.* (2006) suggested that this increased emotional insight contributes to a higher prevalence of depression among individuals with *milder* disabilities. Therefore, clinicians must explore an individual's perceptions regarding what it means to have a disability and how it impacts the person's sense of self-worth, as this will be a pivotal area to address in treatment.

Clinical Vignette #1 (part 1)

Suzy is a 27-year-old female with mild ID, who resides in a group home with three housemates She attends a habilitation workshop with two of her housemates during the day, and there is one residential staff person in her home from 4:00 to 11:00 PM every evening.

Suzy presented in treatment with feelings of anger and resentment, due to the many perceived restrictions in her life. She reported that she wanted to live independently, however her budget could not support it. She wanted to drive a car and attend college. However, she was not able to pass a driver's license examination and was told that the local community college could not provide her with the necessary supports due to her level of cognitive deficits.

Involved care providers noted in the initial referral that Suzy was experiencing increased discord with her housemates; she reported that, while she liked her housemates, she sometimes became irritated with them due to the amount of time they spent together. Suzy often felt isolated and lonely and had a history of attempting to use sexual relationships with men as a way to feel loved and valued by others.

Just prior to entering treatment, Suzy had met strangers via the internet and had exchanged her personal information with them. This had led to frequent calls from unknown men, during which they requested that Suzy send them money. Her multidisciplinary team became aware of this, and residential staff began monitoring her internet usage and providing constant supervision in the community to ensure she was not victimized by others. This fact was a particular source of concern for her in treatment.

Suzy struggled with accepting her disability and with coming to terms with the limitations and structure that were part of her daily life. She frequently reported that having a disability prevented her from being like "normal" people, and that it meant she was "not good enough."

Examples of treatment approaches

Individuals with ID have greater difficulty in acquiring and using important skills of daily life, and they subsequently experience failure at a higher rate and enter new situations with a lower expectation of success. They also often find themselves in situations in which they have little or no choice. In Clinical Vignette #1 (part 1), this was certainly true in Suzy's situation, in which she had no choice in her residential or in her occupational setting. She also felt controlled by those around her due to the many restrictions in various areas of her life.

"Learned helplessness" often develops as a reaction to this chronic sense of failure, as individuals perceive themselves to be powerless to make desired changes in their life and often feel it is futile to try. Individuals also may be dependent upon others for functioning on a daily basis, as assistance may be needed in order to complete many personal and household tasks. At times, individuals who would be capable of completing certain tasks do not do so, as involved caregivers automatically do things for them, simply because it seems easier or quicker. When this occurs on a regular basis, it decreases the individual's sense of self-confidence and contributes to a belief that others are more competent than they are. These experiences can lead to the development of deep-seated views of the self ("core schema") regarding one's presumed inability to navigate successfully through different situations or experiences (Zigler et al., 2002).

Clinicians must be cognizant of these potential concerns and be willing to address openly in psychotherapy the issues relating to the experience of having a disability. A main focus of treatment is assisting the patient in restructuring beliefs about what it means to have a disability, and later helping them to shift the focus of their thinking from the limitations in their lives to the options and possibilities available to them. This can be accomplished by utilizing therapeutic responses and feedback that serve to restore a sense of self-control.

Re-framing events, with an emphasis on the situations in which the individual acted in a competent way, or re-framing distressing events and behaviors as signs of ability to successfully cope with life stressors, will benefit the patient (Keller, 2000). Additionally, using sessions as a forum to role-play, and teaching "scripts" that the individual can use when in situations where they need to assert themselves, can provide a safe place to practice learned skills and will increase the likelihood that these new behaviors will be put into practice.

Clinical Vignette #1 (part 2)

Issues related to Suzy's experience of having an intellectual disability became a main focus of treatment. Time was spent on exploring her feelings of helplessness and hopelessness and exploring her core schemas regarding her disability. The psychotherapist worked to help Suzy to accept herself and to restructure her belief that having a disability meant she was "worthless" and "unlovable," by helping her learn to replace these thought distortions with more rational and self affirming thoughts.

Initially, Suzy struggled to find anything positive about herself. She was asked to choose five people that she cared about and trusted, and then to approach each person and ask them to tell her what they liked about her. She was surprised to learn how others viewed her, and she was willing to accept the possibility that her perceptions about herself were incorrect. She developed affirmation statements in session that were written down on pocket-sized cards that Suzy could carry with her and read through on a daily basis. The psychotherapist also helped her explore how she could begin to empower herself, versus viewing herself as a victim.

In sessions, role-play was instituted that utilized assertive communication strategies, and Suzy began to ask staff for increased opportunities for social outings without her housemates. For Suzy, empowering herself also meant strategizing to widen her peer support network, getting involved in recreational activities, signing up for poetry classes offered by the local literacy council, and joining a peer advocate group. These things helped Suzy feel more in control of her life and helped to increase feelings of self-worth and self-confidence.

Barriers to treatment

The referral process

Typically, individuals with ID are not self-referred. Most often, they are referred to treatment by a concerned care provider who seeks assistance because of some form of maladaptive behavior exhibited by the individual. This makes the referral itself a sensitive matter; the individual may not see the identified problem as an area of concern for them, or they may experience some means of apprehension regarding the referral. In some cases, the referral for psychotherapy may be misconstrued as a punishment or a consequence, and there may be confusion about the purpose of mental health services. In addition, it can lead to confusion regarding the establishment of therapeutic goals, as the person who initiated the referral may want the psychotherapist to focus on an issue that the individual does not view as a problem. Finally, the individual being referred may have no input into either the choice of therapist or the time and/or location of the appointments. In some cases, the person does not even have control over who is present during psychotherapy appointments.

Involvement of multiple care providers

Typically, many professionals are involved in the care of an individual with ID, as these patients are embedded in multiple service delivery systems. They may have case workers, habilitation providers, job coaches and behavior support specialists assigned to them, in addition to a variety of residential providers, which can make the addition of yet another team member confusing. This is particularly true if they have little or no familiarity with mental health services, in which case they may have no understanding of a psychotherapist's role which, by its nature, is inherently different from that of all other members of their multidisciplinary team.

Lack of understanding of purpose of mental health treatment

For the reasons stated above, it is important for the psychotherapist to spend time educating the patient about the purposes of mental health treatment. Individuals with ID may have little or no prior experience with psychotherapy, and may have no knowledge about what to expect. If they were not self-referred, they may need reassurance that they are not being punished and that the clinician is there to support them, rather than acting as an extension of the multidisciplinary team or referral source. Spending time on providing education regarding the purpose of therapy, the role of both the patient and the therapist, and what will occur during a typical session, can dramatically enhance participation and satisfaction with mental health services. It is a critical component of the therapeutic process.

Confidentiality issues

Confidentiality is the cornerstone of psychotherapy. Without the promise of confidentiality, patients would not feel able to share their inner world honestly and openly. Individuals with ID have the same needs for confidentiality as the general population, but they may withhold information out of fear of confidentiality breaches. This actually is of particular concern when working with individuals with ID, due to the fact that many others are intimately involved in their care. Patients frequently witness the free sharing of personal information between multidisciplinary team members, and they may have concerns that information disclosed in psychotherapy will be treated in the same manner. In addition, team members may expect that the psychotherapist will, or should, share sensitive information, regardless of whether the individual has given consent (Lynch, 2004).

This problem is further complicated by the fact that the psychotherapist often does need collateral information from care providers, as individuals with ID are often poor historians and may not accurately report current stressors and problems that should be addressed in treatment. The care providers can also help to ensure that treatment recommendations are followed, such as completion of the homework that is assigned during sessions. Therefore, issues and concerns regarding confidentiality must be identified and addressed on an ongoing basis.

Communication issues

Communication issues impact the provision of mental health services for a variety of reasons. Limited receptive and expressive language skills, if not appropriately addressed,

Clinical Vignette #2

Bob, a 41 year old male with moderate ID, was referred for psychotherapy by his multidisciplinary team due to an increase in aggression and anger outbursts directed at staff and peers. Bob's medical history was significant for seizure disorder, which was well-controlled with medication. However, his legal guardian had become concerned about the potential impact of drinking large quantities of caffeine and, after a consultation with Bob's primary care physician, it was recommended that all caffeine be discontinued.

Bob had enjoyed drinking approximately four cans of a caffeinated beverage a day – two while at work and another two in the evening. Following the physician's order, his team replaced these with a caffeine-free beverage (of the same brand), which resulted in behavioral outbursts and violence directed towards staff.

At the time of the initial referral, the team and guardian requested that the focus of the treatment be to decrease aggression and to increase Bob's willingness to comply with staff requests. They also voiced concern regarding Bob's ability to maintain employment and his current residential placement if his aggressive behavior continued.

Upon meeting Bob, it became clear that he did not view the problem in the same light as his team. He reported that he enjoyed beverages with caffeine and he could taste the difference when staff gave him alternative options. Bob felt that he was being "controlled" and that he should have the right to make his own choices about what he ate and drank. Bob also felt that he was taken to see a psychotherapist because he was "in trouble" due to his recent aggressive behavior, and he expressed anxiety that the psychotherapist would share his thoughts and feelings with the team (mainly around the anger he felt towards them) – which would then lead to negative consequences for him.

The first goal of therapy was to work to establish a therapeutic alliance with Bob and to focus on his wants and needs. It was important to spend time educating Bob regarding the psychotherapist's role in his life and making sure that the boundaries and limitations of confidentiality were understood. The psychotherapist was very specific about what would be shared with the team and the purpose of this collaboration. Once rapport and trust were established, Bob addressed his feelings of anger and resentment and he learned more acceptable ways to communicate his wants and needs to others, as well as strategies to communicate his feelings.

can interfere with the development of the therapeutic alliance and with the individual's ability to benefit from the services provided. Depending on the level of cognitive deficits, the patient may not have the expressive language skills needed to self-report their symptoms. They may know they feel angry or that they are experiencing pain but, without a way to identify and label their feelings, they are unable to understand and communicate their emotional or physical experience. This can make the diagnosis of mental illness much more complicated. The therapist needs to gather collateral information from caregivers to help formulate diagnostic impressions.

Involved caregivers may be able to provide invaluable information, including (but not limited to):

- Sleep records.

- Information regarding changes in weight secondary to appetite changes or medical conditions.

- Documentation of unexplained sadness, crying.

- Isolative behavior or anhedonia.

It is important for the psychotherapist to explore the patient's degree of understanding, and also to ensure that the individual feels comfortable alerting the therapist if, and when, information is presented in a way that is confusing or unclear. This can be done by establishing that the cognitive deficit is a legitimate and neutral topic for discussion and exploration from the beginning, so that issues regarding communication can be negotiated and addressed openly.

Help the patient to feel comfortable when conveying, "I didn't understand what you just said," which would be useful feedback to any instructor. An accurate assessment of language skills is essential to the treatment, since overestimating an individual's abilities will prevent him or her from fully understanding what is being presented. Alternatively, underestimating an individual's abilities may cause them to feel patronized and frustrated, and will negatively impact the development of the therapeutic alliance.

Individuals with ID may struggle with the expression of emotions and feelings, and they may not have the necessary problem-solving skills to manage stressors appropriately when they occur. During sessions, it is important to explore and assess how the person describes feelings, and to provide opportunities to express them. However, before this can occur, the individual must have the ability to recognize and identify what they are feeling. An inability to do this can be extremely debilitating, as individuals can feel overwhelmed and frightened by intense emotional responses that they do not understand.

The ability to identify and label feelings provides a sense of control and comfort that can increase a patient's capacity to appropriately manage their feelings. This ability is also essential in order for a patient to participate actively in, and benefit from, psychotherapy. It is impossible to process emotions and to understand the connection between thoughts, feelings and behaviors without first having the ability to identify them.

Teaching the patient to label feeling states

The psychotherapist can address the labeling of feeling states by facilitating development of a "language" or a means for patients to express their feelings. One strategy is to assist the patient in linking a particular event to the feeling associated with it. For example, to help a patient understand what it means to feel excited or proud, the psychotherapist could explore life events that have elicited those emotional responses, such as graduating from high school or earning an award. This can help the patient to clearly identify, label and communicate the feelings associated with these events.

The psychotherapist may also need to interpret behavior for the patient by identifying and labeling the emotions that are tied to the events discussed in session. For example, "You look sad when you talk about how sick your grandmother is." This helps the patient to identify and acknowledge the feeling, and it opens the door to the possibility of describing similar feelings.

The following are activities that can facilitate the identification and labeling of feelings/emotions:

- Use of pictorial representations of faces to facilitate a patient's identification of emotions.

- Use of journaling, often a useful outlet for those patients with this capacity.

- Use of picture journaling can substitute for writing, i.e. drawing or putting pictures in a journal.

- Expression through music can be an excellent outlet for patients to describe their emotions.

Issues relating to learning and memory

When working with patients with ID, it is important to adjust the complexity of one's techniques to match the patient's level of cognitive development, and to augment these techniques with activities in order to add depth to change and learning. These activities can include art therapy, role-play and therapeutic games. Psychotherapists also should slow down the pace of treatment and lengthen the amount of time spent on each intervention utilized.

Repetition is essential, as repeated review-and-practice of skills that are learned in session helps to facilitate internalization of the material presented. Therefore, the psychotherapist may want to format the psychotherapy session so that repetition of key information occurs, such as reviewing information discussed in the previous session, summarizing skills taught in the current session and discussing how the patient can apply the skills in day-to-day life.

Review homework when it is assigned and after it is completed, to ensure that the patient understands the concept and its value. If the patient has a short attention span, it may be necessary to break down interventions into smaller pieces and utilize shorter session length.

Memory aids

Because of memory limitations, it may be difficult for a patient with ID to remember particular skills learned in psychotherapy or when to use them, particularly when in the midst of an emotional crisis. For this reason, it may be helpful to provide the individual with tools that can be utilized between sessions, in order to provide cues regarding how and when to use the particular coping skill strategies that were learned in treatment.

The use of coping skill cards or stories can be immeasurably helpful with this, as they provide the necessary cues for the implementation of strategies or techniques. Coping skill cards can be easily carried in a wallet or a pocket, making them accessible when needed in the moment. They should be developed with the patient and written in language that is easily understood. Depending upon the reading level of the patient, inclusion of pictures that illustrate the concept being depicted may be necessary. Coping skill cards can also be utilized as homework between sessions, as the patient and/or involved care providers can sit down and review them on a daily basis to help with the internalization of information learned in psychotherapy.

Points to note when creating coping skill cards include:

- Laminated coping skill cards should be small enough to be easily carried around and accessed throughout the day as needed.

- Strategies should be written in positive language that is individualized and geared to the patient's level of understanding. Pictures are often very helpful, particularly with individuals who have minimal reading skills.

- Cards should focus on one issue and should be very specific. For example, if the person wants to talk to "someone" as a coping strategy, the card should include the designated support person's name and phone number.

Collaboration with caregivers

Collaboration with involved caregivers is essential. They can assist with completion of homework assignments between sessions and can prompt the patient to utilize learned skills in his or her natural environment. Caregivers can also provide needed collateral information, as well as information regarding progress made between sessions.

Types of psychotherapy

Although there is limited empirical research available on psychotherapy for persons with ID, the available literature indicates that the efficacy of psychotherapy will be increased dramatically if a flexible and innovative approach is adopted, regardless of the actual type of approach utilized. To date, the literature indicates that techniques that draw from a cognitive behavioral model are the most effective with the ID population. Motivational interviewing, cognitive behavior therapy, dialectical behavioral therapy and supportive psychotherapy are all appropriate approaches to consider when working with a patient with ID, and they are all easily adapted to fit the needs of the patient.

Motivational interviewing

Motivational interviewing (MI) is a counseling approach developed by Miller & Rollnick (2002) and is based on the theory that patients enter psychotherapy with varying levels of acceptance of their problematic behaviors and varying amounts of motivation to change them. MI targets the conflicted feelings that individuals often experience when thinking about making changes, with the psychotherapist working to help the patient identify, explore and resolve his or her ambivalence. Initially developed for the treatment of substance use disorders, it has been utilized as a successful intervention to increase readiness/acceptance of treatment for an array of different disorders, symptoms and circumstances including obsessive compulsive disorder, depression, suicidality, eating disorders and medication compliance problems.

MI is based on the theory that there are five stages of change: pre-contemplation, contemplation, preparation, action and maintenance. The psychotherapist works to facilitate progression through the stages with the use of specific principles and strategies:

- In the pre-contemplation stage, the goal is to raise awareness of the identified problem.

- In the contemplation stage the psychotherapist works to evoke reasons for change and to strengthen self-efficacy.

- In the preparation stage, the focus is on clarifying goals and helping the patient to plan their own course of action to reach them.

- In the action phase, the psychotherapist continues to guide the patient towards change and to prevent relapse.

- In the maintenance stage the therapist works to reinforce the benefit of change and helps the patient to identify and use resources to maintain his/her goals.

MI takes a non-judgmental, non-confrontational approach, targeting the development of insight with regard to acute problems, the consequences of continued engagement in problematic behaviors and the benefits of making changes. Psychotherapists also help the patient to build a sense of hope about their future and their ability to take action that will allow them to reach their goals, thereby increasing their motivation to work through problems.

The objective is to help individuals to restructure their view about their behaviors and to consider the potential gains through change. Psychotherapists accomplish this with the use of "change talk," which is defined as "statements by the patient revealing consideration of, motivation for or commitment to change." Research has indicated that there is a strong correlation between the expression of change talk and positive treatment outcomes. Therefore, in MI, the use of change talk is viewed as a pathway for change.

Examples of strategies that elicit change talk include:

- the use of open-ended questions;

- exploring the advantages and disadvantages of making change, as opposed to maintaining the status quo;

- exploring the patient's beliefs regarding how the future will be different if and when the problem no longer exists;

- exploring goals and values;

- discussing the positives and negatives of making change.

When working with the ID population, using this approach as an adjunct to other psychotherapy should be considered when it is indicated. This is particularly true when the referral was not self-initiated; MI can be a valuable tool to address motivation issues in instances where the patient neither views the identified problem as an issue of concern nor has a desire to change it. It is also possible that the patient will have resentment regarding the referral itself or may view the referral as a consequence or punishment, further decreasing any desire to participate in treatment. In these cases, adding an additional treatment phase, in which multiple sessions are focused on utilization of MI techniques, may help decrease resistance to psychotherapy and serve to increase the patient's motivation to address problematic behaviors.

Research has demonstrated that using MI as an adjunct therapy is an evidenced-based practice that improves patient outcomes, facilitates rapid improvement in symptoms and reduces the length of treatment needed to achieve symptom relief (Merlo *et al.*, 2010).

Miller & Rollnick (2002) developed four basic principles of motivational interviewing:

1 *Expressing empathy.* Psychotherapists ensure that patients believe their perspective is validated and understood, as this will allow them to express their thoughts and feelings openly and honestly.

2 *Development of discrepancy.* Psychotherapists help the patient to develop an understanding of the discrepancy between what the person wants presently and in the future, versus the reality of what is actually happening in the person's day to day life. In time, this can help individuals to understand how actions/behavior may actually move them away from their goals, thus increasing their motivation to make change.

3 *Rolling with resistance.* MI accepts that resistance to change is a natural and understandable reaction. When patients demonstrate resistance in sessions, psychotherapists are non-confrontational with them in order to avoid creating power struggles. Instead, psychotherapists focus on helping patients to define both their problems and potential solutions on their own terms.

4 *Supporting self-efficacy.* MI is a strength-based approach which assumes that the patient has the ability to create positive change. Psychotherapists understand that the power to institute change rests with the patient, and they support the patient's autonomy, regardless of whether the individual decides to make changes or not. This is empowering for the patient, but also ensures that he or she owns the responsibility for his or her actions. Therapists support self-efficacy by emphasizing previous successes as well as pointing out the skills that the patient already possesses.

MI techniques recommended for the general population   In order to accomplish the above objectives, there are four basic techniques that clinicians use in session to help patient gain insight into their problems and to increase motivation to make positive changes. The strategies can be used early in psychotherapy to address issues related to motivation, but also can be reintroduced at any time that motivation issues arise. They are:

- *open-ended questions* – used to help facilitate the flow of communication in order to create forward momentum;

- *affirmations* – used to help restructure the patient's view of him or herself and their ability to make changes;

- *reflective listening* – used to help patients feel that the psychotherapist understands their point of view, as well as to help resolve ambivalence by guiding patients to explore how the current behavior is impacting their overall quality of life and the benefits of making positive change;

- *summaries* – a form of reflective listening that reviews what has occurred in the session, used to draw attention to both sides of the ambivalence that the patient is experiencing, while promoting the development of discrepancy through careful selection of what information is included or excluded.

Modifications of MI techniques for patients with ID   Clinicians may only need to take a more directive approach, helping the patient to identify and express feelings regarding the possibility of change. To address any barriers related to communication issues, clinicians should consider utilization of role-playing, visual prompts, pictures, therapeutic games and activities to help facilitate the patient's involvement.

Cognitive behavioral therapy

Cognitive behavioral therapy (CBT) is an evidence-based and action-oriented form of psychotherapy that is based on the theory that faulty thinking patterns, and the beliefs that underlie such thinking, cause both maladaptive behavior and negative emotions. It incorporates the integration of two distinct psychological theories to form a psychotherapeutic approach which targets both faulty thinking patterns and maladaptive behaviors. Cognitive therapy is designed to help patients resolve symptomatology by learning to identify and change dysfunctional thinking, behavior and emotional responses. Behavioral therapy, or behavior modification, is based on learning theory and is used to train patients to replace undesirable behaviors with new, more appropriate behavior patterns (Romana, 2003).

There are three major levels of cognition that are addressed in the practice of CBT: full consciousness, automatic thoughts and schemas (Wright, 2006):

- Consciousness is a fully alert cognitive state in which rational decisions are made with full awareness.

- Automatic thoughts, on the other hand, are the thoughts that occur in a reflective or habitual manner, which are pre-conscious or subconscious in nature.

- Schemas are the core beliefs that serve as a framework for how information is interpreted, and they are shaped by developmental influences and other life experiences.

Because cognitive schemas play a significant role in how individuals view both themselves and the world around them, addressing maladaptive schemas is an essential component of CBT interventions, because maladaptive schemas can interfere with the development of healthy self-worth and can lead to the development of maladaptive coping strategies. Therefore, the psychotherapist and the patient work together to identify the presence of thinking distortions and maladaptive cognitive schemas. The patient can then learn to test the validity of the beliefs once they are identified, and to make modifications when needed.

CBT utilizes many cognitive techniques to help patients change their maladaptive thinking patterns and learn to alter their perspective of both themselves and the world around them. See Table 1 for summary of CBT techniques.

CBT sessions are goal-oriented and explicitly structured to target specific problems and potential solutions. The therapeutic process is typically completed in 5–20 sessions. However, if the patient has a personality disorder, or if they have chronic illness, the length of treatment is extended as necessary. Each session begins with the psychotherapist and patient working together to set an agenda which determines the particular issues of concern to be addressed. The psychotherapist also spends time assessing target symptoms and reviewing homework assigned the previous session.

The following are the components of a typical CBT session:

- Psychotherapist and patient work together to set an agenda which determines the particular issues of concern to be addressed.

Table 1 Cognitive behavior therapy techniques.

Socratic questioning	Questions that challenge patients' underlying (typically unhealthy) beliefs about themselves.
Guided discovery	This involves gentle questioning about problems designed to help the patient identify dysfunctional thinking patterns that contribute to ongoing problems or exacerbate existing ones.
ABC model (Antecedent, Behavior, Consequence)	This helps patients to identify and label the connections between an activating event, their interpretation of the event, the beliefs or thoughts that occur when the event happens, and the consequences (which are the emotions and actions that are triggered by the beliefs). Once this is accomplished, the clinician can help patients learn to test objectively whether a belief is justified or is based on erroneous assumptions.
Chain analysis	This can help a person to understand the function of a particular behavior by identifying all the factors that led up to it. The individual is able to identify the situation that occurred, their subsequent responses, and all of the thoughts and feelings that occurred just prior to the behavior. Doing this can increase the individual's ability to intervene early on and prevent the behavior or feeling from occurring.
Modeling	This allows the patient and clinician to engage in role-play of different situations.
Journaling	In CBT, individuals are encouraged to keep a diary documenting their thoughts/feelings/reactions in order to demonstrate positive and negative consequences to behavior.

Source: adapted from Beck *et al.*, (1979), pages 10–12, 56, 65, 67, 110, 137, 139.

- Target symptoms are assessed by the psychotherapist.

- Homework assigned the previous session is reviewed.

- Agenda items are explored and worked through.

- Psychotherapist assigns homework.

- Time is spent summarizing the session and getting feedback from the patient.

Modifications of CBT for patients with ID   It may be difficult for patients with ID to identify the abstract concepts, such as thought distortions, which are central components of CBT. However, this issue can be addressed by increasing the number of sessions in order to allow treatment to progress at a slower rate. This enables the psychotherapist to spend additional time providing the necessary education about vital concepts. Repetition of the involved components will help facilitate internalization of the necessary skills.

It is important to elicit the participation of involved care providers, as these can help the patient to recognize and identify when he or she is experiencing cognitive distortions. Care providers can also assist with the completion of homework assignments between sessions, such as documentation in a diary or role-play.

Clinical Vignette #3

Wendy was a 37 year old female with mild ID, who resided in a group home. She had a diagnosis of post-traumatic stress disorder and a history of engaging in self-injurious behavior when under periods of extreme stress.

Wendy struggled with controlling an impulse to steal others people's belongings. Once she took the items (e.g. money, cellphones, clothing, jewelry), she would often become consumed with fear that she would be caught and punished. To avoid this, she would lie about her behavior and attempt to hide her actions by giving the objects away. This typically did little to relieve her anxiety, which would continue to escalate, resulting in anger outbursts or self-injurious behavior (usually in the form of skin picking) as an outlet for her emotional discomfort. Wendy had little understanding of how her actions impacted her relationships with those around her, and she would express confusion and disappointment when peers expressed their anger and frustration with her behavior.

During initial psychotherapy appointments, Wendy would not discuss these issues; although staff were repeatedly reporting incidents of theft, she was adamant that this was not a problem for her. Initially, time and energy were focused on the development of the therapeutic alliance, so that Wendy could feel comfortable enough to open up and share with her psychotherapist. Once this was accomplished, more time was spent in helping Wendy to identify and understand how her actions interfered with the development of healthy friendships with her peers, as well as the potential legal consequences of her behavior. This was important, as she had recently taken a bracelet from a peer at workshop, and this person's family had discussed the possibility of pressing legal charges.

The psychotherapist then targeted her beliefs about the stealing ("I can't help myself"; "It is out of my control") and helped her to identify how these thoughts shaped her feelings and behaviors. She began to complete a journal to document antecedent, behavior and consequence associated with each impulse to steal, and a chain analysis was completed after every identifiable episode of stealing.

This led to Wendy uncovering the factors that precipitated these events. She was able to identify that she was frustrated because her mother picked out all of her clothing, with no input from her, and seldom purchased coveted items such as baseball hats (because her mother did not feel they were "ladylike") or cellphones (because Wendy had a history of calling people excessively when she had had one in the past). Wendy believed she could never purchase the things she desired for herself, so her only option was taking them from others.

Over time, the psychotherapist was able to restructure Wendy's thoughts about this; it was important for her to empower herself and communicate her wants and needs directly to her mother. She was hesitant to do this, however, and several sessions were spent using role-play to illustrate to her how she could present the information to her mother. After a few weeks, she felt ready to discuss the issue with her mother and, although she was not able to have everything she wanted (such as a cellphone), her mother was willing to allow Wendy to participate in shopping trips and to take a more active role in picking out the items that were purchased for her.

In addition, Wendy was able to identify enjoyable behaviors in which she could engage as an alternative when she experienced the urge to steal. She loved playing basketball, and there was a basketball hoop in her back yard, so she decided to "shoot hoops" when the compulsions occurred.

The psychotherapist also discussed the importance of Wendy seeking out assistance and support from involve caregivers as necessary. Wendy identified her group home manager as a trusted support person, so that person was approached to become involved. In psychotherapy, conversation was facilitated between the group home manager and Wendy, in which Wendy agreed to inform her when she felt the urge to steal and the group home manager agreed to facilitate Wendy's treatment recommendations without judgment. Another focus of treatment was expansion of problem-solving skills, and time was spent in practicing relaxation activities to help decrease anxiety; role-playing also was useful in putting all the learned strategies in place.

After several months of treatment, Wendy was able to utilize successfully the coping strategies targeted in treatment on a regular basis. This, in combination with her newfound empowered relationship with her mother, helped to extinguish her stealing behavior.

Dialectical behavior therapy

Individuals with ID are not exempt from the development of personality disorders (see Chapter 10). Exposure to the added environmental stressors mentioned previously, combined with the increased vulnerability to trauma, likely places this specialized population at higher risk. Information on the subject is limited, but a review of the available literature on the topic suggests the prevalence rate of personality disorders among the ID population lies within the range of 7– 90% (Wink *et al.*, 2010).

If a patient with ID is diagnosed with certain personality disorders, particularly borderline personality disorder (BPD), utilization of an evidenced-based model of treatment such as dialectical behavior therapy (DBT), is appropriate and can easily be adapted to meet the needs of the patient with ID. The fact that DBT is a structured, skill-based approach makes it a particularly good fit with this population, as efficacy of treatment is improved when the focus is on building replacement skills rather than merely attempting to eliminate problematic behaviors (Lew, 2011).

DBT is a type of cognitive behavioral treatment that was developed by Linehan (1993) to address the needs of patients diagnosed with BPD. Specifically, it was designed to address the needs of chronically suicidal patients who were not benefiting from traditional treatment models. DBT is based on the premise that the combination of exposure to an invalidating environment, along with unknown biological factions, contributes to the development of affective instability, as evidenced by abnormal reactions to emotional stimulation. It is a complex theoretical approach which combines four different components: CBT, dialectics, mindfulness and validation.

According to Linehan (1993), the theory of dialectics states that everything is composed of opposites and that change is constant and inevitable, and occurs when one opposing force is stronger than the other. In DBT, the focus becomes resolving the apparent contradiction between accepting the "self" (self-acceptance), while allowing change in oneself to occur, in order to bring about symptom improvement and growth in the patient.

"Mindfulness" is a concept that stresses the importance of patients staying present *in the moment* to help minimize thought distortions that are likely based on previous experiences. It is considered a foundation for the other skills taught in DBT, because it helps patients to accept and tolerate the powerful emotions they may feel when challenging their habits or exposing themselves to upsetting situations (Moonshine, 2008). Validation is an essential component, due to the fact that the process of CBT, when used alone, can be quite stressful for patients with BPD; the push for change can be interpreted as an invalidation of their emotional pain and distress. Linehan (1993) found that patients exhibited increased motivation when their emotional experience was validated by the psychotherapist.

The goal of DBT is to validate that the patient's behaviors and reactions are understandable, without agreeing that they are the best or only approach to solve the problem. Individuals with BPD exhibit both emotional dyscontrol, in which the patient is overwhelmed by extremely intense emotions or impulses, and emotional deregulation, in which the person is highly sensitive to stressors and responds to them with poorly modulated emotional responses (e.g. rage, self-mutilation, suicidal behaviors) (Preston, 2006).

DBT focuses on helping patients to learn to regulate their emotions, as well as to improve their ability to cope with stress and their interpersonal relationships. It is an intensive treatment that is comprised of two main components: weekly individual psychotherapy sessions and weekly group therapy sessions.

- Individual psychotherapy focuses on problem solving behavior, quality of life issues, decreasing post-traumatic stress responses secondary to past traumas in the patient's life, and increasing feelings of self-worth and self-esteem.

- The group therapy sessions focus on the internalization of skills from four different modules: core mindfulness skills, distress tolerance skills, emotional regulation skills and interpersonal effectiveness skills.

Standard DBT lasts for approximately one year, or as long as it takes for the patient to learn and implement DBT skills, increase mental health stability and decrease behaviors that are negatively impacting their overall quality of life.

Modifications of DBT for patients with ID   Patients with ID may not have the attention span required to participate in a two-and-a-half hour group session. For this reason, it may be necessary to shorten group sessions to approximately one hour. Charlton & Dykstra (2011) indicate that it may be necessary to shorten the time even further – to 30 minutes – and to compensate for this loss in time by increasing the frequency of group work to twice a week. This ensures that services are provided in a manner that matches the patients' cognitive needs, as well as allowing for increased opportunities to practice and generalize learned skills. It is also important to increase the number of sessions that are spent on each of the four skill modules, as this will help to facilitate internalization of the information presented.

Another valuable strategy is to simplify how information is presented, such as using concrete language and pictures or illustrations on homework and diary cards. This can be particularly helpful with DBT, as the concepts addressed in typical DBT treatment tend to be presented in complex and abstract terms that may not be easily understood by individuals with ID. These concepts will need to be simplified in order to increase comprehension and ability to implement skills learned (Charlton & Dykstra, 2011).

For example, the use of handouts is widely incorporated into the provision of DBT group therapy in the general population. For individuals with ID, the information should be modified so that the language utilized matches the person's level of cognitive ability. Use of pictures may also be helpful to aid in the internalization of the concepts presented. In addition, the psychotherapist should increase the activities that are used, such as therapeutic games, role-play, etc.

When working with patients with ID, it is again essential that there is ongoing collaboration with involved caregivers. Therefore, the psychotherapist should ensure that all involved caregivers receive education and training on the four skill modules, so that they can provide reinforcement of the skills being learned throughout the week.

Supportive psychotherapy

Supportive psychotherapy (SP) is a psychotherapeutic approach that incorporates many specific techniques from a wide variety of psychotherapy theories, including psychodynamic psychotherapy, cognitive behavioral therapy and interpersonal psychotherapy (Gentile & Jackson, 2008). It is an interactive approach, based on a model of conversation rather than silent listening, as the therapist actively engages with the patient. At the core of SP is belief that the positive and supportive relationship developed between the patient and psychotherapist can serve to buttress and repair deficits in the person's self-structure resulting from inadequate early parenting. Therefore, the psychotherapist assumes an intensely empathetic introspective stance with the patient, nurturing positive transference and using this to further strengthen the relationship. Conversely, negative transference is addressed and corrected in order to preserve the therapeutic alliance (Battaglia, 2007).

The psychotherapist uses a more directive approach and frequently provides feedback, suggestions, advice and opinions during session. In a sense, the psychotherapist works to help patients to "re-parent" themselves, as they are provided with the necessary mirroring that will allow for internalization of important psychological functions that are currently deficient. For this reason, fostering and protecting the therapeutic alliance is important, while at the same time taking care not to reinforce or enable destructive behavior patterns.

This can be a delicate balance at times. According to Misch (2006) the psychotherapist serves "as a cheerleader, encouraging, nurturing, validating, praising, or congratulating the patient." The psychotherapist also works to create a safe "holding environment" in which anxiety and other affects are explored but are not allowed to mount to intolerable and debilitating levels. Concurrently, SP seeks to "support" deficient psychological capacities by helping patients to utilize whatever healthy coping skills they possess, while addressing faulty thinking and dysfunctional adaptive defenses.

Self-destructive behaviors are gently challenged and addressed as the psychotherapist works to facilitate improvement in affect regulation, to improve healthy emotional responses to stress and to improve interpersonal skills and relationships (Douglas, 2008). Patients are taught to recognize, acknowledge, identify and label their emotions, as this aids significantly in the ability to develop appropriate coping skills when experiencing painful emotions. This is necessary to help the patient learn to understand the connections between thoughts, feelings and behaviors.

SP can be used with patients who are experiencing a variety of both simple and complex problems. It is a psychotherapeutic approach that is clinically appropriate when working with patients who are unable to tolerate or utilize other types of treatment, and it is sometimes used during periods of decompensation or hospitalization with patients who otherwise are engaged in alternate forms of therapy.

Supportive therapeutic work primarily focuses on the here and now, and on the patient's current functioning. Patients are encouraged to become active and to develop plans to meet life goals and put them into practice. Psychotherapists also ensure that the patient has all the information and education that may be needed to achieve and maintain a stable mood state. This may entail providing education regarding the patient's illness, in which symptoms, course and prognosis are thoroughly explained and discussed.

Patients are given information regarding potential precipitants of decompensation, and what to do to decrease the likelihood of recurrence. With the patient's consent, the psychotherapist may also involve family members or other persons, so that these "concerned others" in the patient's life are able to provide the appropriate supports when necessary. In addition, the psychotherapist may intervene with other people or agencies in order to help the patient, such as communicating with the courts or speaking to an employer or a teacher when needed.

Modifications of supportive therapy for patients with ID   SP inherently includes numerous techniques which are helpful when working with many patients with ID. The fact that it requires a more directive and supportive approach, utilizing techniques such as suggestion, persuasion and reassurance, makes it a good fit for patients with ID. The inclusion of advocacy for patients and encouragement of involvement of concerned others improves outcomes. It is also a very flexible approach, which incorporates many different techniques and can easily be adjusted to meet the needs of the patient.

However, there are some modifications that a psychotherapist utilizing SP should institute in treating patients with ID, including simplifying the interventions that are used. This can be done by reducing the complexity of the techniques and by breaking down interventions into smaller units. As with CBT and DBT, expect a longer length of treatment to allow for repetition of learned skills in order to facilitate retention and generalization. Also, psychotherapists should be sure to augment these techniques with activities, in order to deepen change and learning. Activities could include therapeutic games, drawings, role-plays, etc.

Group therapy

During the last 30 years, research has demonstrated the efficacy of group psychotherapy in various areas of life challenges. Participation in group treatment provides an opportunity to address problems with the assistance and support of other persons who have common issues and goals. This result is a sense of universality, as patients come to realize that they are not alone in the struggles they are facing. In addition, there is immense benefit in witnessing the resourcefulness of group members who are in similar situations, as it provides participants with a sense of reassurance and hope in their own recovery.

Ideally, the group process also can provide a safe forum in which to learn and practice new behaviors without the fear of failure. This treatment modality is effective in patients with ID and can provide them with a unique opportunity to experience validation and normalcy with peers who understand the life stressors they are dealing with. The benefits of group therapy can include:

- improved interpersonal relationships;

- improved ability to effectively utilize problem solving skills;

- improved ability to communicate wants and needs appropriately and effectively to others;

- improved ability to manage symptoms of mental illness and stress;

- improved self-esteem and acceptance of ID.

Modifications of group therapy for patients with ID   While the available research on the provision of group psychotherapy in patients with ID is limited, what studies exist indicate that the Interactive-Behavioral Therapy (IBT) model is the most effective with this population (Tomasulo & Razza, 2009). Over the past 15 years, several studies have been conducted which demonstrated that use of IBT yielded positive outcome measures, and there is empirical evidence that IBT is effective in patients who pose an increased suicide risk (Kirchner & Mueth, 2000). IBT was specifically designed for use with individuals who have some form of cognitive disability, and it incorporates action-based techniques that are drawn from the field of psychodrama. It is theorized that engaging the patient with ID behaviorally and emotionally, as well as verbally, enhances the patient's ability to benefit from the treatment provided (Tomasulo & Razza, 2006).

IBT group sessions are structured into four stages:

1 Orientation stage

2 Warm-up and sharing stage

3 Enactment stage

4 Affirmation stage.

There is also an initial warm-up stage, where the focus is on teaching patients the social skills that are necessary for successful group participation, such as not interrupting and the use of active listening.

During the orientation stage, facilitators work to shape good interpersonal behavior. They may do this by having members repeat what was said to them, ensuring that individuals turn toward the person who is speaking and acknowledge what was said, and/or participate in some way in the group process through interaction.

In the warm-up and sharing stage, participants set agenda items and share what issue(s) they would like to address during the session. At this time, the group selects an issue and a protagonist around whose problems the group therapy session will revolve.

Once this is done, facilitators guide the group into the enactment stage, in which the identified issues are explored. Psychodrama techniques are utilized in order to increase emotional engagement. See Table 2 for frequently used psychodrama techniques.

The final stage is the affirmation stage, in which each member of the group is given feedback about the strengths and gains achieved during that particular therapy session.

Psychotherapy topics and the ID population

Grief and loss issues

Individuals with ID will experience many losses throughout their lifespan. Although they may develop strong bonds with care providers who work with them, there tends to be frequent staff turnover, often without advance notice, which can mean the abrupt end of significant relationships for the individual. They may also experience the illness or death of a parent, who may have been the primary caregiver well into middle-age or even later in life. This can precipitate a complicated grieving process, as it often leads to significant changes that further increase the feelings of loss. For instance, the loss of the caregiver may require the transition to a group home living environment, which most likely means loss of familiar surroundings (home, neighborhood) and of other relationships (neighbors/friends), as well as a change in employment.

The grief of individuals with ID is often disenfranchised (Lavin, 2002), because their experience of loss is not openly acknowledged or supported. In fact, they are often not given the opportunity to mourn or experience openly their feelings about the loss. This can happen

Table 2 Frequently utilized psychodrama techniques

Doubling	During role-play, group members share their view of the identified protagonist. The double acts as an inner voice and reflection of the protagonist.
Role reversal	The protagonist is asked to exchange roles with another person. This enables patients to see themselves from another point of view.
Soliloquizing	The protagonist shares their most intimate thoughts about a crucial situation in their life without addressing other members of the group.
Future projection	The protagonist projects him/herself into their future life.
The mirror	This technique allows the protagonist to step out of the scene and to observe someone else enacting his/her role. The protagonist can then see him/herself as others see them.

Source: adapted from Dayton (1994), pages 26, 34, 35, 71.

for a multitude of reasons, such as a feeling of inadequacy on the part of caregivers to appropriately address feelings of grief, or a desire to "protect" the individual from experiencing emotional pain. In some cases, there may be a misconception that individuals with ID are not capable of understanding grief. As noted before, the severity of cognitive deficits does have an impact on an individual's ability to understand abstract concepts, and this includes death. However, grieving will occur regardless of ability to fully comprehend the finality of death, as individuals with ID will notice the absence of the loved one in their life and will grieve this loss.

When possible, therapeutic interventions should begin while the loved one is ill, rather than waiting until the loss has occurred, in order to avoid the shock of an unexpected death and to address any feelings of grief related to secondary losses that are associated with the illness. For example, if an individual is accustomed to weekly visits from a beloved family member, they will feel the absence or loss of the person as the visits decrease or discontinue altogether.

Research suggests that an individual's level of comprehension of concepts related to death and dying are more related to their cognitive level, as it corresponds to Piaget's stages of development rather than to their chronological age (Dodd *et al.*, 2005; Gentile & Hubner, 2005). However, life experiences that occur as an individual grows older also contribute to a greater understanding of the life cycle and the permanence of death. Therefore, an elderly individual with ID may have a better understanding of the concept of death than a younger counterpart with comparable cognitive abilities. Because an individual's experience of grief and loss will vary depending on the type of loss, and within the developmental framework of the person, it is important for the clinician to provide treatment interventions that are appropriate to their level of cognitive development. The following section may provide some broad guidelines.

Theoretical conceptualization of loss according to likely developmental level   Individuals with profound ID would most likely be functioning cognitively within the sensorimotor stage of development, regardless of their chronological age (Gentile & Hubner, 2005). Individuals in this stage of development will view death as a loss, separation or abandonment. They will lack the ability to comprehend the concept of death, but they will notice and grieve the absence of their loved one, and their reactions will be significantly influenced by the reactions of trusted loved ones and care providers. Individuals functioning in this developmental framework will need reassurance and support as well as adherence to their typical schedule and routines.

Individuals with severe to moderate ID may be functioning in the preoperational stage of cognitive development, regardless of their chronological age. Individuals in this stage of development will see death as temporary and reversible, and will interpret their world in a concrete and literal manner (Gentile & Hubner, 2005). They may believe that the death was caused by their thoughts, or may provide other magical explanations for the loss which can lead them to blame themselves or to believe that they are able to bring a loved one back to life. It is important to provide support and concrete explanations of the loss, and to correct misperceptions. It may be helpful to provide education regarding what the loss means, and to have discussions regarding the fact that the loved one will not return. The psychotherapist will need to spend time helping patients to identify and label their feelings around the loss (e.g. grief, sadness, numbness, anger).

Individuals with moderate to mild ID may be functioning at the cognitive level of concrete operations, regardless of their chronological age. Individuals in this stage of cognitive development will understand that the death is final and irreversible, but may not believe that it is a normal part of life or that it could happen to them (Gentile & Hubner, 2005). The loss may be personalized, and expressions of anger toward the deceased (or toward those believed to have been unable to save the deceased) may occur. The loss may trigger fear regarding the safety of other loved ones, and they may experience anxiety or depression or may exhibit somatic complaints. It is also common to see a demonstration of aggressive behaviors, particularly in males. Providing education regarding death and dying can be helpful, and it is important to allow the individual the opportunity to participate in funeral services. Again, it will be important to facilitate the identification of emotions and the ability to express them. It may be helpful for the psychotherapist to work on activities with the individual, such as creating a memory book or making cards.

Regardless of the level of cognitive ability, it will be important to involve care providers, so that they can understand the tools and strategies that will be helpful for the individual in the moment, and also so that they can assist in long-term support and stabilization.

Attachment theory and its potential relevance for grief and loss in patients with ID   Bowlby (1969) developed the concept of *attachment* several decades ago, and in recent years there is neurobiological research that continues to build support for the relevance of this concept. Bowlby postulated that an individual with an early history of inconsistent and maladaptive relationships is vulnerable later to dysfunctional attachments and is more susceptible to develop psychopathology (Kay, 2005).

The development of sound attachment is theoretically critical to an infant's ability to regulate affect. Bowlby argued that, without a foundation of sound attachment, the individual is left without the capacity to "self-soothe" (Kay, 2005). Although Bowlby focused mainly on the infant's early environmental experiences, the concept of insecure attachment has been expanded to include problems that may occur due to developmental limitations inherent in the child's abilities (Kay, 2005; Hollins & Sinason, 2000). Patients with ID may, in some cases, be predisposed to attachment difficulties related to the cognitive impairment itself, or due to early experiences which affect the ability to develop and navigate relationships.

Hollins & Sinason (2000) outline the following psychic organizing principles which apply to all individuals with ID, regardless of the severity of cognitive deficits:

1 The existence of the disability itself (including the conscious and unconscious fantasies that accompany it).

2 Loss (of the normal self who would have been born).

3 Sexuality (internally distorted by the impact of the disability).

4 Dependency (not being able to live autonomously).

5 Fear of death (being part of a group which society does not reliably accept and protect).

Esterhuyzen & Hollins (1997) describe the effects of an early diagnosis of learning disability on attachment; it is more likely to be insecure and to instigate long-term consequences which may include pathological grief processes and challenging behavior.

Perinatal separation (even if brief) and abuse or neglect, coupled with genetic vulnerability, often seen in individuals with ID, appears likely to be associated with enduring changes in many areas of functioning, including emotional and behavioral regulation which can include attachment, cognitive function, coping style, neuroendocrine response to stress, and brain morphology (Kay, 2005).

Recent research on attachment (in Kay, 2005) has identified a "disorganized/disoriented" type of attachment difficulty, where a person demonstrates "hitting, freezing, unusual posturing, and non-goal directed activity." Externalizing behaviors are often seen in patients with ID as presenting symptoms or either medical or mental health conditions. It is possible that insecure attachment of the disorganized/disoriented type could be the explanation for the emergence of similar behaviors in a situation where a patient with ID, already at risk for insecure attachment, suffers a significant loss.

Clinical Vignette #4

Frances, a 49 year old female with moderate ID, previously resided with her mother until three years ago, at which time her mother passed away from a terminal illness. Her father had passed away 15 years before. After her mother's death, she was uprooted from the home wherein she had spent her entire life, and moved to a group home environment across town from her childhood home.

Frances was an only child, with no other family involvement, so there was no one in her life who could either take her in or assist with the transition to a new home. She struggled with the loss of her parents and with the secondary losses that occurred as a result of their death. Residential staff attempted to help her manage her feelings for approximately one year, but finally made the referral for mental health services after her mood remained depressed, regardless of their attempts to assist her in moving forward following the multiple layers of loss.

Frances's grief was complicated, in that she had never worked through her feelings regarding her father's death; thus, when her mother died, she found herself grieving both losses as if they had both just occurred. In psychotherapy, Frances expressed feelings of anger at her parents for leaving her and stated her belief that if she had been a "better" daughter, they would still be alive. She also shared feelings of anger and resentment regarding the fact that she was now living in a group home, and she had a great deal of distrust for the staff. Her parents had been the only caregivers she had ever previously known, and she felt unable to trust that these "strangers" would take care of her. She was particularly worried that they would steal from her or harm her in some way. Frances spent the majority of her time alone in her room, looking at pictures of her parents and thinking about their deaths.

Initial therapy sessions were focused on developing the therapeutic alliance and giving Frances a safe space in which to express her emotional pain. Time was spent on helping her to process her thoughts and feelings about the loss and exploring her spiritual beliefs. Frances identified that she knew her parents were in heaven, but she was concerned that they were "worried" about her and her adjustment to her new home. In these early sessions, she exhibited multiple crying spells which lasted for several minutes, during which time she was given support and reassurance that she would be able to cope with her overwhelming feelings of grief and loss.

The psychotherapist spent time providing education regarding the life cycle and normalized her parents' deaths. They explored Frances' belief that her parents made a choice to leave her and worked to restructure her thoughts about this. She was taught coping skills to utilize when feeling overwhelmed by her feelings (relaxation techniques, journaling and use of art), and staff were enlisted to help to ensure that homework was completed between sessions. Frances and her psychotherapist worked together to develop a short story book about her experiences with grief and loss. The book reviewed her life with her parents, their death, her experience of grief, her initiation of psychotherapy, coping strategies she was learning in treatment and her hopes and goals for her future. She reviewed the book on a daily basis to help normalize her experiences, to cue her to utilize learned skills and to give her hope about the possibility of recovery.

Time was spent on addressing her fears regarding her new home and staff and examining her distorted thoughts about her move. Frances identified that she was angry with the staff because she blamed them for her move and many of the secondary losses in her life, and once she understood this and was able to accept that her parents' death and her subsequent move were not anyone's fault, her feelings of anger reduced considerably. She begin to keep a gratitude journal, which helped her realize that there were many positive things that she could enjoy about her new life.

As her mood began to lift, Frances experienced feelings of guilt regarding her recovery and what it meant about her love for her parents. The psychotherapist provided reassurance and support and helped her to find ways to incorporate her memories and love for her parents into her life, while also allowing herself to move forward and build a new life on her own.

Eventually, Francis became more active with her housemates and she was able to build close relationships with her staff and increase her participation in recreational activities in the community. As she made progress, her mood continued to improve and psychotherapy was slowly discontinued.

Trauma

The fact that individuals with ID are often dependent upon other people for care and protection makes them particularly vulnerable to a wide range of abuse. Research indicates that they experience abuse, especially sexual and physical abuse, at rates significantly higher than that of the general population. In fact, some studies have indicated that as many as 90% of people with ID will experience some type of abuse during their lifetime (Valenti-Hein & Schwartz, 1995).

This specialized population is particularly at risk for a variety of reasons, which include limited verbal skills, a lack of understanding of what is happening to them, a lack of understanding of appropriate boundaries in relationships, a deep fear of potential consequences for speaking up, and a need to please or be accepted by the abuser. In addition, individuals with ID often learn not to question caregivers or others in authority, making them even more vulnerable if the perpetrator is viewed as an authority figure.

Research suggests that this population also is more vulnerable to the effects of the trauma and more likely to develop post-traumatic stress disorder (PTSD). There are several environmental factors affecting the ID population that can contribute to a predisposition to PTSD, such as early separation from parents due to institutionalization or hospitalizations affecting attachment (see below); a lack of prior experience managing unpleasant or stressful events; and/or a limited system of natural supports (Mevissen & de Jongh, 2010). Once they are exposed to a traumatic situation, difficulties with processing what happened, combined with limited coping skills, can further complicate the situation and increase the likelihood of the development of PTSD (Fernando & Medlicott, 2009).

Research suggests that many, if not most, people with ID have some form of traumatic event in their history (SAMSHA, 2010). *Trauma informed care* is based on the premise that it makes sense to treat everyone with ID as if trauma has possibly occurred. It is based on an understanding of the vulnerabilities or triggers of trauma survivors that traditional mental health approaches may exacerbate. With the use of trauma informed methodologies, these services and programs can be more supportive and avoid re-traumatization. Making sure that someone feels safe and in control of his or her own life will help the individual with trauma history, and will not hurt anyone who does not have a trauma history. It is imperative to treat all individuals with ID as if safety and control is important to them.

Symptoms of PTSD in the ID population   Symptoms of PTSD in the ID population often go unrecognized, because the presentation differs from that of the general population. In patients with ID, reactions to trauma vary according to level of ID and also according to the individual's ability to communicate emotional pain (Mitchell *et al.*, 2005). Without an outlet for expressions of distress, it is common for symptoms to be manifest as behavioral problems such as aggression, insomnia, self-injurious behavior and social isolation.

Psychotherapy with patients with ID who have experienced trauma   Although the research in this area is limited, a review of the available literature indicates that approaches which utilize cognitive behavioral techniques have been effective when treating PTSD in the ID population. In addition, the use of exposure therapy, imagery rehearsal therapy and relaxation training all have a proven efficacy for reducing symptoms (Mevissen & de Jongh, 2010).

When treating an individual with ID who has experienced trauma, it is important to ensure that the individual will feel safe and will have a sense of control regarding participation in mental health services. It may be helpful to discuss these issues openly with the patient.

Asking about preferences regarding the location and time of appointments can avoid unnecessarily exposing patients to triggers which they are unable to tolerate. This is a complicated issue for individuals with ID, due to the fact that, in general, as the level of cognitive disability decreases, so does dependence upon caregivers. This dependence makes it more difficult for more persons with disability to avoid exposure to triggering cues on their own. For this reason, clinicians should try to determine if there are specific triggers for PTSD symptoms for a given patient, and should provide both guidance and support to caregivers in order to help them reduce the patient's exposure to triggers in their environment.

Strategies to remember when treating any person who has experienced trauma

- When working with a trauma victim, it is important to provide education regarding the experience of trauma and to normalize the thoughts and feelings associated with it.

- Because victims have had no power or control over the abuse that occurred, in order to recover, it is essential that they begin to have a sense of control over their lives. Psychotherapy should therefore be an empowering experience for them. This can be accomplished by ensuring that it is a collaborative process, with the patient retaining the power for making decisions in the psychotherapy. This can include: mutually choosing goals for therapy; encouraging the patient to decide some of the content for each session; and teaching skills to assert themselves appropriately in other settings.

- When treating victims of trauma, the psychotherapist should presume that the patients are doing their best and that they want to do well. Use of a "strengths-based" approach that involves building on the strengths of the individuals and their natural support systems will lead to the best patient outcomes.

Summary

Individuals with ID experience mental disorders at rates that are higher than that of the general population, with estimates ranging from 10–85% (Romana, 2003). Although historically it was believed that this population could not benefit from psychotherapy, research produced in the last 10–15 years has demonstrated definitively that this is not the case. It is now understood that the efficacy of treatment improves dramatically when modifications are made to traditional treatment models so that the service delivery matches the developmental and cognitive needs of the patient. There is consensus that when working with patients with ID, the following adaptations are best practices:

- Increase length of treatment to allow for needed repetition and implementation of additional treatment stages.

- Adjust the complexity of the interventions provided to match the patient's developmental framework.

- Reduce the level of vocabulary, sentence structure and length of utterance to match the individual's level of understanding.

- Utilize more directive methods.

- Provide the patient with visual cues to address memory issues.

- Augment interventions with activities to deepen understanding of information presented.

- Involve care providers with the consent of the patient.

References

Ainsworth, M.D.S., Blechar, M.C., Waters, E. & Wall, S. (1978). *Patterns of Attachment: A Psychological Study of the Strange Situation.* Hillside, Erlbaum, NJ.

Arkowitz, H. & Westra, H. (2009). Introduction to the Special Series on Motivational Interviewing and Psychotherapy. *Journal of Clinical Psychology* **65**, 1149–1155.

Aronson, M.L. (1990). Integrating Moreno's Psychodrama and Psychoanalytic Group Therapy. *Journal of Group Psychotherapy, Psychodrama Sociometry* **42**(4), 199–203.

Atkinson, C. (2007). Using Solution-Focused Approaches in Motivational Interviewing with Young People. *Pastoral Care* **25**, 31–37.

Battaglia, J. (2007). Five Keys to Good Results with Supportive Psychotherapy. *Current Psychiatry* **6**, 27–34.

Baxter, J.T. & Cain, N.N. (2006). *Psychotherapeutic Interventions. Training Handbook of Mental Disorders in Individuals with Intellectual Disability*, pp. 115–130. NADD Press, Kingston, NY.

Beck, A.T., Rush, A.J., Shaw, B.F. & Emery, G. (1979). *Cognitive Theory of Depression.* The Guilford Press, New York, NY.

Berry, P. (2003). Psychodynamic Therapy and Intellectual Disabilities: dealing with challenging behaviour. *International Journal of Disability, Development and Education* **50**, 39–51.

Blackman, N.J. (2002). Grief and Intellectual Disability: A Systemic Approach. *Journal of Gerontological Social Work* **38**(1/2) 253–263.

Bowlby, J. (1969). *Attachment and Loss, Vol. 1: Attachment.* Hogarth Press and Institute of Psychoanalysis, London.

Charlton, M. & Dykstra, E.J. (2011). *Dialectical Behavior Therapy for Special Populations: Treatment with Adolescents and Their Caregivers. Psychotherapy for Individuals with Intellectual Disabilities*, pp. 13–36. NADD Press, Kingston, NY.

Clute, M.A. (2010). Bereavement Interventions for Adults with Intellectual Disabilities: What Works? *Omega* **61**(2), 163–177.

Dagnan, D. (2007). Psychosocial Interventions for People with Intellectual Disabilities and Mental Ill-Health. *Current Opinion In Psychiatry* **20**(5), 456–60.

Davidson, P.W. & Cain, N.N. (2006). *Overview. Training Handbook of Mental Disorders in Individuals with Intellectual Disability*, pp. 1–13. NADD Press, Kingston, NY.

Dayton, T. (1994). *The Drama With in: Psychodrama and Experiential Therapy.* Health Communications, Inc., Deerfield, FL.

Dodd, P., Dowling, S., & Hollins, S. (2005). A review of the emotional, psychiatric and behavioral responses to bereavement in people with intellectual disabilities. *Journal of Intellectual Disabilities Research* **49**(7), 537–543.

Douglas, C. (2008). Teaching Supportive Psychotherapy to Psychiatric Residents. *American Journal of Psychiatric* **165**, 445–452.

Esterhuyzen, A. & Hollins, S. (1997) Psychotherapy. In: Read,S. (ed.) *Psychiatry in Learning Disability*, pp. 332–349. W.B. Sanders, London.

Fernado, K. & Medlicott, L. (2009). My Shield Will Protect Me Against the Ants: Treatment of PTSD in a Client with Intellectual Disability. *Journal of Intellectual & Developmental Disability* **34**(2), 187–192.

Gentile, J.P. & Hubner, M.E. (2005). Bereavement in Patients with Dual Diagnosis Mental Illness and Mental Retardation/Developmental Disabilities. *Psychiatry* **2**(10), 56–61.

Gentile, J.P. & Jackson, C.S. (2008). Supportive psychotherapy with the dual diagnosis patient: co-occurring mental illness/intellectual disabilities. *Psychiatry* **5**(3), 49–57.

Haddock, G., Lobban, F., Hatton, C. & Carson, R. (2004). Cognitive-Behaviour Therapy for People with Psychosis and Mild Intellectual Disabilities: A Case Series. *Clinical Psychology and Psychotherapy* **11**, 282–298.

Hollins, S. & Sinason, V. (2000). Psychotherapy, learning disabilities and trauma: New perspectives. *British Journal of Psychiatry* **176**, 32–36.

Hurley, A., Tomasulo, D.J. & Pfadt, G. (1998). Individual and Group Psychotherapy Approaches for Persons with Intellectual Disabilities and Developmental Disabilities. *Journal of Developmental and Physical Disabilities* **10**, 365–386.

Jahoda, A., Dagnan, D., Jarvie, P. & Kerr, W. (2006). Depression, Social Context and Cognitive Behavioural Therapy for People who have Intellectual Disabilities. *Journal of Applied Research in Intellectual Disabilities* **19**, 81–89.

Kay J. (2005). Attachment and Its Disorders. In: Klykylo, W.M. & Kay, J. (eds.) *Clinical Child Psychiatry, 2nd Edition*. John Wiley and Sons.

Keller, E.M. (2000). Points of Intervention: Facilitating the Process of Psychotherapy with People who have Developmental Disabilities. In: Fletcher R. (ed). *Therapy Approaches for Persons with Mental Retardation*, pp. 27–47. NADD Press, Kingston, NY.

Kirchner, L., & Mueth, M. (2000). Suicide in individuals with developmental disabilities. In Fletcher, R. (ed.) *Therapy approaches for persons with mental retardation*, pp. 127–150. NADD Press, Kingston, NY.

Lavin, C. (2002). Disenfranchised grief and individuals with developmental disabilities. In Doka, K.J. (ed.) *Disenfranchised Grief: New directions, challenges, and strategies for practice*, pp. 307–322. Research Press, Champaign, IL.

Leichsenring, F., Hiller, W., Weissberg, M. & Leibing, E. (2006). Cognitive-Behavioral Therapy and Psychodynamic Psychotherapy: Techniques, Efficacy, and Indications. *American Journal of Psychotherapy* **60**(3), 233–259.

Lew, M. (2011). *Dialectical Behavior Therapy for Adults Who Have Intellectual Disability. Psychotherapy for Individuals with Intellectual Disability*, pp. 37–66. NADD Press, Kingston, NY.

Linehan, M.M. (1993). *Cognitive-Behavioral Treatment of Borderline Personality Disorder*. Guilford, New York.

Lynch, C. (2004). Psychotherapy for persons with mental retardation. *Mental Retardation* **42**(5), 399–405.

Maerov, P. (2006). Demystifying CBT: Effective, easy-to-use treatment for depression and anxiety. *The Journal of Family Practice* **5**. (8)

Martin, A. (2010). Intellectual Disability, Trauma and Psychotherapy. *Journal of Applied Research in Intellectual Disabilities* **23**(3), 301–301.

McCarthy, J. (2001). Post-Traumatic Stress Disorder in People with Learning Disability. *Advances in Psychiatric Treatment* **7**, 163–169.

Merlo, L.J., Storch, E.A., Lehmkuhl, H.D., Jacob, M.L., Murphy, T.K., Goodman, W.K. & Geffken, G.R. (2010). Cognitive behavioral therapy plus motivational interviewing improves outcome for pediatric obsessive-compulsive disorder: a preliminary study. *Cognitive Behavioral Therapy* **39**(1), 24–27.

Mevissen, L. & de Jongh, A. (2010). PTSD and its treatment in people with intellectual disabilities: a review of the literature. *Clinical Psychology Review* **30**(3), 308–316.

Miller, W.R. & Rollnick, S. (2002). *Motivational Interviewing: Preparing People for Change.* Guildford Press, New York.

Misch, D.A. (2006). Basic Strategies of Dynamic Supportive Therapy. Influential Publications. *Focus* **4**, 253–268.

Mitchell, A., Clegg, J. & Furniss, F. (2006). Exploring the Meaning of Trauma with Adults with Intellectual Disabilities. *Journal of Applied Research in Intellectual Disabilities* **19**, 131–142.

Moonshine, C. (2008). *Acquiring Competency and Achieving Proficiency with Dialectical Behavioral Therapy: Volume I. The Clinicians Guidebook.* Pesi, LLC, Eau Vlaire, WI.

Murphy, G.H., O'Callaghan, A.C. & Clare, I.C.H. (2007). The Impact of Alleged Abuse on Behaviour in Adults with Severe Intellectual Disabilities. *Journal of Intellectual Disability Research* **51**(10), 741–749.

Preston, J.D. (2006). *Integrative Treatment for Borderline Personality Disorder: Effective, Symptom-Focused Techniques, Simplified for Private Practice.* New Harbinger Publications, Inc., Oakland, CA.

Prout, H.T. & Browning, B.K. (2011). The Effectiveness of Psychotherapy with Persons with Intellectual Disabilities. In: Fletcher, R. (ed.) *Psychotherapy for Individuals with Intellectual Disabilities*, pp. 265–287. NADD Press, Kingston, NY.

Razza, N.J. & Tomasulo, D.J. (2011). Group Psychotherapy with Trauma Survivors Who Have Intellectual Disabilities. In Fletcher, R. (ed.). *Psychotherapy for Individuals with Intellectual Disabilities*, pp. 195–208. NADD Press, Kingston, NY.

Romana, M.S. (2003). Cognitive-behavioral therapy. Treating Individuals with Dual Diagnoses. *Journal of Psychosocial Nursing* **41**(12), 30–35.

Sakdalan, J.A., Shaw, J. & Collier, V. (2010). Staying in the Here-and-Now: a Pilot Study on the Use of Dialectical Behaviour Therapy Group Skills Training for Forensic Clients with Intellectual Disability. *Journal of Intellectual Disability Research* **54**(6), 568–72.

Substance Abuse and Mental Health Services Administration (SAMSHA) (2011). Trauma Informed Care and Trauma Services. http://www.samhsa.gov/nctic/trauma.asp Access Date 08/31/11.

Taylor, J.L., Lindsay, W.R. & Willner, P. (2008). CBT for People with Intellectual Disabilities: Emerging Evidence, Cognitive Ability and IQ Effects. *Behavioural & Cognitive Psychotherapy* **36**(6), 723–733.

Tomasulo, D.L. & Razza, N.J. (2006). Group Psychotherapy for People with Intellectual Disabilities: The Interactive-Behavioral Model. Journal of Group Psychotherapy, *Psychodrama and Sociometry* **59**(2), 85–93.

Tomasulo, D.L. & Razza, N.J. (2009). Empirical Validation of IBT for Clients with Intellectual Disabilities. *The Group Psychologist* **19**(3).

Turk, J., Robbins, I. & Woodhead, M. (2005). Post-traumatic stress disorder in young people with intellectual disability. *Journal of Intellectual Disability Research* **49**, 872–875.

Valenti-Hein, D. & Schwartz, L. (1995). *The Sexual Abuse Interview for Those with Developmental Disabilities.* James Stanfield Company, Santa Barbara, CA.

Weiner, H.B. & Sacks, J. (1969). Warm-Up and Sum-Up. *Group Psychotherapy* **22**(1–2) 85–102.

Whitehouse, R.M., Tudway, J., Look, R. & Kroese, B. (2006). Adapting Individual Psychotherapy for Adults with Intellectual Disabilities: A Comparative Review of the

Cognitive-Behavioural and Psychodynamic Literature. *Journal of Applied Research in Intellectual Disabilities.* **19**, 55–65.

Willner, P. (2005). The Effectiveness of Psychotherapeutic Interventions for People with Learning Disabilities: A Critical Overview. *Journal of Intellectual Disabilities Research* **49**(1), 73–85.

Wink, L.K., Erickson, C.A., Chambers, J.E. & McDougle, C.J. (2010). Co-morbid intellectual disability and borderline personality disorder: a case series. *Psychiatry* **73**(3), 277–287.

Wright, J. (2006). Cognitive Behavior Therapy: Basic Principles and Recent Advances. *Focus* **4**, 173–178.

Zerler, H. (2009). Motivational Interviewing in the Assessment and Management of Suicidality. *Journal of Clinical Psychology* **65**, 1207–1217.

Zigler, E., Bennett-Gates, D., Hodapp, R. & Henrich, C.C. (2002). Assessing personality traits of individuals with mental retardation. *American Journal on Mental Retardation* **3**, 181–193.

14

Behavioral Assessment and Interventions

Betsey A. Benson, PhD, Associate Professor, The Ohio State University, Columbus, Ohio

Introduction

Behavioral assessment and intervention is a long-standing method for achieving behavior change with persons with intellectual disabilities (ID). It has been demonstrated to be an effective approach to teach adaptive skills as well as to reduce problem behavior (Jacobson & Holburn, 2004). Behavioral interventions can be implemented concurrently with other treatments. Continuing data collection is a hallmark of the behavioral approach and is a valuable tool for tracking the response to interventions.

It is beyond the scope of this chapter to provide a complete account of behavior interventions with persons with ID. There are many excellent sources of information available on applied behavior analysis (Cooper *et al.*, 2007) and on behavioral interventions in persons with ID (Matson *et al.*, 2004). In this chapter, the methods and process of behavioral assessment are described, as well as the elements of behavior support plans. Considerations for integrating behavioral interventions with other treatments are discussed. Behavioral intervention occurs in the context of other services and supports received by the individual with ID. These approaches can complement one another and work in concert to achieve positive outcomes.

Behavioral assessment

The foundation of behavioral assessment and intervention is the A-B-C model of behavior, where A = antecedents, B = behavior and C = consequences. The antecedent conditions

Psychiatry of Intellectual Disability: A Practical Manual, First Edition.
Edited by Julie P. Gentile and Paulette M. Gillig.
© 2012 John Wiley & Sons, Ltd. Published 2012 by John Wiley & Sons, Ltd.

include characteristics of the physical environment as well as the social environment. The behaviors of concern need to be defined clearly and in observable, concrete terms in order to facilitate assessment and intervention. The consequences are events that regularly follow the occurrence of the problem behavior. Behavioral assessment gathers information on each part of the A-B-C model. Behavioral support plans direct changes in the antecedents and/or the consequences in order to change behavior.

The functions of behavior are the consequences that are related to maintaining the occurrence of a behavior. Some behavior functions are:

- Tangible (to obtain desired items or activities)

- Escape (from attention or activities)

- Social (to obtain attention)

- Sensory (to obtain stimulation).

Behaviors can serve multiple functions for an individual. If an individual does not have speech, behavior may serve a communication function. Once the functions of the behavior are identified, interventions can be selected with a higher likelihood of success.

Frequent behaviors of concern that may result in referral for behavioral assessment of a person with ID include verbal aggression, physical aggression, property destruction, self-injury, sexually inappropriate behavior, pica (eating non-food items) and non-compliance. Noncompliance with medical instructions, such as not taking prescribed medications or not following dietary restrictions, may result in a referral for behavior support services.

Behavioral assessment is a process that identifies the antecedents of the behavior and the consequences of behavior within the context of the individual's environment. The goals of behavioral assessment are to gather information on the behaviors of concern, identify the environmental influences on behavior and learn the functions of those behaviors for the individual and their likely consequences.

During behavioral assessment, information is obtained on the individual's current skills. The assessor needs to determine if the individual has a current level of skill to perform in an appropriate manner but is not doing so frequently enough – or, alternatively, if the individual needs to acquire a skill to replace the behavior of concern. If skill acquisition is needed, then plans for training appropriate behavior need to be made. One type of training that could be included is functional communication training; for example, a nonverbal individual who responds with aggression following a demand can learn to request a break through use of a gestural sign or other method.

Behavioral assessment considers environmental influences on behavior by gathering information from multiple settings, including those in which the individual is reported to have no problems or less significant problems. Comparing settings with different frequency of behaviors of concern helps to identify the environmental supports that assist the individual and, conversely, situations in which those supports are lacking. Environments also vary in terms of the expectations and demands placed on individuals. It is not unusual for an individual with ID to be reported to have no problems at home, but significant problems in an employment setting, or vice versa.

Identifying the factors that underlie such behavioral variations is part of the assessment process. It is also important to assess whether the expectations and demands placed on the individual are consistent with their developmental level. If tasks are too difficult (resulting in frustration) or too easy (resulting in boredom), then problem behaviors may be more likely to occur.

There are several methods of behavioral assessment. These include direct observation of the individual in the environment; interviewing the individual and others who know the person well; rating scales completed by informants; and functional analysis, in which the individual is placed in carefully structured analogue situations. Most behavioral assessment uses multiple methods.

When directly observing the individual in an environment, data can be collected on the frequency, the latency or the intensity of the target behavior. The individual can be observed continuously and problem behavior recorded throughout the observation period, or a time sampling approach can be used, in which segments of time are selected for recording data. An advantage of direct observation as an assessment method is that the behavior is observed in context, within the flow of typical events and interactions. A disadvantage of this method is that it is labor-intensive.

The completion of an A-B-C chart (see Table 1) is an assessment method in which observers record a description of events that happen immediately before and after the occurrence of problem behaviors. The information obtained from the A-B-C chart can be used to develop hypotheses about likely functions of problem behaviors, and also to develop more detailed assessment tools.

Individuals who know the person well are an important source of information for a behavioral assessment. There are structured behavioral interview formats that have been developed to assist in gathering the necessary information for a behavioral assessment (O'Neil *et al.*, 1997). The interview is structured to obtain information about how the problem behavior is defined and where, when, how often a behavior occurs. It also addresses environmental antecedents and daily schedules. There are questions about the situations that predict the occurrence of the behavior by time of day, setting or activity, and what the typical consequences for the behavior are. The individual's primary method of communication, as well as the availability of alternative behaviors and the previous interventions that were used, are also included.

An advantage of the structured interview method is that similar information from multiple informants can be obtained. This method requires that the informant knows the individual well and can extrapolate from his or her experience. The assessor needs to keep in mind the various roles that informants hold in relation to the individual, and how their perspective influences the information provided in the interview.

The individual referred for assessment should also participate in the assessment process as much as possible. Obtaining first-hand information about the individual's interests and preferences is useful in identifying potential reinforcers that could be incorporated into the behavior

Table 1 A-B-C chart.

Date: Time: Location	What happened before?	Behavior – what did the individual do? Possible behaviors: (list)	What happened afterwards?	Initials

plan. In addition, referred individuals can provide their own perspective on how the behavior of others influence them. For example, the individual may discuss ways in which specific expectations are not being met, share that there are perceived inequities in treatment in comparison to others, or that he or she wants staff or family to show respect in their interactions.

Rating scales completed by others can provide information on the behaviors of interest as they provide a standardized method of comparing one informant's report to another. Rating scales for identifying behavioral functions include the Motivational Assessment Scale (MAS) (Durand & Crimmins, 1988) and the Questions About Behavior Functions (QABF) (Paclawskyj *et al.*, 2000). For each behavior of interest, the individual rates the frequency with which the statement is true.

Some questions from the MAS are:

- "Does the behavior occur following a command to perform a difficult task?"

- "Does the behavior occur whenever you stop attending him or her?"

- "Does the behavior occur to get something that he or she has been told he or she can't have?"

Several statements refer to each of the typical behavior functions such as tangible, escape, demand and attention. A score for each function is obtained and indicates the relative degree to which a function influences the behavior of concern.

Rating scales for problem behavior that were created for individuals with intellectual disabilities can also provide useful information for the behavioral assessment. Two behavior problem rating scales for individuals with ID are the Aberrant Behavior Checklist (ABC) (Aman & Singh, 1986) and the Behavior Problems Inventory (Rojahn *et al.*, 2001). The ABC is a 58-item checklist of problem behaviors that are rated on a scale of 0–3 to indicate the severity of the problem. The Behavior Problems Inventory is a 52-item rating scale for self-injury, stereotypic and aggressive/destructive behavior. Items are rated on a 0–4 frequency scale and a 0–3 severity scale.

Both rating scales have established reliability and validity. Informant ratings using these scales may be useful in identifying the specific target behaviors and the severity of the problem.

Functional analysis of behavior is an assessment method that was developed by Iwata *et al.* (1982). In this method of assessment, the individual participates in a structured series of brief sessions in which the environment is manipulated to simulate conditions that are thought to affect the occurrence of the target behavior. The sessions present the conditions for assessing the primary functions of behavior.

Common conditions that are presented in a functional analysis are escape, demand, tangible, alone, and play or leisure. For example, in one session, if the individual engages in the target behavior, the experimenter responds with attention. In another session, the same behavior will be followed by no attention. Higher rates of problem behavior in one condition in comparison to another are interpreted as evidence for the function of the problem behavior. Functional analysis is most applicable to the study of behaviors that occur frequently and can be assessed in a controlled environment.

An example of a functional analysis demonstrates the method, results and application of the findings. A nonverbal, young adult with ID engaged in self-injurious behavior that consisted of scratching behind his ears, resulting in open wounds and a risk of infection. He was introduced to five standard functional analysis conditions, including demand, social attention, alone, tangible, and a control condition in a clinic setting.

- In the demand condition, he was prompted to complete habilitation goals, including wiping tables or shredding paper.

- In the social attention condition, the therapist provided a verbal reprimand at the first instance of self-injury.

- In the alone condition, he was alone in the session room with no materials.

- In the tangible condition, he received a small piece of a preferred food item after he engaged in self-injury.

All sessions were terminated at the first instance of self-injury, or after five minutes if no self-injury occurred. The bar graph (Figure 1) shows the average latency in seconds to self-injury for the five conditions.

In this example, the alone condition was associated with the shortest average latency to self-injury. The individual refrained from self-injury for longer periods of time in the demand and tangible conditions. However, self-injury occurred in all conditions, suggesting that it is maintained in part by its own sensory consequences. As a result of the functional analysis, it was recommended that the patient be given many opportunities to engage in activities in the day program. Other functional analysis sessions were conducted later to examine the relative effectiveness of alternative blocking procedures for self-injury, which were subsequently piloted in his day program by the staff.

There has been some criticism of the functional analysis method, on the grounds that it is an analogue approach. In addition, there have been some reports that other methods of assessment that are less labor-intensive compare favorably to the functional analysis method for high-frequency behavior (Yarborough & Carr, 2000). Many problem behaviors are found to have multiple functions, indicating that, to be most effective, behavioral interventions cannot focus on just one function (Matson & Boisjoli, 2007).

Potential reinforcers are identified as part of a behavioral assessment. A reinforcer is defined by its effect on behavior; it increases the future likelihood of a behavior occurring.

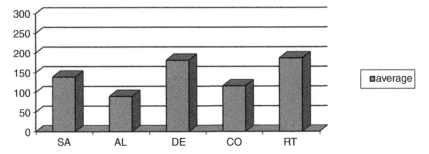

Figure 1   Results of a functional analysis of self-injury in terms of latency (sec.) to response. Conditions: SA = Social attention, AL = Alone, DE = Demand, CO- Control, RT = Tangible. (V. Rodriguez, K. Sikora, J. Gallaway, personal communication, 4/15/11)

Reinforcers can be tangible items, such as special food items, movie tickets or toys. They can also be activity-based, such as gaining access to a preferred activity. In addition, tokens, points, or stickers can be awarded immediately and later exchanged for other, preferred things.

The selection of reinforcers should be individualized. Potential reinforcers can be identified through interview or observation. The effectiveness of any reinforcer for an individual can change and should be re-assessed periodically. Some considerations in selecting reinforcers are their ease of use and portability, their age-appropriateness and the potential for satiation, i.e. whether the individual will tire of them easily. When incorporated into a behavior plan, access to a reinforcer should be controlled so that it is only available as programmed, and not available otherwise.

Behavioral assessment thus involves the assessment of multiple settings, with multiple informants. In addition, information is gathered on the referred individual's medications and side effects, history and background information, including trauma history, psychological evaluation reports, the individual's educational plan (IEP) and individual service plan, as well as incident reports. Behavioral assessment should also include information on the individual's eating, sleeping, and activity levels. The results of a behavioral assessment are consistent with the biopsychosocial model.

Behavior versus psychiatric problem

There is frequent discussion in the ID and mental health fields as to whether an individual's maladaptive behavior is a behavior problem or a psychiatric illness. Some behaviors reflect symptoms of mental illness or are made worse by mental illness. The presence of a psychiatric disorder can lead to or exacerbate a behavior problem, e.g. if an individual with a depressive disorder becomes aggressive when prompted to participate in activities.

Some symptoms of depression include lack of energy, loss of interest and wanting to be alone. If the response to the person's aggression is to develop a behavior plan, it may be ineffective if the depressive illness is not treated. The psychiatric illness in this case is a setting event or antecedent for the challenging behavior. Psychiatric conditions interact with environmental and learning variables in people in ways that vary across individuals (Sigafoos et al., 2003). Not all individuals with a depressive disorder engage in aggressive behavior, as in the example described above.

Psychiatric symptoms can interfere with the individual's typical behavior. For example, a young woman's work productivity declines when she is hallucinating. A thorough assessment is key. The assessor should look for clusters of symptoms, the history and change of behavior over time, reports of sleep, appetite and activity, and consistency of behavior across settings. One should consider how psychiatric stability or instability affects the behavior. If there is little or no improvement in the individual's behavior in spite of high-quality behavior intervention, then psychiatric or medical issues may have been missed or not adequately addressed.

Behavioral assessment can help clarify whether there is a psychiatric and/or behavioral issue. For example, a young woman with mild ID was referred for behavioral assessment because she told her staff at work that her sister was talking to her from inside the ceiling. The results of the behavioral assessment indicated that the report of hearing her sister's voice occurred only when she was confronted about taking items that belonged to someone else. The identification of this pattern in her behavior increased the likelihood that her report of hearing voices was a behavioral issue, not a psychiatric one.

When trying to determine if problem behavior is a behavioral and/or a psychiatric issue, close cooperation between psychiatric and behavioral services is an efficient and effective method for achieving results.

Experiencing stress in one's life can influence behavior in a negative way. People with ID experience many of the same stressors as other individuals, as well as some additional ones (Rush & Frances, 2000). Further, they may have fewer coping skills to manage or to adapt to stress (Hartley & Maclean, 2005). During a behavioral assessment, consideration should be given to the temporal relationship between possible stressors and the emergence or worsening of problem behaviors. Reducing or eliminating stress may be a part of the total intervention package for problem behaviors.

Once the behaviors of concern have been defined in specific, concrete terms, baseline data are collected. The term "baseline data" refers to information collected on the occurrence of the target behaviors prior to any new intervention. The frequency, intensity or severity of the target behaviors can be recorded at various intervals (e.g. hourly, daily, each work shift, etc.). Baseline data provide a pre-treatment point of comparison for gauging the effectiveness of the behavior plan. The data should be collected for a sufficient amount time to obtain stable results and it should be examined for patterns, e.g. by day of week, time of day, location, etc.

Information obtained from baseline data collection is useful in planning the interventions to be included in the behavior plan, and also in developing the initial criteria for defining improvement. Data collection is an ongoing process in the behavioral approach and it continues throughout the assessment and intervention periods.

The result of a functional assessment is the development of hypotheses about the influence of antecedents and consequences on the problem behaviors. The selection of interventions is based on the identified functions of the behaviors of concern.

Behavioral intervention

The goals of behavioral intervention with individuals with ID are to reduce problematic behavior and to increase appropriate behavior in a context that promotes the independence of the individual. The behavior support plan should provide the individual with the opportunity for self-determination and choice as much as possible. It should incorporate the least restrictive interventions necessary to influence behavior, while protecting the health and safety of the individual and those around him or her (Carr *et al.*, 2002; Kazdin, 2001). The individual, their guardian (if appropriate) and the members of the interdisciplinary team should provide input into the development of the behavior support plan.

A behavior support plan includes the behavior goals and intervention strategies. It specifies who implements the behavior plan, the data collection process and procedures, and how the plan is monitored. The behavior plan is not a static document, but should adjust to the growth and change of the individual and should state the criteria for its discontinuation.

While behavioral assessment, as an intervention, is specific to an individual and their unique strengths and needs, some general guidelines have been offered for the treatment of psychiatric and behavioral problems of persons with ID. A panel of national experts rank-ordered seven psychosocial interventions for a number of psychiatric disorders and behavior problems for children and adults with ID. In all cases, regardless of the diagnostic condition or developmental level, the first-line treatments recommended by the experts were client and family education, applied behavior analysis and managing the environment (Rush & Frances, 2000). Client and family education included helping clients and families to understand more about the individual's behavioral and psychiatric problems and how to manage them.

Antecedent control

An initial consideration in the construction of the behavior support plan is whether there are environmental modifications that could reduce or prevent the occurrence of the target behavior or increase the likelihood that appropriate behavior occurs (Luiselli & Cameron, 1998). These modifications might include changes in activities, social groupings or routines, or changes in the physical environment.

For example, from a review of the assessment results, it may be apparent that problem behaviors often occur during transition periods from one activity to another, or from one setting to another. Developing specific routines to occur during the transition periods could be helpful. This might involve using verbal or visual prompts to prepare in advance for transition, such as posting a sign or providing a verbal prompt when there are 15 minutes remaining, until it is time to board the bus. It also may be the case that the number of demands placed on the individual shortly after making a transition could be reduced for a period of time, to allow the individual to adjust to the transition. For example, when arriving home from school or from day services, the individual has the opportunity to select an activity or to relax in their room prior to being asked to take medications, make lunches or go on an errand.

Individuals with ID may benefit from the use of visual schedules or other visual displays as aids to prompt tasks to complete (or steps in a task). A visual schedule shows activities or events in order, using symbols, words or pictures. If the individual can use the visual display to guide their behavior, it can reduce the number of requests made by others and, in turn, reduce noncompliance with demands.

Rule reminders are another approach to antecedent control of problem behavior. These are prompts that remind an individual what the rules or expectations are in a particular setting. They can be provided verbally or in written form. Rule reminders might be used to review with an individual, prior to an outing, what the behavioral expectations are during that outing. Rule reminders could also be used at the start of the school day or the work shift, to remind the individual what behaviors are permitted or not permitted in the setting. Rule reminders could also include details of the goals that the individual is working on for the day, such as completing a certain number of work pieces or school assignments, and the reinforcer that he or she will earn for meeting those goals.

Focus on consequences

The least restrictive alternative guideline for providing behavioral treatment states that the procedure which is least intrusive, yet most likely to be effective, should be used first. Restrictive intervention strategies are used only when the problem behavior has not responded to positive approaches and if they are a threat to the safety of the individual or others (Association for Behavior Analysis International, 1993).

Differential reinforcement is a positive behavioral intervention that has been found to be effective in reducing a wide range of problem behaviors in adults with ID, either alone or in combination with other interventions (Chowdhury & Benson, 2011). It involves reinforcing one type of behavior and withholding reinforcement for another type of behavior. There are several types of differential reinforcement:

- In differential reinforcement of incompatible behavior (DRI), the behavior that is reinforced is incompatible with the problem behavior. For example, appropriate verbalizations are reinforced, while inappropriate verbalizations are not.

- Differential reinforcement of alternate behavior (DRA) is similar to DRI, except that the behavior reinforced is a desirable alternative to the problem behavior but not necessarily incompatible with it. The individual might be reinforced for staying on task, as an alternative to inappropriate verbalizations. When the assessment of a problem behavior indicates that the function of the behavior is attention, the behavior plan will remove or limit attention for the problem behavior, while prescribing that attention is given instead for more appropriate behavior.

- In differential reinforcement of other behavior (DRO), a reinforcer is provided when the problem behavior has not occurred within a pre-specified period of time. For example, if inappropriate verbalization does not occur for one hour, a reinforcer is made available.

- Finally, differential reinforcement of low rates (DRL) requires that reinforcement be delivered if the problem behavior occurs at a lower rate than a pre-determined criterion. This method is selected when a problem behavior occurs too frequently, but the goal is not to eliminate the behavior entirely. For example, an individual who makes repeated approaches to staff of up to 140 times per shift could be reinforced for approaching staff 100 times or fewer per shift.

Restrictive or aversive interventions are used after reinforcement-only procedures are tried and found to be inadequate, or when the problem behavior presents danger to self or others. When these procedures are used to decrease problem behaviors, it is important also to use reinforcement procedures at the same time in order to encourage the development of appropriate behaviors. Two types of restrictive procedures are response cost and financial restitution:

- In response cost, an individual loses points, tokens or access to preferred activities as a consequence for engaging in a target behavior.

- If an individual engages in property destruction or takes items belonging to others, then financial restitution might be included in a behavior plan. The individual would be held responsible for payment to repair damages or to replace the item. Financial restitution as a behavioral intervention should be used only with individuals who have an understanding of the value of money.

Time out from positive reinforcement involves interrupting the reinforcement obtained by the individual following the occurrence of target behavior. Time out is exclusionary if the person is removed from the environment for a period of time, whereas it is inclusionary if the person remains in the setting but reinforcers are removed following the occurrence of a target behavior. Time out is an intervention that might be considered if the individual is endangering others through aggressive or destructive behavior. Strict limits are kept on the duration of time out, and supervision of the individual is required during the time out period. Time out is not an appropriate intervention for a problem behavior whose function is escape.

The individual who is learning relaxation or coping skills could practice them during the time out period. Coping skills could be prompted prior to aggressive acts if precursors of impending aggression are identified. The goal would be for individuals to be able to calm themselves prior to engaging in aggression and without leaving the environment.

Manual restraint is an intervention that should have very limited use with people with ID in the community. It is sometimes used as a crisis intervention technique when the danger to self or others is imminent. The use of manual restraint might be contraindicated by a person's trauma history. When it is included in a behavior support plan, detailed instructions must be provided for the circumstances in which restraint can be used, the type of restraint permitted, the duration of the restraint allowed and a detailed fading procedure for elimination of the restraint.

Close oversight of restraint use is required, and intensive training in safe restraint practices must be done with all individuals who implement this intervention. Debriefing of the staff and the client following a restraint should be completed to identify triggers of the event and other possible de-escalation methods that could have been used prior to the use of restraint. Manual restraint is a controversial procedure, and some states have prohibited the use of particular types of restraint with persons with ID (Ohio Department of Mental Retardation and Developmental Disabilities, 2008).

Training, implementation and monitoring of behavior support plans

The training of individuals who will implement the behavior plan is of critical importance. To be effective, a behavior plan must be implemented consistently. In addition to training on the specifics of the behavior plan, training should also address the individual's mental health diagnoses and symptoms, and any considerations related to intellectual disability characteristics, if appropriate.

Once all implementers have been trained, the behavior support plan can be initiated. Frequent checks on implementation should be made, especially in the initial stages, and troubleshooting of any issues encountered. The behavior support plan should be given time to achieve effects. Data collection continues throughout the implementation period. Graphing of the data can be useful, along with notations of any medication changes or environmental factors.

The behaviors monitored during the implementation of a behavior support plan can also include tracking of behaviors not directly addressed in the plan. These might include the individual's mood, sleep patterns, menstrual cycle, etc. This information can be useful in the evaluation of the effectiveness of the behavior support plan and, with appropriate consent, it can be shared with other professionals who are working with the individual. Revisions to the behavior plan are made as progress occurs.

Coordination of behavior support services with other interventions

Individuals with ID and mental health or behavior problems frequently present a complex picture. Coordination among the many professionals working with the individual is strongly recommended (American Academy of Child and Adolescent Psychiatry, 1999). A behavior support plan and the ongoing monitoring associated with it can provide information on the individual's progress and can also promote the integration of services. The examples shown in the clinical vignettes illustrate different types of collaboration between the behavior support service and other services provided to the individual.

Clinical Vignette #1

Coordination between psychiatric and behavioral services can be promoted through the identification and tracking of an index behavior. In this instance, a specific behavior is tracked through the monitoring of the behavior support plan and, with appropriate consent, reported to the physician on a regular basis.

For example, a young woman with a diagnosis of bipolar disorder and Williams syndrome was receiving psychiatric care and behavioral services. The support staff in her home noticed that the woman's swearing seemed to increase in frequency, prior to the emergence of other manic symptoms. The behavior support plan tracked the frequency of swearing, as well as other behaviors that were addressed in the plan, and they shared the monthly behavior data with the psychiatrist.

The psychiatrist adjusted medications when warranted by a change in the individual's mental status.

Clinical Vignette #2

In a second case, a young man with a diagnosis of psychotic disorder NOS was referred for behavioral services. One behavior of concern was that he had stored his urine in a jar in his bedroom closet. This problem was considered a health and safety issue in the home.

The behavior plan tracked the unsafe behavior and included the intervention of regular room searches for inappropriate items. The behavior plan also tracked the frequency of talking out loud to himself, which was a behavior that fluctuated with his mental status.

The behavior data was shared with the prescribing physician, and medication information was in turn shared with the behavior specialist.

At a second level of integration between behavioral and psychiatric interventions, the behavior plan incorporates interventions to manage mental health symptoms and behaviors.

Clinical Vignette #3

Miss A. was a young woman with mild ID and bipolar disorder. She had multiple psychiatric hospitalizations and had been prescribed several different medications or combinations of medications since adolescence. Her treatment plan included psychiatric care, a behavior support plan, and family and caregiver education. The family and caregiver education included information on Miss A.'s mental health diagnosis and her ID. It also included ways for staff to encourage skill development to promote more independent living, and symptom reporting for relapse prevention.

One target behavior in Miss A.'s behavior plan was verbal aggression. The antecedents of verbal aggression were being told "No" and sleeping too much or not enough. Functional analysis interviews indicated that verbal aggression occurred to avoid demands and also to express anger. Verbal aggression was often a precursor to physical aggression. Sleep issues seemed to be related to psychiatric symptoms and medication changes, but they were also thought to be due to a lack of productive activities.

Prevention procedures in the behavior plan included establishing schedules and routines, including a daily activity and daily menu developed with her input the day before. Staff working in her home did not start sentences with the word "No," but gave her an explanation and offered alternatives. Redirection and reassurance were also given. When Miss A. was agitated, she was reminded of consequences and other alternatives were suggested. She was encouraged to go to bed by midnight and to wake up in the morning in time for the chosen activity.

Replacement behaviors included in the behavior plan were to speak respectfully to staff, follow the menu, and complete 2–3 household tasks per day that she had previously been able to complete. If she met the established behavior criteria three days per week, then she earned a wrapped "grab bag" surprise, such as nail polish, stationery, or colored pencils that were provided by her mother.

When verbal aggression occurred, staff first tried to talk to her about the problem. If verbal aggression continued, then staff withdrew for ten minutes before re-engaging with her. The criteria for earning the weekly reward were gradually increased as progress was made.

Miss A. participated in individual counseling, in which she learned relaxation techniques and anger management. She later resumed participation in a vocational program.

At a third level of integration, the behavior support plan incorporates elements of other treatments and adjusts to changes in mental health status (Esbensen & Benson, 2003). The behavior plan can be designed to promote the practice or use of skills that are addressed in psychotherapy. These can be incorporated into the behavior plan and included in staff training.

Clinical Vignette #4

Miss B., a young woman with mild ID and a diagnosis of borderline personality disorder, was receiving psychiatric services, counseling and behavior support. Her target behaviors included self-injury, property destruction and running away. She had a history of many psychiatric hospitalizations and crisis care in the community. She was known to the local police and had spent time in jail.

The behavior plan was based on Wilson's (2001) four-stage model for borderline personality disorder, and it provided specific staff supports to match each stage. The stages were defined in terms of observable behaviors.

- Stage 1 = optimal functioning. When in this stage, Miss B. appeared happy and she was engaged in activities. Staff encouraged her to practice coping skills and relaxation, to keep busy and be productive, to write in her emotion journal and to discuss feelings with them daily.

- In Stage 2, antecedents or precursors to problems are observed. Her behavior included reporting auditory hallucinations and an increase in depressive statements. She had poor eye contact and seemed withdrawn. Staff encouraged her to use coping strategies; they made calls for support to a supervisor or others as previously arranged, and suggested that she move to a quiet area.

- Stage 3 is Crisis. Her behaviors were self-abuse, cutting, barricading herself in her room and requesting calls to 911. Staff monitored her from a safe distance and kept her safe, with minimal interactions. They stayed calm, did not try to reason with her and watched for signs of resolution.

- Stage 4 is resolution. She appeared calm and tired, not threatening to hurt herself or to run away, not expressing feelings of sadness or depression. Staff engaged her in conversation, validated her feelings and concern and prompted the use of coping strategies. The goal was to return to Stage 1 functioning.

The behavior plan specified that Miss B. receive points daily for writing in a journal, attending work as scheduled, following telephone guidelines, taking medications and having a discussion about emotions with staff in her home. When a pre-determined number of points were earned, she received a special outing that she selected in advance.

The behavior plan monitoring included recording the amount of time she was in each stage, as well as frequency data on the target behaviors and interventions. The data were shared with the counselor and the psychiatrist. Significant improvements were observed overall. However, brief periods of worsening of symptoms, followed by return to stability for several months, continued to be observed.

Table 2 Behavior support plan data summary form.

Name: Miss B.		Location: Home		Plan Monitor: Jane Smith					

Behavior Support Summary Data Form									

		Review dates and data (month)							
Target Behaviors	Previous Year	M:1	M:2	M:3	M:4	M:5	M:6	M:7	M:8
TO DECREASE									
Self-injury	.75×/mo.	0	0	3	1	0	0	0	0
Para suicidal behavior	.17×/mo.	0	0	3	1	0	0	0	0
Barricading self in room	.08×/mo.	0	0	3	1	0	0	0	0
Physical aggression	.47×/mo.	0	0	3	3	0	0	0	0
Verbal aggression	.86×/mo	2	0	8	11	0	0	0	0
Property destruction	.25×/mo	0	0	3	5	0	0	0	0
Calling 911 for non-emergency	.33×/mo	0	0	2	0	0	0	0	0
AWOL	.25×/mo.	0	0	1	1	0	0	0	0
Went to ER, hospital or jail	.45×/mo	0	0	2	1	0	0	0	0
INTERVENTION USE									
Verbal praise given		84	82	85	59	79	78	73	86
TO INCREASE									
Took medications (%)		100	100	98	98	100	98	100	100
Followed telephone guidelines (%)		99	100	99	97	100	100	100	100
Went to work as scheduled (%)		94	93	80	62	95	95	95	95
Wrote in journal (%)		94	100	87	77	97	100	94	100
Emotion discussion with staff (%)		94	93	87	90	97	100	90	100
Earned reinforcer (%)		64	91	62	27	92	90	91	100
Time in Stage 1		100	100	75	60	100	96	100	98

A sample form (Table 2) shows a summary of the behavior plan data, displayed by month, for Clinical Vignette #4.

Keys to successful coordination

Designing, implementing and monitoring behavioral interventions for people with ID and psychiatric disorders can be a complex task. However, when the various services and supports provided to the individual with ID work in concert, they can jointly contribute to the success of the interventions and the progress of the individual (Sevin *et al.*, 2001).

These elements contribute to successful coordination of psychiatric, psychotherapeutic and behavior interventions:

- Staff and family education on psychiatric diagnoses, ID syndromes, medical issues, and relevant background information such as trauma history.

- Ongoing tracking of target behaviors and symptoms.

- Appropriate interventions that are based on a thorough assessment.

- Routine communication among team members, including psychiatrist, counselor and behavior specialist.

- Effective intervention comes from a unified approach and timely response to changes in mental status and behavior.

As progress is made, the need for a behavior support plan may decrease, but the need for active coordination of services continues. The planned interaction of team members may be successfully reduced in frequency, but ongoing communication is still needed. The members of the interdisciplinary team and its resources need to be available to respond to changes in mental health status or behavior, and to assist the individual in coping with stressful life events.

References

Aman, M.G. & Singh, N.N. (1986). *Aberrant Behavior Checklist – Community*. Slosson Educational Publications, East Aurora, NY.

American Academy of Child and Adolescent Psychiatry (1999). Practice parameters for the assessment and treatment of children, adolescents, and adults with mental retardation and comorbid mental disorders. American Academy of Child and Adolescent Psychiatry Working Group on Quality Issues. *Journal of the American Academy of Child and Adolescent Psychiatry* **38**, 5–31.

Association for Behavior Analysis International (1993). Understanding behavior analysis. Retrieved June 10, 2010 from: http://www.abainternational.org/BA/FAQ13.asp.

Carr, E.G., Dunlap, G., Horner, R.H., Koegel, R.L., Turnbull, A.P., Sailor, W., Anderson, J., Albin, R.W., Koegel, L.K. & Fox, L. (2002). Positive behavior support: Evolution of an applied science. *Journal of Positive Behavior Interventions* **4**, 4–16.

Chowdhury, M. & Benson, B.A. (2011). Use of differential reinforcement to reduce behavior problems in adults with intellectual disabilities: A methodological review. *Research in Developmental Disabilities* **32**, 383–394.

Cooper, J.O., Heron, T.E. & Heward, W.L. (2007). *Applied behavior analysis*. Pearson/Merrill-Prentice Hall Upper, Saddle River, NJ.

Durand, V.C. & Crimmins DB. (1988). Identifying the variables maintaining self-injurious behavior. *Journal of Autism & Developmental Disorders* **18**, 99–117.

Esbensen, A.J. & Benson, B.A. (2003). Integrating behavioral, psychological and pharmacological treatment: A case study of an individual with borderline personality disorder and mental retardation. *Mental Health Aspects of Developmental Disabilities* **6**(3), 107–113.

Hartley, S.L. & Maclean, W.E. (2005). Perceptions of stress and coping strategies among adults with mild mental retardation: Insight into psychological distress. *American Journal on Mental Retardation* **110**, 285–297.

Iwata, B.A., Dorsey, M.F., Slifer, K.J., Bauman, K.E. & Richman G.S. (1982). Toward a functional analysis of self-injury. *Journal of Applied Behavior Analysis* **27**, 197–209. (Reprinted from *Analysis and Intervention in Developmental Disabilities* **2**, 3–20, 1982).

Jacobson, J.W. & Holburn S. (2004). History and current status of applied behavior analysis in developmental disabilities. In: Matson, J.L., Laud, R.B.,& Matson, M.L. (eds.) *Behavior modification for persons with developmental disabilities: Treatments and supports (vol. 1)* pp. 1–32. NADD, Kingston, NY.

Kazdin, A.E. (2001). *Behavioral modification in applied settings* (6th ed.). Thomson Learning, Belmont, CA.

Luiselli, J.G. & Cameron, M.J. (1998). *Antecedent control: Innovative approaches to behavioral support.* Paul H. Brookes, Baltimore, MD.

Matson, J.L. & Boisjoli, J.A. (2007). Multiple versus single maintaining factors of challenging behaviors as assessed by the QABF for adults with intellectual disabilities. *Journal of Intellectual Developmental Disabilities* **32**, 39–44.

Matson, J.L., Laud, R.B. & Matson, M.L. (eds.) (2004). *Behavior modification for persons with developmental disabilities: Treatments and supports (vol. 1)* NADD, Kingston NY.

O'Neil, R.E., Horner, R.H., Albin, R.W., Storey, K. & Sprague, J.R. (1997). *Functional assessment of problem behavior: A practical guide.* Brooks/Cole, Pacific Grove, CA.

Ohio Department of Mental Retardation and Developmental Disabilities (2008). Information Notice 08-11-03.

Paclawskyj, T.R., Matson, J.L. & Rush, K.S. (2000). Questions about Behavioral Function (QABF): A behavioral checklist for functional assessment of aberrant behavior. *Research in Developmental Disabilities* **21**, 223–9.

Rojahn, J., Matson, J.L., Lott, D., Esbensen, A.J. & Smalls, Y. (2001). The Behavior Problems Inventory: An instrument for the assessment of self-injury, stereotyped behavior, and aggression/destruction in individuals with developmental disabilities. *Journal of Autism and Developmental Disorders* **31**, 577–587.

Rush, A.J. & Frances, A. (eds.) (2000). Expert Consensus Guideline Series: Treatment of psychiatric and behavioral problems in mental retardation. *American Journal of Mental Retardation* **105**, 159–228.

Sevin, J.A., Bowers-Stephens, C., Hamilton, M.L. & Ford, A. (2001). Integrating behavioral and pharmacological interventions in treating clients with psychiatric disorders and mental retardation. *Research in Developmental Disabilities* **22**, 463–485.

Sigafoos, J., Arthur, M. & O'Reilly, M. (2003). *Challenging behavior and developmental disability.* Whurr Publishers, London.

Wilson, S.R. (2001). A four-stage model for management of borderline personality disorder in people with mental retardation. *Mental Health Aspects of Developmental Disabilities* **4**, 68–76.

Yarborough, S.C. & Carr, E.G. (2000). Some relationships between informant assessment and functional analysis of problem behavior. *American Journal on Mental Retardation* **105**, 130–151.

15

Legal Issues for Treatment Providers and Evaluators

Jeannette Cox, JD, Associate Professor, University of Dayton School of Law, Dayton, Ohio

Introduction

The law related to intellectual disability (ID) reflects ongoing debates about the appropriate balance between competing impulses to protect and to empower persons with intellectual disabilities. Historically, the law focused almost exclusively on sheltering persons with ID from abuse and poor decisions. Recent reforms led by the disability rights movement, however, have recognized that this protective impulse has too often resulted in the law treating adults with ID as perpetual children – a status that often results in disempowerment, isolation and the underdevelopment of functional abilities. These reforms have also recognized that simple adjustments to standard operating procedures (often termed "reasonable accommodations" or "reasonable modifications") frequently eliminate the need to exclude persons with ID from the privileges and responsibilities of citizenship.

In response to the disability rights movement, nearly all areas of the law now recognize that a diagnosis of ID, standing alone, has no legal significance. For example, an ID diagnosis does not automatically mean that a court may appoint a guardian to make financial decisions for the individual. Similarly, an ID diagnosis does not automatically mean that an individual accused of a crime is not competent to stand trial. Instead, the law requires an individualized determination of how a specific individual's functional abilities interact with the demands of the relevant activity, such as managing a particular set of assets or

Psychiatry of Intellectual Disability: A Practical Manual, First Edition.
Edited by Julie P. Gentile and Paulette M. Gillig.
© 2012 John Wiley & Sons, Ltd. Published 2012 by John Wiley & Sons, Ltd.

participating in a particular criminal trial. This detailed inquiry into an individual's need for protective legal action aims to maximize the self-determination of persons with ID.

The law's individualized inquiry into the particular strengths and limitations of a person with ID is relevant to mental health practitioners in two ways:

- First, the need to make individualized determinations of a particular person's abilities will arise in a mental health treatment practice. A treating professional must comply with civil rights laws, which frequently require modifications to typical practices in order to ensure that persons with disabilities have access equal to the benefits available to persons without disabilities. A treatment provider must also comply with the law of informed consent, which requires an assessment of the patient's ability to understand and weigh the risks and benefits of a proposed treatment.

- Second, the need to make individualized determinations of a person's abilities may arise in a forensic mental health context. Persons with ID, as well as caregivers and courts, frequently request mental health professionals to assess an individual's functional abilities for a legal purpose.

In light of these two distinct points of contact with the law – as a treatment provider and as a forensic expert – this chapter proceeds in two parts. Part I describes legal issues relevant to providing mental health treatment to persons with ID. This discussion includes a brief survey of civil rights laws, the law of informed consent and the law of guardianship and other forms of substituted consent. Part II, which focuses on forensic issues, surveys some of the legal contexts in which a psychiatrist or other mental health provider may be asked to provide information about an individual's functional abilities. Focusing on the legal issues that a mental health practitioner is most likely to encounter, this part discusses applications for disability benefits, petitions for guardianship and evaluations of competency to stand trial.

Please note that this chapter is for general information purposes only. It is not intended to be comprehensive and should not be considered legal advice for a specific case or set of facts. Please contact an attorney in your area for more detailed information about how the specific provisions of your state's law apply to your practice.

Part I   Law related to the mental health treatment of persons with intellectual disability

a) The right to reasonable modifications

Although good treatment practices will naturally reflect the nondiscrimination and empowerment goals embodied by civil rights laws, treatment providers should nonetheless be mindful of civil rights laws that prohibit disability-based discrimination. These statutes, most notably Section 504 of the Rehabilitation Act of 1973 and the Americans with Disabilities Act of 1990, prohibit "covered entities" (which include hospitals, professional offices of health care providers and treatment centers) from denying an individual with a disability an equal opportunity to enjoy the services that the covered entity provides (29 U.S. C.S. 794, 2006; 42 U.S.C.S. 12101, 2006). In order to provide equal access to services, covered entities must make reasonable modifications to their architecture, policies, practices and procedures. These reasonable modifications remove barriers that would otherwise prevent persons with disabilities from accessing the services enjoyed by persons without disabilities.

Reasonable modifications for a person with ID may include adjusting the manner in which information is communicated. For example, a person with limited ability to digest written informed consent materials may require an oral explanation. Reasonable modifications may also include speaking at a slower place and using simple and concrete terminology whenever possible. It may also include using visual materials (e.g. charts and photographs) to aid communication. Another modification that may facilitate communication between the individual and the treatment provider is to permit an individual with an ID to involve a trusted friend or family member in his discussions with the treatment provider.

While a treatment provider's obligation to provide reasonable modifications is normally triggered by a request from the individual, the nature of ID may prevent some individuals from making a request for modifications. In such a circumstance, the civil rights laws require a treatment provider to initiate a discussion about the need for reasonable modifications. Although the treatment provider may not force an individual to accept an unwanted modification, the treatment provider can offer options designed to enable the individual to benefit from the treatment provider's services. The law does not mandate, however, that a treatment provider must implement the particular modification preferred by the individual, so long as the offered modification offers enables the individual to enjoy the benefits provided to persons without disabilities and is "reasonable."

Although the civil rights statutes do not define "reasonable," judicial treatment of the term suggests that determinations about whether a particular modification is "reasonable" will involve weighing the individual's need for the modification against the cost to the treatment provider that would implement it. The treatment provider may avoid making reasonable modifications only if they can demonstrate that these would impose an "undue burden" on the treatment provider or "fundamentally alter" the nature of their facilities or the goods and services provided.

b) Informed consent and substitute decision-makers

While compliance with disability nondiscrimination laws should naturally accompany good treatment practices, compliance with informed consent law poses unique challenges. Before proceeding to treat an individual with an ID, a treatment provider must determine whether the individual's limited capacity to understand the risks and benefits of the treatment renders the individual unable to provide informed consent.

The law of informed consent requires health care providers to establish that the patient understands the risks, benefits and possible side effects of a proposed treatment, as well as reasonable alternatives. In addition to understanding the proposed treatment, the patient must also freely consent to it, without coercion or manipulation from the treatment provider or others. In the absence of a significant medical emergency, a health care provider who provides treatment without first obtaining informed consent will be liable to the patient for battery or medical negligence.

The law of informed consent does not require that the patient fully understand the technical aspects of the proposed treatment, such as how a particular medication affects

brain chemistry. Many patients without ID lack sufficient education or training to understand the technical aspects of particular medical treatments, and yet the law regards them as
able to provide informed consent. The patient's understanding must simply be sufficient
to enable him or her to make a reasoned choice about whether to accept or reject the
proposed treatment.

A person's ability to give informed consent will often vary, depending on the type of
treatment proposed. While a person with significant ID may be able to consent to a routine
examination, the same person may be unable to consent to the administration of a
medication that entails significant risks. The degree of risk involved in a particular
treatment, as well as the number of treatment options and the complexity of the information
about possible side effects, will affect whether an individual can give informed consent.

Assessing the capacity to provide informed consent   To assess whether a patient has
sufficient understanding to provide informed consent, the health care provider should ask
the patient open-ended questions. The practitioner should avoid questions that elicit a "yes"
response, because a patient with ID may give "yes" as a default response in order to disguise
a lack of understanding. In keeping with civil rights laws that require health care providers to
modify procedures in order to ensure equal opportunities to persons with disabilities, the
practitioner should either modify written materials or orally translate them in order to
effectively communicate their content to the patient. If, after modifying the informed
consent procedure as much as possible, the treatment provider is still uncertain about
whether a patient may give informed consent, it may be appropriate to obtain an independent
evaluation.

If the patient's understanding is sufficient to enable informed consent for purposes of the
treatment proposed, the health care provider must also carefully assess the voluntariness of
the patient's consent. Because persons with ID are vulnerable to coercion and manipulation
from family members and other support persons, the health care provider should speak with
the patient privately to determine whether his or her consent is, in fact, freely given. Also, to
reduce the possibility that the patient will be unduly influenced by the health care provider's
views, the provider should encourage the patient to consult relatives, caregivers and other
members of the support network to help the patient to think through their decision.

Obtaining informed consent via a substitute decision-maker   When a patient is unable to
provide informed consent to a particular medical procedure, the treatment provider cannot
proceed without obtaining informed consent from a substitute decision-maker who provides
informed consent on the patient's behalf. Even when a patient is unable to provide consent
him/herself, the law protects the patient's right to bodily integrity by requiring that the
treatment provider obtain consent from a substitute decision-maker. This person is obliged
to make decisions based on the patient's best interests, which will involve honoring the
patient's wishes whenever possible.

In some circumstances, the substitute decision-maker will be a guardian. Guardianship is
a legal mechanism whereby a court determines that a person is unable to make certain
decisions for him/herself and grants the legal authority to make such decisions to another
person, called the guardian, who acts on the person's behalf. If an individual is subject to a
guardianship order that has granted the guardian legal authority to provide informed
consent, the health care provider must obtain the guardian's consent to treatment.

Even when the medical practitioner believes that the individual has the functional capacity to provide informed consent, the health care provider must obtain the guardian's consent, because a court has extinguished the individual's legal authority to provide consent and has transferred this right to the guardian.

Not all guardians have the authority to provide informed consent, however, because modern guardianship statutes encourage courts to tailor a guardian's responsibilities to the individual's specific needs. For example, some individuals have a guardian only for the limited purpose of handling their financial affairs; the individual retains all other legal rights, including the right to make medical treatment decisions. To determine whether the guardian has legal authority to provide consent to medical treatment, the treatment provider may ask the guardian to provide a copy of the court's guardianship order, which outlines the scope of the guardian's authority. Guardianship law is discussed in more detail later in this chapter.

If a patient does not have a guardian, one option for obtaining substituted consent is for the patient's caregiver to file a petition for guardianship. However, because the appointment of a guardian can take a significant amount of time, it is often not an appealing vehicle for obtaining informed consent. Additionally, because a guardianship order extinguishes one or more of an individual's legal rights and is difficult to undo, most disability rights advocates urge caregivers first to explore less intrusive and permanent options for obtaining substituted consent.

The least intrusive method to obtain substituted consent is for the individual to voluntarily give someone legal authority to make health care decisions on her behalf by executing a "health care power of attorney." In some states, an individual may be able to execute a health care power of attorney even though she is unable to give informed consent to a particular medical procedure because a decision about whom the person trusts to make medical decisions is less intellectually difficult than a decision about whether the benefits of a medical procedure outweigh the risks (Hurley & O'Sullivan, 1999). In some states, a health care power of attorney may be oral rather than in writing.

For persons who do not have sufficient mental capacity to appoint a health care agent, most states have laws that allow relatives and close friends to provide informed consent to treatment for a person who is unable to understand the issues involved in a medical decision. These statues normally list those persons – often called "surrogate decision-makers" – in order of priority. The patient's spouse, if any, is usually named first, then any adult children, then parents or domestic partner, then siblings, and then close friends.

The law requires a surrogate decision-maker to make treatment decisions based on his or her understanding of what the individual would want if the individual were able to understand the applicable information. A surrogate decision-maker cannot provide in-formed consent if the patient resists treatment, however, because surrogacy statutes do not formally transfer a patient's right to make decisions to the surrogate.

In some states, obtaining substituted consent for certain types of treatments (such as the administration of psychotropic medication, electroconvulsive therapy, behavior modifica-tion programs involving aversive stimuli, or admission to a mental health care facility) may require additional measures, even if the patient does not object. Some states specifically prohibit surrogate decision-makers from authorizing these types of treatments. Some states also prohibit health care agents and guardians from doing so in the absence of a specific grant of authority to consent to these particular types of treatment (405 Ill. Comp. Stat. 5/2-107(a), 2008). Accordingly, these treatments may require an individual's physician or caregiver to obtain a special court order determining that the patient lacks the capacity to make the decision and that the benefits of the treatment outweigh any harm (Vars, 2008).

In summary, providing mental health treatment to persons with ID requires compliance with disability discrimination laws and the law of informed consent. A treatment provider may not rely on an ID diagnosis alone, but must assess an individual's functional abilities in the context of the particular treatment that the practitioner seeks to provide.

The interaction between the individual's functional abilities and the treatment may require the provider to modify normal procedures in order to provide the individual access to the provider's services. Similarly, the interaction between the individual's functional abilities and the complexity of treatment decisions may require the provider to obtain the assent of a substituted decision-maker in order to comply with the law of informed consent.

Part II Legal questions requiring evaluation of persons with intellectual disability

Legal issues related to ID also arise in a consultative forensic practice, because the legal system frequently relies on mental health practitioners to assess persons' intellectual abilities. As the foregoing discussion indicates, one legal question that mental health practitioners frequently encounter is whether an individual's level of understanding is sufficient to satisfy the law of informed consent. While this question will arise in a mental health practitioner's own practice, it may also arise in a consultative role when other doctors require mental health practitioners' special expertise to help make judgments about informed consent.

Part III of this chapter surveys three other contexts in which a mental health practitioner may be asked to assess an individual's intellectual abilities for a legal purpose: eligibility for disability benefits; petitions for guardianship; and competency to stand trial. While these three questions are not the only legal questions that may require a mental health practitioner to assess a person's intellectual ability, they represent the breadth of legal questions for which a person's intellectual ability may be relevant.

Although, in the past, many areas of the law relied heavily on diagnosis of ID to determine whether an individual was eligible for special treatment under the law, today most legal questions require a deeper inquiry into the individual's functional abilities. Also in contrast to the past, when persons with ID were frequently deemed "disabled" or "incompetent" for all legal purposes, today each legal question involves a different standard for determining "disability" or "incompetency." Accordingly, many persons' intellectual limitations will be legally significant in some contexts, but not others.

Before evaluating individuals for a legal purpose, treating practitioners should carefully consider whether conducting such an evaluation may prevent them from providing effective treatment to the individual. While the law rarely prohibits mental health practitioners from evaluating persons that they simultaneously treat, ethical and pragmatic considerations frequently militate against performing this dual role. Some examinations, for example, may result in the examinee losing significant legal rights. If the examinee opposes guardianship, conducting an evaluation that results in a guardianship may generate conflict between the examiner and examinee that will irreparably damage the treatment relationship.

Conducting an evaluation may also damage a treatment relationship, even when an evaluation results in the examinee obtaining a benefit (s)he desires, such as Social Security Supplemental Income (SSI). Because most legal inquiries related to ID require proof of limited intellectual functioning, evaluators must collect detailed information about an individual's weaknesses and past failures. Conducting an evaluation and preparing a report that emphasizes a person's deficiencies can easily conflict with treatment goals of building the individual's sense of competence, control and autonomy.

The damage to the treatment relationship can be particularly great when a court or agency requires the evaluator to testify orally about the person's limitations. Re-framing questions to focus on abilities, rather than inabilities, may be therapeutically beneficial to the individual, but it may result in an inaccurate legal determination because court and agency adjudicators are more accustomed to a limitations-focused approach.

For all types of assessments, it is important to keep in mind that some persons with ID may attempt to minimize their limitations by adopting a compliant and cooperative attitude with authority figures. In order to counteract this tendency and to assess accurately an individual's level of understanding, an evaluator should avoid questions that may elicit a simple "yes" response. Conversely, an evaluator should also keep in mind that some persons with ID may have developed a "learned passivity" due to a submissive relationship with a caregiver or another perceived authority figure. Taking time to make an individual feel comfortable and empowered to speak for his- or herself may help to reveal an individual's true abilities more accurately.

a) Disability benefits

One context in which a mental health practitioner may be asked to provide information about an individual's functional limitations is for purposes of the individual's eligibility for disability benefits. For example, the Social Security Administration has two programs that may be applicable.

The first program, Social Security Disability Insurance (SSDI), is available for persons who have a significant work history but are now unable to "engage in any substantial gainful activity by reason of [a] medically determinable physical or mental impairment" (42 U.S.C. S. 423(d)(a(A)(2000). For individuals over 55, the standard is whether the person is unable to perform past relevant work. Most persons with significant ID are eligible for little or no SSDI benefits, because they do not have sufficient work history to be considered "insured" under this program. However, in certain circumstances, disabled individuals without sufficient work history may receive disability benefits based on the work history of a deceased spouse, a deceased parent or a living parent currently receiving social security benefits (Social Security Administration: www.ssa.gov).

The Social Security Administration's other disability benefits program, Supplemental Security Income (SSI), is more commonly applicable to persons with significant ID. Unlike SSDI, receipt of SSI payments does not require that an individual have a significant work history. Instead, it requires that the individual have limited income and assets. The standard for adult "disability," however, is the same for SSI and SSDI. An adult must be unable to "engage in any substantial gainful activity by reason of any medically determinable physical or mental impairment."

A person under age 18 can receive SSI disability benefits if he or she meets the stricter disability standard of "marked and severe functional limitations" that "very seriously limits his or her activities." Because the disability standard is stricter for persons under 18, some persons unable to qualify for SSI disability benefits as a child may qualify at age 18 when the broader disability definition applies.

A person automatically meets the Social Security Administration's adult disability definition if the individual has an ID that manifested prior to age 22 and has either:

1 a valid verbal, performance, or full-scale IQ of 59 or less; or

2 severe mental limitations, evidenced by inability to complete an IQ test and dependence upon others for personal needs such as toileting, eating, dressing or bathing.

The Social Security Administration assumes that persons falling into these categories are unable to engage in substantial gainful activity without any further assessment of their functional limitations.

Persons with less severe ID may also meet the Social Security Administration's adult disability definition if their ability to work is significantly limited. For example, a person may meet this definition if they have an IQ of 60 through 70 and an additional impairment, physical or mental, "imposing an additional and significant work-related limitation of function." Similarly, a person with an IQ of 60 through 70 may meet the disability definition if their IQ results in at least two of the following:

1 Marked restriction of activities of daily living.

2 Marked difficulties in maintaining social functioning.

3 Marked difficulties in maintaining concentration, persistence, or pace.

4 Repeated episodes of decompensation, each of extended duration.

b) Petitions for guardianship

Another legal context in which a mental health practitioner may be asked to assess an individual's functional limitations is a petition for guardianship. Guardianship is a legal mechanism whereby a court determines that a person is unable to make certain decisions for him/herself and grants the legal authority to make such decisions to another person, called the guardian. Because the law presumes that persons who have reached 18 years of age are competent to make their own decisions unless they are proven incompetent, an individual's 18th birthday often provides the impetus for an individual's relatives or other interested persons to consider petitioning a court to establish a guardianship (Millar, 2003).

Historically, guardianship orders used to transfer *all* legal decision-making authority to the guardian. However, the disability rights movement critiqued this "plenary guardianship" – which resulted in a near-total loss of the legal rights that accompany adulthood – as unduly restrictive for many individuals who are able to handle some, but not all, of their personal affairs. In response to this criticism, most states have revised their guardianship statutes to permit courts to tailor a guardian's authority to the needs of the individual. A guardianship order that permits an individual to retain decision-making authority over matters within his or her abilities is often termed a "limited guardianship."

Prior to the guardianship reform movement, an ID diagnosis was often sufficient to justify the appointment of a guardian. Today, however, most states take a functional approach that focuses less on diagnostic labels and more on the person's strengths and weaknesses related to the particular decision-making areas that the proposed guardian seeks to control. Emphasizing that guardianship is appropriate only in extreme circumstances, the model guardianship statute suggests that guardianship is appropriate for an individual who "lacks the ability to meet essential requirements for health, safety, or self-care, even with appropriate technological assistance" (National Conference of Commissioners on Uniform State Laws, 1997).

The guardianship reform movement also strengthened the procedural safeguards designed to protect individuals from unnecessary loss of decision-making authority. Many states require any court that rules on a petition for guardianship to hold a hearing first. The individual has the right to speak at the hearing and, in most states, also has the right to an attorney or advocate to assist him/her in raising objections. The individual may object to the particular person proposed as guardian, the proposed scope of the guardian's authority, or to the need for a guardian altogether.

Another reform recently incorporated into many states' guardianship laws is the involvement of a "neutral evaluator" who facilitates the gathering of information relevant to the court's decision. A mental health expert may serve as a "neutral evaluator." A mental health expert may also serve as a witness on behalf of a party to the guardianship proceeding (either for or against guardianship) (Perlin et al., 2008).

When conducting an examination for purposes of a guardianship proceeding, it is important to ensure that the examinee understands, to the greatest extent possible, that the evaluation may result in a significant loss of rights, e.g. the right to make autonomous health care choices, the right to make independent financial decisions, or the right to enter into a contract. The examiner should also explain that the examination results will be shared with the court, and that the examiner may testify at the guardianship hearing (Drogin & Barrett, 2010).

While it is not strictly necessary that the examinee's level of understanding meet the legal requirements of "informed consent" (because the person's ability to provide such consent may be one focus of the examination), the APA Ethics Code nonetheless mandates that "psychologists inform persons with questionable capacity to consent . . . about the nature and purpose of the proposed assessment services, using language that is reasonably understandable to the person being assessed" (American Psychological Association, 2002, amended 2010).

An examiner should tailor the assessment to the specific powers that the guardian seeks to assume. For example, if the guardian seeks to control where the individual resides, the court will need information about the degree of assistance the individual needs with domestic tasks, such as meal preparation and personal hygiene. The court will also require information about the individual's ability to respond appropriately to an emergency situation such as a fire in the home. In addition to interviewing the examinee and administering functional skills tests, it is also important to interview friends and relatives, particularly those who have been caretakers, in order to understand the individual's skill level. The examinee's medical history, educational records and work history may also provide useful information.

If the guardian seeks to control the individual's finances, the court will need information about the individual's ability to manage his or her finances. This assessment will require an understanding of the individual's financial situation. If the individual has limited assets and no income aside from a monthly SSI check, it is probably unnecessary for a court to appoint a guardian to control their finances. If the individual needs help managing his/her SSI funds, their caregiver may petition the Social Security Administration to become the individual's representative payee. However, if the individual has a significant portfolio of investments that are not already managed by a trustee or other fiduciary, but is unable adequately to understand and manage his or her finances, it may be necessary to appoint a guardian for this purpose.

When discussing a proposed petition for guardianship with an individual's caregivers, an evaluator should keep in mind that the appointment of a guardian is a dramatic step which removes the autonomy that the law confers on individuals when they reach adulthood. It may also profoundly influence an individual's sense of control and self-determination. Because of the risk that guardianship may unduly deny individuals with ID the opportunity to direct their own lives, many disability rights advocates urge caregivers to consider alternatives (Salzman, 2010).

One alternative is for family and friends to provide a supportive environment in which the individual can make his or her own decisions with assistance in identifying and weighing the options (Millar, 2007). Another alternative to guardianship is for individuals to authorize someone to make certain decisions on their behalf by executing a "power of attorney." Although this option requires individuals to understand the consequences of appointing someone to act as their agent, some persons unable to make complicated decisions about their medical treatment or finances may nonetheless be able to understand the consequences of appointing someone else to do so (O'Sullivan, 1999).

A mental health practitioner who evaluates an individual with a dual diagnosis of ID and mental health disorder should also keep in mind that persons who lose legal rights in a guardianship proceeding rarely regain them (Stancliffe *et al.*, 2000). Accordingly, if it appears that some of the individual's current limitations are the result of a mental health condition which may significantly improve over time, rather than the individual's more static underlying ID, it is important to provide this information to the court. Sharing this information may lead the court to craft a temporary guardianship order that will prevent an individual from permanently losing his/her decision-making rights.

c) Competency to stand trial

The criminal justice system also frequently requests mental health practitioners to assess individuals' functional limitations. The most common legal question about a criminal defendant's mental capacity is whether the individual is competent to stand trial. This inquiry focuses on the defendant's mental abilities at the time of trial and plea bargaining.

Assessments of competency to stand trial reflect the legal principle that criminal defendants should have a fair opportunity to defend themselves from criminal charges. The adversarial nature of the criminal justice system assumes a fair contest between the prosecutor and the defendant. In order for this contest to be fair, criminal defendants must have sufficient mental acuity to understand the criminal adjudication process and to assist counsel in preparing their defense. In the words of the United States Supreme Court, "it is not enough for the district judge to find that the defendant is oriented to time and place and has some recollection of events." Instead, the criminal defendant must have "sufficient present ability to consult with his lawyer with a reasonable degree of rational understanding," "a rational as well as factual understanding of the proceedings against him," and the capacity to "assist in his defense" (Dusky v. United States, 1960); Drope v. Missouri, 1975).

An ID diagnosis, by itself, does not automatically establish that an individual is incompetent to stand trial. The factual and legal complexity of the proceedings is also relevant. Some cases may involve complicated choices about defense strategy, while other cases do not. Accordingly, an individual may be competent to stand trial for the purposes of some criminal charges but not others. Conversely, the lack of an ID diagnosis does not automatically establish that an individual is legally competent to stand trial. The experience of a trauma or mental disturbance may lead a person who was formerly considered competent to be currently incompetent for the purposes of standing trial. Similarly, mental illness or substance abuse may temporarily render an individual with an average or above-average IQ incompetent to stand trial.

Before conducting a competency evaluation, it is important to consult with the individual's criminal defense attorney. This consultation serves three purposes:

- First, it permits the examiner to confirm that the defendant has had an opportunity to consult with counsel prior to the evaluation. In the rare circumstance in which a court orders a competency evaluation before the defendant has obtained counsel, the evaluation should be postponed until the defendant has had the opportunity to discuss the evaluation request with his/her attorney.

- Second, consultation with defense counsel enables the examiner to obtain information about the complexity of the defendant's case and the types of defense strategy decisions that the defendant will have to make. This information will help the examiner tailor the evaluation to elicit information relevant to whether the defendant is competent to understand the specifics of his/her case.

- Third, defense counsel may also help the examiner collect information relevant to the competency evaluation, such as mental health and educational records, as well as contact information for relatives and other persons who may have pertinent information.

An evaluation of an individual's competency to stand trial should attempt to measure the following:

1 The person's ability to understand the criminal process, especially the roles of prosecutor, judge, jury, and defense counsel.

2 The person's ability to accurately perceive the likelihood (s)he will be found guilty and the likely success of available defense strategies.

3 The person's ability to communicate with defense counsel about the facts of the case and legal strategy (Scott, 2010).

In addition to a clinical interview, a forensic assessment tool designed specifically for persons with ID may be helpful. The Competence Assessment for Standing Trial for Defendants with Mental Retardation (CAST*MR) is one available tool (Zapf & Roesch, 2009). Before commencing the examination, it is essential for the examiner to communicate clearly to the examinee that the purpose of the examination is not therapeutic, but instead is to determine whether the examinee's current mental limitations prevent him from standing trial. Although it is not strictly necessary to obtain informed consent when a court has ordered the competency evaluation, good ethical practices demand that the examiner carefully explain the evaluation's purpose. Most crucially, the defendant should understand that the court will receive the evaluator's report.

In addition to evaluations related to an individual's competency to stand trial, the criminal justice system may also rely on mental health practitioners to assess an individual's mental functioning at the moment the crime occurred. The most familiar (although rarely applicable) criminal responsibility inquiry is the "insanity defense," which excuses an individual from criminal responsibility for actions taken when they were unable to understand what they were doing or that what they was doing was wrong.

ID alone is seldom used to establish an insanity defense, because an ID severe enough to establish that a person was unable to understand the significance of his/her actions would also easily establish that the person was incompetent to stand trial. Because ID is usually fairly static, persons whose ID were severe enough to meet the standard for legal insanity at the time of the crime will often be incompetent to stand trial. However, an ID not severe enough to prevent an individual from standing trial may, when combined with a psychotic episode at the time of the crime, establish an insanity defense.

Persons not able to establish an insanity defense may introduce evidence of ID and mental health disorders in an attempt to receive a lesser penalty. Many offenses carry different penalties depending on the perpetrator's state of mind, or *mens rea*, at the time of the offense. For example, evidence of an ID or mental health disorder may help a defendant to establish that a crime was not premeditated, but was instead an impulsive act.

In summary, conducting forensic evaluations of persons with ID usually requires an individualized inquiry into a person's functional abilities, similar to the assessments required to comply with civil rights and informed consent laws. Each inquiry is unique, however, because the legal question – such as the individual's ability to understand the criminal defense strategy used in a particular trial – is often extremely context-dependent. An evaluator must not only determine the individual's functional abilities, but must also consider how those functional abilities interact with the demands of the individual's current legal situation.

Conclusion

This chapter has surveyed the most common legal issues that mental health practitioners encounter when working with persons with ID. Part I surveyed the law relevant to providing mental health treatment to persons with ID. In the course of this practice, a treatment provider must comply with civil rights laws as well as the law of informed consent. Part II briefly surveyed three legal questions for which mental health practitioners are frequently asked to provide information about an individual's intellectual abilities: applications for disability benefits; petitions for guardianship; and assessments of criminal competency.

The concern overarching these disparate areas of the law is that, rather than relying on an ID diagnosis, the law requires an individualized inquiry into each individual's unique needs and circumstances. The law may regard an individual to be "disabled" or "incompetent" for one purpose but not for others. Each legal inquiry requires an individualized determination of how a person's mental abilities interact with the specific context. The complex and time-consuming task of determining how the individual's mental abilities interact with the specific context aims to maximize his or her right to exercise the privileges and responsibilities of citizenship to the full extent of his or her abilities.

References

29 U.S.C. §794 (2006); 42 U.S.C. §12101 (2006).

405 Ill. Comp. Stat. 5/2-107(a) (2008).

42 U.S.C. §423(d)(1)(A) (2000).

American Psychological Association (2002, amended 2010). Ethical principles of psychologists and code of conduct. *American Psychologist* **57**, 1060–1073.

Drogin, E.Y. & Barrett, C.L. (2010). *Evaluation for Guardianship*. Oxford UP, New York.

Dusky v. United States, 362 U.S. 402 (1960); Drope v. Missouri, 420 U.S. 162 (1975).

Hurley, A.D. & O'Sullivan, J.L. (1999). Informed Consent for Health Care. In: Dinerstein, R.D., Herr, S.S. & O'Sullivan, J.L. (eds.) *A Guide to Consent*, pp. 39–55. American Association on Mental Retardation, Washington, DC.

Millar, D.S. (2007). "I Never Put it Together": The Disconnect Between Self-Determination and Guardianship: Implications for Practice. *Education and Training in Developmental Disabilities* **42**, 119–129.

Millar, D.S. (2003). Age of Majority, Transfer of Rights and Guardianship: Considerations for Families and Educators. *Education and Training in Mental Retardation and Developmental Disabilities* **38**, 378.

National Conference of Commissioners on Uniform State Laws, Uniform Guardianship and Protective Proceedings Act of 1997, *Uniform Laws Annotated* **8A**, 312.

O'Sullivan, J.L. (1999). Adult Guardianship and Alternatives. In: Dinerstein, R.D., Herr, S.S. & O'Sullivan, J.L. (eds.) *A Guide to Consent*, pp. 39–55. American Association on Mental Retardation, Washington, DC.

Perlin, M.L., Champine, P.R., Dlugacz, H.A. & Connell, M.A. (2008). *Competence in the Law: From Legal Theory to Clinical Application*. John Wiley & Sons, Hoboken, NJ.

Salzman, L. (2010). Rethinking Guardianship (Again): Substituted Decision Making as a Violation of the Integration Mandate of Title II of the Americans with Disabilities Act. *University of Colorado Law Review* **81**, 157–245.

Scott, C.L. (2010). Competency to Stand Trial and the Insanity Defense. In Simon, R. & Gold, L. (eds.) *Textbook of Forensic Psychiatry* 2nd ed pp. 337–372. American Psychiatric Publishing, Arlington, VA.

Social Security Administration: www.ssa.gov.

Stancliffe, R.J., Abery, B.H., Springborg, H. & Elkin, S. (2000). Substitute Decision-Making and Personal Control: Implications for Self-Determination, *Mental Retardation* **38**, 407–421.

Vars, F.E. (2008). Illusory Consent: When an Incapacitated Patient Agrees to Treatment. *Oregon Law Review* **87**, 353–400.

Zapf, P. & Roesch, R. (2009). *Evaluation of Competence to Stand Trial*. Oxford University Press, New York.

16

Syndromes of Intellectual Disability

Kelly M. Blankenship, MD, Assistant Professor of Psychiatry, Indiana University, Indianapolis, IN
Christina Weston, MD, Associate Professor, Wright State University, Dayton, Ohio

Introduction

The etiology of intellectual disabilities (ID) can be uncertain in the majority of cases. In approximately half of individuals with moderate-to-profound ID a genetic etiology can be identified (Raynham et al., 1996). The most commonly known disorder is Down syndrome, but other genetic syndromes and syndromes acquired through prenatal exposure to toxic substances are commonly seen, including Williams syndrome, Fragile X syndrome and fetal alcohol syndrome. Psychiatrists and community providers need to become familiar with these syndromes so that these disorders can be screened, identified and treated for psychiatric and other medical disorders that may be associated with the particular syndrome. Identification of syndromes also helps families, because they can link with national support groups and have a better understanding of what to expect for their child with regard to health and development.

Down syndrome

Down syndrome (DS) occurs in one of every 700–1000 births, and it is the most common congenital disorder associated with intellectual disability (Dykens et al., 2000). In the

Psychiatry of Intellectual Disability: A Practical Manual, First Edition.
Edited by Julie P. Gentile and Paulette M. Gillig.
© 2012 John Wiley & Sons, Ltd. Published 2012 by John Wiley & Sons, Ltd.

majority of cases, it is caused by the non-dysjunction of chromosome 21, causing trisomy 21. The risk of occurrence increases with maternal age, from a rate of 1 in 200 at age 25 to 1 in 20 at age 45 (Benke, 2004). However, since most children are born to younger women, the majority of cases are born to younger mothers. It is the disorder most people visualize when they think of intellectual disability, largely due to typical facial characteristics which make the syndrome recognizable at birth. Because of its obvious genetic features, it is usually diagnosed at birth. It has been widely studied and is well known to society at large. A 1990s TV show *Life Goes On* featured an adolescent with DS (played by Chris Burke) and his family.

Medical issues

The characteristic dysmorphic features of DS include a small head with a flat-looking face, slanted eyes with epicanthal folds, a flattened nasal bridge, small ears and mouth, and enlarged protruding tongue, a broad neck, single palmar crease and short stature (Dykens *et al.*, 2000; Martin, 2010). In addition to these characteristic physical features, individuals with DS are at risk for several medical conditions. For example, congenital heart defects are found in up to half of all infants with DS but, fortunately, most cases are mild or corrected easily with surgery (Dykens *et al.*, 2000).

DS individuals frequently have hearing loss (66–89% of the time), vision impairments (60% of the time), dental crowding and other dental conditions (60–100% of the time). They are also susceptible to thyroid dysfunction, with hypothyroidism occurring in 10–40% of the DS population (Smith, 2001). Since the symptoms of hypothyroidism can be confused with the features of DS, the onset can be missed and annual screening is recommended. Obesity is also frequently seen in individuals with DS (50–60% of the time). It is possible that sedentary lifestyle, hypothyroidism, low metabolism and lack of exercise contribute to obesity in this population (Dykens *et al.*, 2000).

Individuals may also have atlantoaxial instability (which can be seen on standard neck x-rays) and which occurs in up to 14% of individuals with DS (Pueschel & Scola, 1987). It is recommended that all children with DS get a neck x-ray when three years old to screen for this condition. This screening is required for them to participate in Special Olympics (AAP, 2001). When atalantoaxial subluxation occurs (in 1–2% of DS individuals), it causes cervical spinal cord compression. Signs and symptoms include gait disturbance, spasticity, increased reflexes, weakness, clonus, neck pain, loss of upper or lower body strength and changes in bowel or bladder function (Smith, 2001).

Recognition and treatment of the medical problems described above have led to increased life expectancy for individuals with DS. In a study of mortality rates associated with DS from 1983 to 1997, Yang *et al.* (2002) found that the median age of death has improved from 25 years in 1983 to 49 years in 1997. As expected, congenital heart defects, dementia, hypothyroidism and leukemia were listed as causes of death more frequently in individuals with DS than in those without DS. Surprisingly, the authors found that the rate of non-leukemia malignancy was less than one-tenth that of the general population in persons with DS (Yang *et al.*, 2002).

Another study (Esbensen *et al.*, 2007) compared the mortality of adults with DS living with their families to that of adults with ID from other causes who were living with their families. Those persons with DS had a higher mortality rate than those without. Age, functional level, decline in functional abilities and worsening behavior were predictive of mortality. Unexpectedly, the study found that both ID and DS were often listed as causes of death on the death certificate, rather than, or in addition to, the specific medical cause of death.

Genetics

DS is caused by the presence of all, or part, of an extra copy of chromosome 21. In 95% of cases of live-born infants, this occurs when a whole extra chromosome 21 is present in all cells, as a result of nondysjunction of chromosome 21 during formation of the ovum. It is estimated that as many as 75% of trisomy 21 conceptions result in miscarriage (Dykens *et al.*, 2000).

Another 3–4% of DS cases occur from translocation, where part of chromosome 21 breaks off during cell division and attaches to another chromosome, usually chromosome 14 (NDSS, 2011). In 75% of such cases, this is a new mutation, but 25% can represent an inherited familial translocation. If this is discovered, the parents need to be screened for this chromosomal anomaly and genetic counseling initiated.

In 1–2% of DS cases, the cause is a "mosaic" form of DS, where only some of the cells show the trisomy 21 pattern. Individuals with the mosaic cause of DS may be phenotypically less severely affected than those with the other etiologies of DS (AAP, 2001). Methods exist to screen for risk of DS *in utero* and are routinely offered to most pregnant women. These methods involve examining serum markers during the first and second trimester, in conjunction with a fetal ultrasound. When elevated risk is found by these screening methods, chorionic villus sampling and amniocentesis can be performed. These studies are 100% accurate for the diagnosis of DS, but unfortunately they carry a 1% risk of spontaneous termination or miscarriage (NDSS, 2011). Due to these risks, some couples decide not to have the procedure performed.

Cognitive functioning

Individuals with DS have IQ levels in the moderate to severe ID range, although there is significant variability in level from individual to individual. A downward trajectory of intellectual development has been noted in DS, with a decline during childhood. The highest IQ measurements are found in infancy, but scores become lower as a child ages (Hodapp, 1999). In the latter study, IQs of individuals with DS which averaged 50 at 5–7 years decreased to an average of 41 in 7–9 year olds and to 37 in 13–15 year olds. This slowing appears to be related to several factors. Children with DS have difficulty mastering new developmental skills, such as Piaget's sensorimotor tasks, and attaining stage III grammar which features longer sentences (Dunst, 1988; Fowler *et al.*, 1994).

Individuals with DS have significantly impaired expressive language and impaired receptive language, but they have strengths in the pragmatics of language (Moldavsky *et al.*, 2001). However, in most cases, individuals with DS are able to engage in conversation (Dykens *et al.*, 1994), and their visuospatial abilities are spared relative to their IQ. As they age, they develop impaired memory associated with dementia of the Alzheimer's type (Moldavsky *et al.*, 2001).

Behavioral phenotype

The personalities of children with DS are sometimes described as "placid and good tempered," as well as "stubborn, hyperactive, aggressive and impulsive" (Moldavsky *et al.*, 2001; Dykens *et al.*, 2000). They often have fewer serious problem behaviors when compared with children with other forms of ID, and they show relative strengths in social functioning (Fidler, 2005).

Fidler *et al.* (2006) examined toddlers with DS on measures of visual processing, expressive language, receptive language, fine and gross motor functioning and social function. She found that they showed strengths in areas of visual processing and receptive language, but relative weaknesses in gross motor and expressive language skills. Their deficits were only 2.5 months behind age-equivalent scores, which is much less than is seen as individuals with DS get older. When socialization scores were compared to those of children with other forms of ID and to children with typical cognitive development, the DS children and typical children had similar scores and were significantly higher than the ID group. The authors suggest that with targeted educational and intervention programs for the specific deficits of toddlers with DS, it may be possible to develop treatments that can prevent future functional delays (Fidler *et al.*, 2006; Fidler, 2005).

Psychopathology

Despite their relative strengths in socialization, individuals with DS are susceptible to mental illness. As with the general population, individuals with DS can have a range of mental disorders, including mood disorders, psychotic disorders, anxiety disorders, developmental disorders, disruptive disorders and dementia. Perhaps due to their socialization strengths, children with DS are at a lower risk of psychopathology when compared with other groups of children with ID (Dykens, 2007; McCarthy & Boyd, 2001). Depression is the most frequently seen mood disorder in the adult DS populations (McCarthy & Boyd, 2001; Mantry *et al.*, 2007). However, most studies have had difficulty identifying any individuals with DS and co-occurring mania or bipolar disorder.

When compared to other ID populations, adults with DS have higher rates of depression, with a prevalence range of 2.7–11.4%, compared with adults with other ID, who have a depression range of 1.1–1.7% (Dykens, 2007; Mantry *et al.*, 2007). However, when the two-year incidence of depression was examined, it was found to be 5.2%, which was the same as seen in the general population (Mantry, 2007), suggesting that depression may last longer in the DS patient. When an individual with DS becomes depressed, the person presents more often with biological and behavioral problems, such as withdrawal, mutism, psychomotor retardation, low mood, passivity, decreased appetite and insomnia. In terms of differential diagnosis, it is important to distinguish the onset of depression from the prodromal features of dementia in patients with DS (Deb, 2007).

Anxiety disorders are also seen in adults with DS, with a prevalence rate of 2.7% in one survey (Mantry, 2007). Obsessional slowness in daily living routines was attributed, in one study, to obsessive compulsive behaviors and not to hypothyroidism or depression (Charlot *et al.*, 2002). Despite the findings of this study, elevated rates of obsessive compulsive disorder have not been identified in adults with DS (Dykens, 2007).

The link between Alzheimer's disease (AD) and DS is well known. AD affects the areas of the brain that control thought, memory and language abilities, and it contributes to a significant decline in an individual's ability to carry out activities of daily living. Most individuals with DS aged 40 or older show signs of dementia. Clinically remarkable symptoms of dementia are seen in only about half of individuals with DS over 50, however (Zigman *et al.*, 1993). In a review of the literature, Zigman & Lott (2007) conclude that approximately 50–70% of individuals with DS develop dementia by the age of 60–70, and that some individuals with DS survive dementia-free into their mid-to-late 70s.

A large population study of 506 individuals with DS that examined the rates of AD in DS patients found the overall prevalence of dementia to be 16.8%, with no significant gender difference (Coppus *et al.*, 2006). As this population aged, the prevalence increased from 8.9% of 45–49 year olds to 32.1% of 55–59 year olds and 25.6% of the over-60 population.

Adults with DS present with AD 20–30 years earlier than does the general population (Courtenay *et al.*, 2009). Several genetic factors are believed to lead to the association between AD and DS, especially the triplication of the APP gene on chromosome 21, which leads to increased deposition of amyloid in plaques (Dykens, 2007). It is important to be mindful of the increased risk of AD in the DS population and to monitor for it when caring for these individuals.

Clinical Vignette #1

RM was born to a mother in her 40s. RM had the dysmorphic features of Down syndrome. Her family chose to have her remain in the home which, at the time (the 1950s), was rather rare, as most similar children were institutionalized. RM was born without any heart defects, but did have some mild hearing loss and strabismus. She had significant delays and never developed any speech other than the word "no" and grunts. Although it was difficult to obtain, psychological testing found her IQ to be in the mid-30s. She did have some verbal comprehension and could comply with most simple requests or commands.

RM needed assistance with most activities of daily living (ADLs) and she was incontinent at night and needed frequent toileting reminders during the day. In adolescence and adulthood, she developed stereotypic behaviors. She would knock two small bells on a string together repeatedly and appeared to enjoy the activity. She would smile when other family members showed interest in this behavior. She also enjoyed sweeping and would sweep the porch repeatedly – so much so that she would wear out the straw brooms. She attended school in adolescence in a separate classroom, and participated in a few outside enrichment outings as an adult. She never participated in a workshop setting, but she did perform numerous repetitive tasks on the family farm.

As her parents aged, RM was able to transition to the care of a sibling's family living next door to her parents. However, after several years, she began to lose some of her ability to perform ADLs and her family members were unable to care for her. At 52, she was placed in an institutional setting. At that time, she had significant difficulty adjusting and she developed some aggressive behaviors towards staff, which was a new presentation for her. She also refused to eat, and no medical etiology for her refusal could be found. She had always been thin, but her weight loss became significant.

The situation became so dire that several crisis hospitalizations were required, and her physician recommended that a feeding tube be placed. At this point, she was started on an selective serotonin reuptake inhibitor (SSRI) antidepressant for presumed depression by her family physician. No significant change in her behavior was noticed as she was switched to a variety of different placements until a private residential home specializing in ID populations was found and she was transferred there. At that facility, she was placed under the care of a psychiatrist, who started her on olanzapine to treat her aggression and contribute to weight gain. Once there, her aggressive behaviors stopped and she resumed eating.

Since then, RM has had some decline in her ability to perform self-care and she has been placed on donepezil for presumed Alzheimer's disease. In her 60s, she remains in the nursing home, is friendly with the staff and appears to recognize family members when they come to visit her. She still continues her stereotypic behaviors when allowed.

This vignette illustrates the course of DS for an individual with more severe intellectual disability. RM's stereotypic behaviors are similar to that seen in autism. When faced with the significant change in her living situation, for which there was no adequate transition, she decompensated significantly and became life-threateningly ill upon her refusal to eat. Her apparent depression was the first time she had been placed on psychotropic medications. As is frequently the case, it is unclear whether the psychotropic medications helped her or if the change in environment was more helpful to her recovery.

Also highlighted here are the diagnostic challenges in distinguishing dementia from depression. It appears that RM developed dementia, which led to her need for institutional care, and then she subsequently developed depression in relation to the stress of the environmental changes. RM's vignette also illustrates the increasing lifespan of adults with DS, as she has surpassed the average life expectancy of the mid-50s for individuals with DS. Only 13.5% of individuals with DS are alive at 68 (Baird & Sadvonick, 1989). RM has been fortunate to have avoided experiencing obesity or any other of the more severe medical problems common to individuals with DS.

Williams syndrome

Williams syndrome (WS) is another genetically caused form of ID, which occurs in approximately 1 in 10,000 births. It is caused by the micro-deletion on the long arm of chromosome 7 at 7q11.23, which includes the gene for elastin, a protein in connective tissue (Ewart et al., 1993). This insufficiency of elastin is likely related to the medical and physical features of WS, such as premature skin aging, hoarse voice, full cheeks and increased likelihood of hernias and bladder diverticulae (Dykens et al., 2000).

WS occurs sporadically and has a low recurrence rate. The dysmorphic features of WS present in childhood with "elfin-like" facies. Facial findings include stellate irises, epicanthal folds, a flat nasal bridge, short upturned nose, anteverted nostrils, long philtrum, full lips, macrostomia, full lower cheeks and a small, delicate chin. The facial features do not become recognizable until infants are six months of age. Features can become coarser over time and can be subtle in many individuals (Pober & Dykens, 1996; Dykens et al., 2000). The former term "Elfin-Facies" syndrome has become out-dated and is considered pejorative (Dykens et al., 2000).

Medical issues

WS is a "multisystem" disorder and can cause severe medical complications. Cardiac complications are caused by elastin arteriopathy, which results in thickened arterial walls. Complications include supravalvular aortic stenosis in 60% of individuals with WS (Dykens *et al.*, 2000). Severe cardiac disease is seen in 30% of WS children and requires surgical correction (Bruno *et al.*, 2003). Hypertension is also common in WS, and blood pressure should be checked in both arms at medical visits and treated when necessary (Mervis & Morris, 2007). WS requires monitoring by a cardiologist over the patient's lifespan due to potential cardiac complications.

Musculoskeletal symptoms include hyperextensible joints and decreased muscle tone, which leads to motor delays. Older individuals with WS are prone to joint contracture, clumsiness and gait problems, which are found in up to 85% of individuals with WS (Chapman *et al.*, 1996). WS is also associated with elevated blood calcium in a minority of individuals, which can lead to constipation and abdominal pain (Dykens *et al.*, 2000). Growth is often stunted, with short stature seen in 50% of individuals with WS.

Vision problems are also common. Up to 54% have strabismus ("crossed eyes") that is correctable (Winter *et al.*, 1996). Up to 75% of individuals with WS have a distinctive "starburst" stellate iris pattern. Although it is unrelated to vision, it aids in the diagnosis of WS (Winter *et al.*, 1996). Up to 95% of individuals with WS have hyperacusis or hypersensitivity to sound. They often cover their ears when confronted with loud noises, and this can lead to behavioral disturbances. Fortunately, the hyperacusis decreases as children age (Van Borsel *et al.*, 1997).

Cognitive functioning

Most people with WS function in the mild to moderate range of ID, with the mean IQ range falling between 50–60. Occasionally, some have only borderline intellectual functioning (Dykens *et al.*, 2000; Moldavsky *et al.*, 2001). Individuals with WS have a number of cognitive and linguistic strengths and weaknesses. They have strengths in vocabulary, linguistic affect, auditory short-term memory, facial recognition and memory, musicality and "theory of mind" (the ability to interpret the mental states of others) (Dykens *et al.*, 2000). Their weaknesses are in visual-spatial construction, perceptual planning and fine motor control.

Behavioral phenotype

Children with WS are often described as friendly, charming and lovable. In a study of parents' descriptions of their children with WS, nearly all rated them as kind-spirited, caring and seeking the company of others (Dykens *et al.*, 2000). These behaviors can produce social and behavioral vulnerability. Individuals with WS can be too friendly and can approach others indiscriminately. In one study, 82% were seen to be overly friendly towards strangers; however, this improved as children became adults (Gosch & Pankau, 1997).

While individuals with WS have a social orientation, they have difficulty keeping friends. In one study, 76–96% of subjects report difficulties making and keeping friends

(Dykens *et al.*, 2000). This may be related to their low tolerance for frustration and teasing, their tendency toward excessive chatter and their strong desire to have friends (Dykens *et al.*, 2000), which make it difficult for them to engage in the reciprocal interactions commonly seen in friendships. The social disinhibition of WS, along with their impulsivity, may leave these individuals susceptible to abuse or exploitation (Dykens & Hodapp, 1997).

Psychopathology

Individuals with WS have been found to have difficulty with anxiety, ADHD and depression. In the most extensive study of psychopathology in WS, Leyfer *et al.* (2003) interviewed parents of 119 children ages 4–16 years with WS using a structured diagnostic interview. They found that 80.7% of children with WS met the criteria for at least one psychiatric diagnosis. The most prevalent diagnosis was ADHD, with almost 65% meeting diagnostic criteria. Of those with ADHD, 68.8% had the inattentive type and 27.3% had the combined type (Leyfer *et al.*, 2006). Unlike normotypic children, where there is a male predominance of ADHD, there was no sex difference in children with WS.

In another survey of members of the WS association, 190 parents of WS children aged 6–18 years completed several symptoms measures. Parents reported that anxiety-related symptoms increased as children aged (Switaj, 2000). Dykens (2003) conducted semi-structured interviews of caregivers of individuals with WS ages 5–49 years, which found a 35% prevalence rate for specific phobias, 16% prevalence for generalized anxiety disorder, 4% prevalence for separation anxiety and 2% prevalence for obsessive compulsive disorder (OCD). This study did not screen for symptoms of ADHD or oppositional defiant disorder, however.

In a smaller study, which compared 25 boys with WS to boys with Fragile X syndrome and boys with ID of non-specific etiology, the subjects with WS were found to have more significant anxiety, depression and attention problems (Pérez-García *et al.*, 2010). Leyfer *et al.* (2006) found that 53.8% of children with WS had a specific phobia, with 11.8% meeting criteria for generalized anxiety disorder, 6.7% having separation anxiety and only 1.7% having a social phobia. When specific phobia data were analyzed, the most common phobia was of loud noises (27.7%), which was likely due to the hyperacusis seen in WS. Only 3.4% of the sample met criteria for oppositional defiant disorder (ODD).

Fetal alcohol spectrum disorder

Prenatal exposure to alcohol has been widely recognized as a cause of birth defects which include a range of physical, mental, intellectual and behavioral abnormalities. It is a significant public health concern as it is a preventable form of ID. Medical expenditures for children with fetal alcohol syndrome (FAS) in the United States were nine times higher than children without any ID (Amendahh *et al.*, 2011).

The term "fetal alcohol spectrum disorders" (FASDs) refers to the range of difficulties seen in the offspring of women who drank while pregnant. It includes children with mild to severe levels of morphological and behavioral problems, but this term is not intended for use as a clinical diagnosis (Bertrand *et al.*, 2004). At the severe end of the spectrum is fetal alcohol syndrome, which includes distinctive facial anomalies and central nervous system anomalies (Jones & Smith, 1973).

Many children with prenatal alcohol exposure do not meet full criteria for FAS as they have few, if any, of the physical dysmorphic features but they do still have some impairment. The 1996 Institute of Medicine report on FAS (Stratton *et al.*, 1996) recommended the use of the terms *partial fetal alcohol syndrome* to refer to youths who do not meet full FAS criteria, *alcohol-related birth defects* (ARBD) to describe youths with malformations in the skeletal and major organ systems, and *alcohol-related neurodevelopmental disorders* (ARND) to describe youths with functional and mental impairments. The terms *fetal alcohol effects* (FAE) and *partial fetal alcohol syndrome* (pFAS) have also been used to describe children who have some symptoms but do not meet full criteria for FAS.

In their review, Sampson *et al.* (1997) estimated that between 1.3–4.8 of every 1,000 births meet criteria for FAS, and the combined incidence of FAS and ARND in Seattle was 9.1 in every 1,000 live births. A higher incidence of FAS is seen in disadvantaged populations such as those living in poverty and in Native American populations (Egeland *et al.*, 1998; Abel, 1995).

Diagnosis of FAS

In an effort to aid the recognition and diagnosis of FAS, the Institute of Medicine (IOM) (Stratton *et al.*, 1996) proposed criteria to clarify the diagnosis of FAS. Diagnosis is complicated because, given the current awareness of the birth defects caused by drinking and the shame associated with having an alcohol use disorder, many mothers are reluctant to report their alcohol use honestly. Also, in other situations, children have been removed from their parents and thus the mother's history of prenatal substance use is unavailable. The IOM has proposed criteria to allow for the inability to confirm maternal alcohol use and make the diagnosis of FAS, but they note that maternal alcohol use has been unconfirmed. The diagnosis of FAS otherwise requires:

1 confirmation of maternal alcohol exposure;

2 the presence of "a characteristic pattern of facial anomalies," which include short palpebral fissures, flat upper lip, flattened philtrum and flat midface;

3 growth retardation (low birth weight for gestational age, decreasing weight over time not due to nutrition or disproportional low weight to height);

4 central nervous system neurodevelopmental abnormalities as evidenced by at least one of the following:
    (a) decreased cranial size at birth;
    (b) structural brain anomalies (e.g. microcephaly, partial or complete agenesis of the corpus callosum and cerebellar hypoplasia);
    (c) neurologic hard or soft signs (e.g. impaired fine motor skills, neurosensory hearing loss, poor tandem gait, and poor eye-hand coordination).

The diagnosis of pFAS is made when some of the characteristic facial anomalies occur and either item 3 or 4 above, or there is evidence of a complex pattern of behavior or cognitive abnormalities *"that are inconsistent with developmental level and cannot be explained by familial background or environment alone, such as learning difficulties, deficits in school performance, poor impulse control, problems in social perception, deficits in higher level receptive and expressive language, poor capacity for abstraction or metacognition; special deficits in mathematical skills or problems in memory, attention or judgment"* (Stratton *et al.* (IOM), 1996).

The criteria for diagnosis of FAS have been further clarified to include more specific measures of facial anomalies, growth deficiency and central nervous system abnormalities in the 2004 National Task Force on FAS/FAE guidelines (Bertrand *et al.*, 2004). Stoler & Holmes (2004) summarized the research related to the amount of alcohol required to see specific abnormalities:

- It is estimated that the amount of alcohol required for development of FAS is over 4 ounces of absolute alcohol/day, which is equivalent to over eight standard drinks a day.

- Decreased birth weight is seen with 2–3 ounces of alcohol per day.

- Decreased IQ (5–7 points) is seen with 1.5 ounces of alcohol per day.

- Spelling and reading difficulties can be seen with over half an ounce of alcohol per day.

- Functional deficits can be seen with binge drinking of five drinks or more in a single occasion once a week.

- Hyperactivity and inattention can be seen with 0.45 ounces of alcohol per day (Stoler & Holmes, 2004).

It is important to realize that there is a wide variety of possible effects, and these can be different from individual to individual; they can also vary based on the type of prenatal alcohol exposure, genetic factors and the adverse postnatal environment.

Medical conditions

Prenatal exposure to alcohol affects multiple organ systems, depending on dose and timing of alcohol consumption, and a variety of birth defects are seen. Alcohol-related birth defects are outlined in the IOM report (Stratton *et al.*, 1996).

- Cardiac defects include atrial septal defects, ventral septal defects, aberrant great vessels and tetralogy of fallot.

- Skeletal abnormalities include hypoplastic nails, clinodactyly, shortened fifth digits, pectus excavatum and scoliosis.

- Renal problems include aplastic, dysplastic or hypoplastic kidneys, hydronephrosis and horseshoe kidneys.

- Ophthalmic problems include strabismus, small globes leading to refractive problems and retinal vascular anomalies.

- Auditory problems include conductive hearing loss and neurosensory hearing loss (Stratton *et al.* (IOM), 1996).

It is important to examine infants with FAS for these alcohol related birth defects, and also to be aware that, as with the neurodevelopmental effects, they can occur in instances where characteristic facial anomalies are not present.

Cognitive deficits

Researchers have consistently found diminished intellectual performance in children with FAS. Diminished intellectual functioning was found in children with heavy prenatal alcohol exposure, irrespective of the presence or absence of physical features of FAS (Mattson *et al.*, 1997). Researchers have been unable to find specific verbal or performance IQ strengths, and it is likely that children with FAS display deficient performance on complex intellectual tasks across the board (Kodituwakku, 2007).

Attentional deficits are frequently seen in children with FAS. In a comparison of attention deficit hyperactivity disorder (ADHD) and individuals with FAS, Coles (2001) examined four factors of attention: ability to focus; ability to shift focus; ability to sustain attention; and the ability to learn new material, problem solve or encode. The FAS group showed greater deficits in encoding and shifting focus, and the ADHD group displayed greater deficits in alerting and sustaining attention. Subsequent studies found that children with FAS performed less well in visual tests of sustained attention than controls, especially the Digit Span and Arithmetic tests which involve an auditory modality (Lee *et al.*, 2004). This most probably occurred because these two tests also involve intellectual ability, and it is likely that more complex tests of attention distinguish children with FAS from controls more readily than simple tests (Kodituwakku, 2007).

Executive functioning refers to the abilities involved in goal-oriented behavior. Executive functioning requires the specific skills involved in planning, inhibition and mental representation. In a review of the studies involving executive function in children with FAS, Kodituwakku (2007) noted impairment in cognitive planning, deficient cognitive set shifting and the use of ineffective strategies during problem solving, as well as deficits in verbal and non-verbal fluency and working memory.

Behaviors frequently seen which can indicate an executive function deficit include: poor organization, planning or strategy use; lack of inhibition; concrete thinking; difficulty grasping cause and effect; inability to delay gratification; difficulty following multistep directions; difficulty changing strategies or thinking of things in a different way; poor judgment; and inability to apply knowledge in new situations (Kodituwakku *et al.*, 1995; Connor *et al.*, (1999, 2000); Carmichael-Olson, 1998).

Behavioral deficits

As children with FAS develop, they frequently have significant behavioral dysfunction, as well as impairments in academic performance, emotional functioning and social skill deficits. In one study, the life outcomes of a cohort of individuals with FAS were interviewed. The cohort had significant prevalence rates of adverse life outcomes: 61% had disrupted school experiences; 60% had trouble with the law (of which 50% were detained/incarcerated); 49% had inappropriate sexual behaviors; and 35% had drug or alcohol problems (Streissguth *et al.*, 2004). The authors also found that a stable home environment and receiving a diagnosis of FAS or FAE at an earlier age were associated with better life outcomes, presumably due to targeted intervention.

Spohr *et al.* (2007) examined individuals with FAS and FAE 20 years after initial assessment. They found that many symptoms of FAS reduced over time, but that a significant number of individuals still had growth retardation, microcephaly, developmental delay and hyperactivity. The facial features present in early life had disappeared, but a thin upper lip and elongated philtrum were prominent. Males were found to have more growth deficiency than females. Career development review found that only 13% of these individuals had held "ordinary" jobs, 27% lived in institutions and 35% were in dependent-living situations where they received assistance from others. Assessment of emotional and behavioral problems in this study found that significant externalizing, aggressive, delinquent and disruptive difficulties were present.

When rates of psychiatric disorders in individuals with fetal alcohol spectrum disorders have been examined, up to 87% of individuals meet criteria for a psychiatric disorder, with 61% having a mood disorder (major depressive disorder, 26%; and bipolar disorder, 35% – O'Connor *et al.*, 2002). In a study of 25 year olds born to mothers who had been identified as binge drinkers during pregnancy, higher risks of Axis I substance dependence or abuse and of Axis II passive-aggressive and antisocial disorders or traits were found (Barr *et al.*, 2006).

Attentional problems are found in persons with FASD. Although the diagnosis of ADHD is frequently given, as described above, the attention problems in these patients differ from those seen in other individuals with ADHD (O'Malley & Nanon, 2002). Also, one retrospective case study found that children with FAS had a 79% response rate to dextroamphetamine and only a 22% response to methylphenidate (O'Malley *et al.*, 2000). This differs from the response seen in individuals with ADHD, in which both medications generally have a 70% response rate.

Social skill deficits are frequently seen in FASD. Social functioning is multifaceted and the intellectual and executive functioning deficiencies seen in FAS can lead to poor peer and social interactions. Individuals with FAS often have mental representation problems, leading to social perception or social communication deficits that make it harder for them to grasp the subtle aspects of human interactions (Carmichael-Olson, 1998; Thomas *et al.*, 1998). Difficulty in understanding the consequences of behavior and inappropriate behavior are often seen in these individuals (Streissguth *et al.*, 1991).

Behaviors often seen in clinical settings which represent social difficulties include: lack of stranger fear; naïveté and gullibility; being easily taken advantage of; poor choice of friends; preference towards younger friends; immaturity; superficial interactions; adaptive skills being significantly below cognitive potential; inappropriate sexual behaviors; difficulty in understanding the perspective of others; and poor social cognition (Coles & Platzman, 1993; Kelly *et al.*, 2000; Roebuck *et al.*, 1999).

A study which examined the neurodevelopmental functioning of children who met criteria for FAS, pFAS and ARND found that children who meet criteria for FAS had significantly poorer outcome than the children with pFAS and ARND. The children with pFAS and ARND had similar neurodevelopmental functioning (Chasnoff *et al.*, 2010).

Clinical Vignette #2

JX was first evaluated in juvenile detention when he was 16 years old. At that time, he was noted to be thin and small for his age, despite having completed puberty. He had a small head and a thin upper lip, and a flattened, elongated philtrum. His mental health history included a diagnosis of ADHD as a child, but no medication treatment. More recently he had began attending a school for youths with behavioral problems and he had received treatment with atamoxetine and risperidone. His mother had a current history of alcohol and cannabis dependence, but history of prenatal alcohol use could not be confirmed. JX's early developmental history could also not be obtained. He was placed on an IEP when he started kindergarten and currently had a 3rd grade reading level.

During the subsequent two years, JX returned to the juvenile detention center frequently with minor charges of domestic violence or probation violations. He was observed to have poor peer interactions. At times he would pretend to act tough, like a gangster, but when violent situations would occur he would be fearful. He would often lie and exaggerate the degree of his criminal activity in order to fit in with his peers in detention. He would report excessive daily cannabis use, but would have negative drug screens.

He was treated for ADHD with lisdexamfatamine (Vyvanse) when he was in a long-term secure residential treatment program for juvenile offenders, and where his compliance with the medication could be monitored. While there, he was found to be very anxious; no improvement was found in his ability to focus on school work was noted, so the lisdexamfatamine was discontinued. He was later started on an selective serotonin reuptake inhibitor antidepressant to treat anxiety. He had some improvement but, after a riot occurred at his facility and some youths escaped, his behavior changed. He began to act bizarrely and smeared feces and broke sprinklers in an effort to return to juvenile detention, so he would appear "tough."

He did return to detention, where he had difficulty interacting with his peers and would frequently annoy them, but he was able to get along well with boys who were several years younger than him when they were on his unit. He annoyed some of his same-age peers so much that he was attacked and sustained a black eye. He was eventually placed in another program with a social skills emphasis. Although he was able to complete it he was noted to have significant difficulty understanding when his peers were annoyed with him, and difficulty in giving helpful feedback to them. When school and vocational issues were discussed, he had unrealistic expectations such as being able to start a record label to support himself. He was screened for local intellectual disability services while he was in this program. He was found eligible and was linked to them when he was released shortly before his 18th birthday.

This case vignette illustrates the challenges seen when treating FAS (or suspected FAS) individuals. In this case, prenatal alcohol use and developmental history were unavailable. At 16, JX still had some facial features, growth abnormalities and neuro-developmental problems that were strongly suggestive of FAS. In his case, he had not been identified as having the disorder when he was younger. His involvement with the juvenile justice system and poor response to treatment highlights his difficulty with social skills, especially his inability to plan and understand the consequences of his negative behaviors. Fortunately for him, his providers were able to recognize his cognitive delay and link him with intellectual disability services upon his release.

Fragile X syndrome

Fragile X syndrome (FXS) is the most commonly inherited cause of ID. It affects mostly men, but can occur in women (Cornish *et al.*, 2008). The disorder is due to an expansion of the trinucleotide sequence CGG within the FMR1 gene on the X chromosome (Panagarikano *et al.*, 2007). This expansion leads to a decrease in the amount or absence of fragile X mental retardation protein (FMRP). Greater than 200 repeats of the CGG sequence defines a full mutation at the FMR1 gene. A smaller expansion of the trinucleotide sequence (55–200 CCG repeats) is termed a pre-mutation. This typically results in an increase in the amount FMRP produced.

Common features of FXS include poor eye contact, shyness, impulsivity, inattention, hyperactivity, long facies, larger ears, prominent jaw, soft skin, high arched palate, narrow inter-eye distance and larger testes (Hagerman *et al.*, 2009; Hayes & Matalon, 2009; Reiss & Hall, 2007; Tsiouris & Brown, 2004). Pre-mutation carriers often exhibit clinical features not found in individuals with a full mutation including primary ovarian insufficiency and fragile X-associated tremor/ataxia syndrome (FXTAS) (Hagerman *et al.*, 2009).

Medical issues

Most individuals diagnosed with FXS do not have major medical concerns. Recurrent otitis media and sinusitis are commonly diagnosed in young children with FXS, however. One third of infants are diagnosed with gastro-esophageal reflux disease after presenting to the pediatrician with recurrent vomiting or fussiness. Epilepsy is commonly diagnosed in children with FXS. The incidence of epilepsy in this population is between 13–18% of boys and 5% of girls. Joint laxity that leads to joint hyperextenisibility and pes planus (flat feet) is common in children with FXS. Improvement is usually noted with age (Garber *et al.*, 2008). There have been some reports of neuroendocrine dysfunction in individuals with FXS which can include increased birth weight, macrocephaly and large stature. Enlarged testes (macroorchidism) and mitral valve prolapse have been recorded (Penagarikano *et al.*, 2007). Poor motor coordination and strabismus has been reported in this population as well (Zingerevich *et al.*, 2009).

The pre-mutation carriers have more concerning medical issues. Twenty percent of the women who are carriers for the pre-mutation have premature ovarian failure (Cornish *et al.*, 2008). Women with premature ovarian failure experience infertility and termination of their menses prior to 40 years of age (Bibi *et al.*, 2010). Additional studies have reported that carriers who have normal cycles also exhibit endocrine dysfunction. Welt *et al.* (2004) studied eleven 23–41 year old normally ovulating women and observed shortened cycles, elevated follicle-stimulating hormone, elevated inhibin B within the follicular phase and elevated inhibin A and progesterone in the luteal phase when compared with controls (Cornish *et al.*, 2008).

In pre-mutation carrier males, a disorder termed fragile X-associated tremor/ataxia syndrome (FXTAS) has been reported. The prevalence rate of FXTAS has been reported to affect 30% of male carriers of the premutation allele. It is characterized by an action tremor starting in the fifth decade, with an increase of symptoms that eventually incorporates ataxia. Individuals can develop loss of sensation in their lower extremities, autonomic dysfunction and cognitive decline that can result in dementia. Females usually do not develop FXTAS and, when symptoms of this disorder are observed in females, they are less severe (Terracciano *et al.*, 2005).

Genetics

FXS is typically due to an expansion of the trinucleotide sequence CCG found within the FMR1 gene on the X chromosome. The expansion of the trinucleotide sequence causes hypermethylation, leading to silencing of the FMR1 gene (Penagerikano *et al.*, 2007). Because the fragile X mutation is carried on the X chromosome, it follows the classic X-linked pattern of inheritance. Mothers will pass the genetic mutation to 50% of their offspring, and men will pass the mutation to all of their daughters (Martin & Arici, 2008).

Most cases of FXS are caused by the trinucleotide repeat reaching over 200 copies. This causes the FMR1 gene to stop transcribing. If 55–200 copies are present, this is termed a pre-mutation allele. The allele can expand slightly to produce a larger pre-mutation allele or can expand to a full mutation. The expansion into a full mutation occurs only in females, as the full mutation becomes unstable during spermatogenesis (Garber *et al.*, 2008; Terracciano *et al.*, 2005). Thus, the mutation can expand from mother to child. Because the expansion only occurs in oocytes and not in sperm, women with pre-mutation can have children with full mutations, but men will only pass the pre-mutation to their daughters (Martin & Arici, 2008).

Individuals with FMR1 alleles with repeats ranging from 45–55 are termed the "gray zone" because unstable alleles with these numbers of repeats have been reported but the expansion of the allele is unlikely (Garber *et al.*, 2008). Women who are premutation carriers are at risk for premature ovarian failure and males are at risk for FXTAS. Male pre-mutation carriers typically do not develop the neurodevelopmental problems that those with the full mutation develop. However, the condition FXTAS has been reported to develop in 30% of males with the premutation (Terracciano *et al.*, 2005). In the general population, pre-mutation alleles occur in 1 in 130–250 women and 1 in 250–810 men. Testing for the full allele and pre-mutation is performed through an accurate and inexpensive blood spot screening test (Hagerman & Hagerman, 2009).

Cognitive functioning

The common cognitive profile for individuals with FXS includes difficulties with attention/executive function, visual memory and perception, difficulties interpreting visual-spatial relationships, deficits in visual-motor coordination and abstract reasoning. Children with FXS do not lose skills over time, but do not develop at the same trajectory as their age-matched peers.

Females with FXS exhibit the same deficits as males with this disorder, but usually function at a higher intellectual level and exhibit less severe deficits (Reiss & Hall, 2007). Only 25% of females with a full mutation exhibit IQs less than 70 (Hagerman *et al.*, 2009). Boys usually exhibit IQs within the mid to severe range of ID and females' cognitive deficits range from sub-clinical learning disabilities to the 25% of females with FXS that develop mild to moderate ID (Cornish *et al.*, 2008). The average IQ in adult males with the methylated full fragile X mutation is 40. IQs in males with full mutation tend to range from 20 to 70. Males without a complete inactivation of the FMR1 gene suffer fewer cognitive deficits. Delayed speech is frequently observed (Garber *et al.*, 2008; Terracciano *et al.*, 2005).

Behavioral phenotype

Boys with FXS usually experience delayed developmental milestones, such as sitting at ten months without support and walking at 20 months. Behavioral difficulties are noted at an early age and include problems with attention, hand flapping, hand biting and gaze aversion (Wattendorf & Muenke, 2005). Other behaviors attributed to males with FXS include hyperactivity, stereotypic movements and unusual speech. At a young age, boys with FXS tend to exhibit tactile defensiveness and sensitivity to noise and taste.

Males with FXS tend to be shy, socially withdrawn and emotional. They also tend to be less energetic than other males with ID that do not have FXS. Females and males with FXS tend to exhibit shyness, social avoidance, inattention, aggression, tantrums and self-injurious behaviors during tantrums (Tsiouris & Brown, 2004).

Most boys with FXS exhibit autistic behaviors, and about 30% of boys diagnosed with FXS meet the Diagnostic and Statistical Manual of Mental Disorders, Fourth Edition (DSM-IV) criteria for autistic disorder (American Psychiatric Association, 2000). Having a comorbid diagnosis of autism typically entails more deficits in social inter-actions, lower cognitive functioning, lower abilities to adapt and more language deficits (Hagerman *et al.*, 2009).

Reports suggest that females with FXS have more discrepancies in their presentations. Females with FXS who exhibit a lower IQ are more likely to have a long face, mandibular prognathism and large everted ears (Terracciano *et al.*, 2005). Females with a full FXS mutation are more likely to exhibit social anxiety, shyness, social avoidance, withdrawal, problems with language, mood lability and depression (Garber *et al.*, 2008).

Psychopathology

The most consistent behavioral trait in young individuals with FXS is inattention, hyperactivity and impulsivity. Many young boys with FXS are diagnosed with ADHD. Eighty percent of boys with FXS and 35% of girls with FXS are noted to exhibit inattention and hyperactivity (Tsiouris & Brown, 2004). When boys with FXS are compared with age-matched controls with ID of unknown etiology, they exhibit similar levels of motor activity; however, those with FXS exhibit higher levels of inattention, restlessness, fidgeting, distractibility and impulsivity. Evidence has suggested that, in contrast to other age-matched controls, these traits of inattention and hyperactivity do not improve with age. Further, Cornish *et al.* (2004) have suggested that individuals with FXS can be differentiated from those with DS in regards to their signs and symptoms of ADHD. Individuals with FXS exhibit "signature" strength in sustained attention (the ability to continue focus over a period of time), with moderate deficiencies in selective attention and severe deficits in the ability to switch their attention and/or inhibitory control.

Frequently, symptoms of repetitive behaviors, speech deficits and difficulties within social interactions are seen in individuals with FXS. One or more of the following symptoms are exhibited by up to 90% of those with FXS: perseveration; self-injury; hand flapping; poor eye contact; and social avoidance (Roberts *et al.*, 2009). Autistic disorder is diagnosed in 30% of those with FXS, with evidence to suggest that "autistic behavior" increases over time (Roberts *et al.*, 2009). FXS accounts for 2–6% of all cases of autistic disorder (Cornish *et al.*, 2008).

Reports suggest that 75% of those with FXS exhibit high level of anxiety. Merenstein *et al.* (1996) reported that 50% of individuals with FXS have reported panic attacks. It has also been reported that two-thirds of those with FXS meet DSM-IV criteria for Avoidant Personality Disorder (Roberts *et al.*, 2007).

Clinical Vignette #3

CB is a 25 year old Caucasian male. He has multiple physical features of FXS, including large, protruding ears, high-arched palate, prominent forehead, a long narrow face and narrow inter-eye distance. His mother had testing performed *in utero*, and prior to his birth he was diagnosed with FXS. After his mother was informed of this diagnosis and she was tested and was found to be a carrier of the premutation.

CB's difficulties started within the first year of his life. He was delayed in his sitting and walking. He started to walk prior to two years old, but still was not speaking. By two years of age he was engaged in physical, occupational and speech therapy. Shortly after turning 2, he started to use sign language to communicate his wants and needs but he still failed to use verbal communication.

At 4 years of age, he started to exhibit speech that was mostly preservative in nature. He would exhibit significant tantrums if his schedule were disrupted, or if he made a request that was not granted. He failed to make eye contact even when prompted. He did not like to engage in social interactions and preferred to play alone. When excited, he would jump up and down and exhibit hand flapping. He had significant difficulties with inattention and his parents reported significant problems with hyperactivity.

He started school at age 5 years. IQ testing was performed through the school system and his IQ was reported at 60. Through the testing performed by the school, he was given a comorbid diagnosis of autistic disorder. When he entered school, more demands and schedule changes were placed on him. He had difficulties with these and his tantrums increased.

He started to exhibit aggressive behavior and self-injurious behaviors while having the tantrums.

CB's mother made an appointment with a child psychiatrist for a medication evaluation. The psychiatrist agreed with the diagnosis of autism and FXS. He prescribed risperidone for the aggressive outbursts and irritability associated with the autistic disorder. He also referred CB to psychologist who specialized in behavioral modification therapy for children with autistic disorder.

Autism spectrum disorders

Autism spectrum disorders (ASDs) are neurodevelopmental disorders that entail impairments in social interactions, communication and restricted repetitive and stereotyped behaviors and interests. These disorders are diagnosed in children three years and older (American Psychiatric Association, 2000). ASDs consist of autistic disorder, Asperger's disorder and pervasive developmental disorder not otherwise specified (PDD NOS) (Blankenship et al., 2010). Asperger's disorder is differentiated from autistic disorder by lack of language delay, lack of ID, development of age-appropriate self-help skills, adaptive behavior and inquisitiveness regarding the environment. PDD NOS is diagnosed when there is a pervasive deficiency in an individual's ability to engage in reciprocal social interaction using verbal or nonverbal communication skills, or the presence of stereotyped repetitive behaviors or interests (American Psychiatric Association, 2000).

ASDs occur in about one in 150 children. Males are diagnosed three to four times more often than females (Landa, 2008). ASDs are inheritable, but the genetics surrounding them is multifarious. Historically, approximately 75% of children who are diagnosed with autistic disorder also have comorbid ID. However, more recent data suggests the prevalence of ID in individuals with ASDs to be between 40–55% (Newschaffer et al., 2007). Children with these disorders often exhibit other significantly interfering behaviors including hyperactivity and inattention, irritability and aggression and interfering repetitive behaviors (Blankenship et al., 2010).

Medical issues

There are multiple genetic syndromes that have been described in children with ASDs. These include tuberous sclerosis complex, FXS, DS, neurofibromatosis type 1, Angelman syndrome, Prader-Willi syndrome, Charge syndrome, Goldenhar syndrome, chromosome 2q37 deletion syndrome, chromosome 13 deletion syndrome, Cohen syndrome, Cole-Hughes macrocephaly, Cowden syndrome, De Lange syndrome, Duchenne muscular dystrophy, Giles de la Tourette syndrome, hypomelanosis of Ito, Lujan-Fryns syndrome, mitochondrial disease, phenylketonuria, Smith-Lemli-Opitz syndrome, Smith-Magenis syndrome, Sotos syndrome, Steinert's myotonic dystrophy, Timothy syndrome, Turner's syndrome, velocardiofacial syndrome, Williams syndrome and 47,XYY syndrome (Zafeiriou et al., 2007).

Children with ASDs have higher rates of seizure disorder then the general population. Seizure disorders in those with ASDs range from 11–39%, and 42% of children with both ID and motor deficits have seizure disorders. Children diagnosed with an ASD but normal range IQ, no motor deficits and an associated etiologic medical condition or a positive family history have seizure rates of 6–8%.

A study performed by Parmeggiani *et al.* (2007) comparing 77 autistic children with 77 children diagnosed with PDD NOS, matched for age and gender, found epilepsy rates of 35.1% in children with PDD NOS, with no statistical difference in the rate of seizures in children with autism. They found that seizure outcome was better in the children with autism (Parmeggiani *et al.*, 2007). Another study found that 10% of children with autism and no diagnosed seizure disorder had abnormal electroencephalograms (EEGs) (Dover & Couteur, 2008).

Although the literature regarding gastrointestinal (GI) problems in children with ASDs is somewhat ambiguous, some studies have found GI disorders at rates of 46–85%. GI disorders typically consist of diarrhea or chronic constipation. Another study performed in the United Kingdom failed to find a difference in the GI disorders between children with ASDs and a control population. However, a cross-sectional study that was performed recently found a lifetime history of GI symptoms in 70% of those with ASDs, 42% of those with other developmental delays and 28% in children with no developmental delay (Myers *et al.*, 2007). At least in part, GI symptoms could be contributed to "dietary obsessions" or pica, both of which have been reported in children with ASDs (Rutter, 2006).

Frequent ear infections and immune system dysregulation in children with ASDs has also been reported (Rutter, 2006; Newschaffer *et al.*, 2007).

Sleep disorders are frequently diagnosed in children with ASDs. Some reports suggest an abnormality in melatonin regulation. Some studies have found melatonin to be effective for improving sleep in children with ASDs, as well as for children with other developmental delays (Myers *et al.*, 2007).

Genetics

Research suggests that ASDs are 90% heritable, and most evidence suggests a multi-factorial inheritance. ASDs are four times more likely to occur in boys than girls. Depending on the definition used, there is a 70–90% concordance rate in twins (Mendelsohn & Schaefer, 2008). Because the concordance rate of monozygotic (MZ) twins is not 100% and the severity of deficits differs between MZ twins, environmental factors are considered to be etiologically significant as well (Newschaffer *et al.*, 2007). There seems to be a range in the forms of genetic susceptibility from atypical (Mendelian causes) to complex interactions between several genes and environmental stressors (Geschwind, 2009).

The National Institute of Health has located a gene on chromosome 7 linked to families that have more than one child with autism (Twedell, 2008). Other chromosomes that have been found to have one or more "autism-associated abnormality" include chromosomes 2, 3, 15, 16, 17, 22 and X (Charles *et al.*, 2008). No candidate genes have been identified. This is a strong area of continued interest and research (Dover & Couteur, 2008).

The risk of autism in a second sibling when one is affected is 6%, with a risk of 20% for the broader-range phenotype including all ASDs. This is significantly greater than the general population risk of 0.5% (Dover & Couteur, 2008).

The male predominance as discussed above has led to consideration of the role of the X chromosome and imprinted genes. However, the reason for male predominance continues to be unknown (Johnson & Myers, 2007).

Cognitive functioning

The reported prevalence of ID in ASDs has appeared to change over time. Before 1990, the rate of ID was estimated to be approximately 90% of individuals with ASDs. Studies published after 1990 reported rates between 70–75%. The most recent studies suggest rates of ID in ASDs to be less than 50% (Johnson & Myers, 2007).

The cognitive functioning in ASDs is considered to be "uneven." Some areas of cognitive ability in those with ASDs are significantly advanced, while others areas are significantly delayed. Advanced abilities often include exceptional focusing, memory, calculation, music and/or art abilities (Johnson & Myers, 2007). Children with autism often exhibit selective attention. They appear to have difficulty giving attention to multiple aspects of stimuli, especially auditory stimuli. Children with autism tend to attend more to objects than to people (Volkmar *et al.*, 2005).

Executive functioning in autism differs from typical development. Those with autism tend to be rigid and exhibit a strong preference for sameness. Tests in those with autism show significant deficits in planning and mental flexibility. Some theories believe that the deficit in theory of mind exhibited in those with autism is due to deficits in executive functioning (Elsabbagh & Johnson, 2008).

Behavioral phenotype

Atypical behavior can be seen prior to the age of two years in children with ASDs. In many children, deficits in social functioning and communication are present by 14 months of age (Landa, 2008). Frequently, these children will exhibit a speech delay or atypical speech. Children with ASDs will often exhibit echolalia. They tend to repeat words or phrases with the exact same intonation in which they heard them. Other children exhibit extreme sensory over- or underactivity (Martinez-Pedraza & Carter, 2009).

Often, children with ASDs appear to have no desire to communicate. They often fail to use nonverbal cues or gestures. One of the earliest clues is the lack of alternating vocalization that infants start to exhibit at six months with their caregiver. They also appear to have no preference for their primary caregiver's voice. They can exhibit a disregard for human voices, but appear very tuned in to environmental sounds (Johnson & Myers, 2007). Many individuals with autism fail to develop the ability to have conversation or to speak for social purposes (Carr & LeBlanc, 2007).

There are several early social deficits that are often exhibited by small children with ASDs. These include absence of "joint attention" to other people and lack of inherent drive to connect with others. Joint attention is the engagement of one person by another to share excitement or amusement (e.g. a toddler pointing out a plane to their parent as a way of sharing the experience). They are often content to be alone, make little eye contact and ignore attempts for their attention. In older years, they exhibit difficulties with emotional reciprocity and often have few friends. They often focus on parts of the situation and miss "the big picture." They often lack theory of mind (the ability to understand others' perspective), something which begins at age four years in typically developing children. Because of this, they struggle with empathy, sharing and comforting (Johnson & Myers, 2007). Play behaviors are often noted to be repetitive and lacking in imagination (Carr & LeBlanc, 2007).

Children with ASDs can start to develop one or more repetitive behaviors prior to age two years (Landa, 2008). Common repetitive behaviors include flapping, or walking and rocking. Restricted interests can often center around several or unusual items, and individuals can become very upset when these items are not available for them. Individuals with ASDs often exhibit a strong preference for sameness and routines. They often exhibit rituals and routines within their daily activities. They can exhibit significant distress if there is a schedule change or if an action performed out of sequence (Carr & LeBlanc, 2007).

Psychopathology

Frequent interfering symptom clusters that are exhibited in individuals with ASDs include inattention and hyperactivity, stereotypical and repetitive behaviors, as well as aggression and self-injurious behaviors (Blankenship *et al.*, 2010).

Inattention, hyperactivity and impulsivity are very common within the ASD population. However, the DSM-IV-TR excludes ADHD diagnosis in those with an ASD (American Psychiatric Association, 2000). Studies have reported that between 40–50% of children diagnosed with ASDs also meet DSM-IV-TR diagnostic criteria for ADHD (Blankenship *et al.*, 2010). A retrospective chart review by Goldstein & Schweback (2004) found that, of 27 children studied with PDD, 26% met DSM-IV criteria for ADHD (combined type) and 33% met DSM-IV criteria for ADHD (inattentive type).

Repetitive behaviors are a core feature of ASDs. Many children with ASDs exhibit the need for sameness, lining up objects and rituals (e.g. in going to bed or eating). Many individuals with ASDs will object to furniture being moved out of place or to driving a different way to a school or other frequent destination. Repetitive movements can include toe walking, spinning, side walking, lunging, flapping, head-banging and rocking. In a small study of 14 males with autistic disorder (McDougle *et al.*, 2000), 86% exhibited repetitive movements.

Studies have compared the repetitive thoughts and behaviors of those with autistic disorder and those individuals diagnosed with obsessive compulsive disorder (OCD). One study by McDougle *et al.* (1995) found that those diagnosed with autism were less likely than those with OCD to exhibit obsession of contamination, sexual, religious, symmetry or somatic substance and compulsion of cleaning, checking and counting. Individuals diagnosed with autism exhibited compulsions of ordering, hoarding, telling or asking, touching, tapping or rubbing more commonly than those with OCD (Blankenship *et al.*, 2010).

Irritability, aggression and self-injurious behavior (SIB) are frequently significantly interfering symptoms in those with ASDs. Studies have reported that approximately 30% of children diagnosed with ASDs exhibit significant irritability. SIB seen in the population often includes head-banging, which can place a child at risk for subdural hematoma or retinal detachment (Blankenship *et al.*, 2010). The irritability and tantrums frequently interfere with the individual's ability to learn in an educational setting and to benefit from therapy interventions (Stigler & McDougle, 2008). See Chapter 11 for more detail on the medical and mental health work-up to determine etiology.

Clinical Vignette #4

David was a 7 year old male diagnosed with PDD-nos. His pediatrician first became concerned with his significant irritability, speech delay and frequent ear infections at his two-year well visit. The pediatrician noted that his mother had voiced frustration at each visit that David cries "all the time" and seemed exceptional upset by "loud noises." At the time of his two-year well visit, he vocalized two words – "mom" and "dad" – but possessed no other speech. He had tympanostomy tubes placed at 18 months of age due to multiple ear infections. The pediatrician diagnosed him with an expressive speech delay and referred him to speech therapy.

By the time David turned four, he was exhibiting multiple other interfering symptoms. He would flap his hands whenever he was excited or upset. He had significant difficulties with inattention and hyperactivity. In his first few days in a typical preschool, he had difficulty remaining seated and he walked around the room flapping his hands and hitting other children as a way of interacting. He was subsequently placed in a special needs preschool.

His eye contact was abnormal. His eye contact was poor. He did not respect personal boundaries or respond to social or emotional cues. He did not return "hello" or "goodbye" waves. If children became upset because he was entering their personal space, he was not able to interpret their emotion and would continue his action unabated, even if the other child began to cry. The number of words he was able to speak improved, but he continued to exhibit difficulty in his use of language. He exhibited frequent echolalia and pronoun reversal. He would exhibit significant tantrums if his schedule were changed or if tasks were completed out of their normal order.

By his 7th birthday, David had been in speech therapy for almost five years, in a social skills group for three years and in behavioral management therapy for three years. He was learning pragmatics of speech and appropriate social behavior, and his parents were learning appropriate ways to discipline him. Although he showed great improvement, he still lagged behind his typical peers, as social skills and pragmatics of speech are innate to those children. In addition, generalizing was somewhat difficult for David. He would have to think through his actions and responses first, making them appear awkward and rehearsed.

Summary

The syndromes of ID have a variety of causes, from the known genetic mutation of DS to the suspected candidate genes of ASD, to the prenatal toxin exposure of FAS. Only the most commonly occurring syndromes of ID are discussed in this chapter, but there are many others of great clinical and research interest. While the disorders have ID in common, they have unique medical conditions, etiologies, behavioral phenotypes and psychopathology.

Becoming familiar with the specifics of each syndrome will assist the clinician in identifying and formulating treatment plans for each individual. Future research in this area will lead to improved understanding of the disorders and can focus on improving recognition and interventions to improve the functioning of individuals with these syndromes.

References

Abel, E.L. (1995). An update on incidence of FAS: FAS is not an equal opportunity birth defect. *Neurotoxicology and Teratology* **17**, 437–443.

Amendah, D.D., Grosse, S.D. & Bertrand, J. (2011). Medical expenditures of children in the United States with fetal alcohol syndrome. *Neurotoxicology and Teratology* **33**, 322–324.

American Academy of Pediatrics (AAP) (2001). *Health Supervision for children with Down syndrome Pediatrics* **107**, 442–449.

American Psychiatric Association (2000). Diagnostic and Statistical Manual of Mental Disorders, 4th ed., text revision (DSM-IV). APA, Washington, DC.

Baird, P.A. & Sadovnick, A.D. (1989). Life tables for Down syndrome. *Human Genetics* **82**, 291–292.

Barr, H.M., Bookstein, F.L., O'Malley, K.D., Connor, P.D., Huggins, J.E. & Streissguth, A.P. (2006). Binge drinking during pregnancy as a predictor of psychiatric disorders on the structured clinical interview for DSM-IV in young adult offspring. *American Journal of Psychiatry* **163**, 1061–1065.

Benke, P.J. (2004). Down syndrome. In: Dambro, M.R. (ed.) *Griffith's 5-Minute Clinical Consult*. Lippincott Williams & Williams, Philadelphia, PA.

Bertrand, J., Floyd, R., Weber, M., O'Connor, M., Riley, E., Johnson, K.A., Cohen, D.E.& National Task Force on FAS/FAE (2004). *Fetal alcohol syndrome: Guidelines for referral and diagnosis*. Centers for disease Control and Prevention, Atlanta, GA.

Bibi, G., Malcov, M., Yuval, Y., Reches, A., Ben-Yosef, D., Almog, B., Amit, A. & Azem, F. (2010). The effect of CGG repeat number on ovarian response among Fragile X permutation carriers undergoing preimplantation genetic diagnosis. *Fertility and Sterility* **94**, 869–874.

Blankenship, K., Erickson, C.A., Stigler, K.A., Posey, D.J. & McDougle, C.J. (2010). Autism spectrum disorders and mental retardation. In: Stolerman, I. (ed) *Encyclopedia of Psychopharmacology*, Springer-Verlag, Heidelberg, Germany.

Bruno, E., Rossi, N., Thuer, O., Cordoba, R. & Alday L.E. (2003). Cardiovascular findings, and clinical course in patients with Williams syndrome. *Cardiology in the Young* **13**, 532–536.

Carmichael-Olson, H., Feldman, J.J., Streissguth, A.P., Sampson, P.D. & Bookstein, F.L. (1998). Neuropsychological deficits in adolescents with fetal alcohol syndrome: Clinical findings. *Alcoholism, Clinical and Experimental Research* **22**, 1998–2012.

Carr, J.E. & LeBlanc, L.A. (2007). Autism spectrum disorders in early childhood: an overview for practicing physicians. *Primary Care: Clinics in Office Practice* **34**, 343–359.

Chapman, C.A., De Plessis, A. & Pober, B.R. (1996). Neurologic findings in children and adults with Williams syndrome. *Journal of Child Neurology* **11**, 63–65.

Charles, J.M., Carpenter, L.A., Jenner, W. & Nicholas, J.S. (2008). Recent advances in autism spectrum disorders. *International Psychiatry in Medicine* **38**, 133–140.

Charlot, L., Fox, S. & Friedlander, R. (2002). Obsessional slowness in Down's syndrome. *Journal of Intellectual Disability Research* **46**, 517–524.

Chasnoff, I.J., Wells, A.M., Telford, E., Schmidt, C. & Messer, G. (2010). Neurodevelopmental functioning in children with FAS, pFAS, and ARND. *Journal of Developmental and Behavioral Pediatrics* **31**, 192–201.

Coles, C.D. (2001). Fetal alcohol exposure and attention: Moving beyond ADHD. *Alcohol Research & Health* **25**, 199–203.

Coles, C.D. & Platzman, K.S. (1993). Behavioral development in children prenatally exposed to drugs and alcohol. *International Journal of the Addictions* **28**, 1393–1433.

Connor, P.D., Streissguth, A.P., Sampson, P.D., Bookstein, F.L. & Barr, H.M. (1999). Individual differences in auditory and visual attention among fetal alcohol-affected adults. *Alcoholism, Clinical and Experimental Research* **23**, 1395–1402.

Connor, P.D., Sampson, P.D., Bookstein, F.L., Barr, H.M. & Streissguth, A.P. (2000). Direct and indirect effects of prenatal alcohol damage on executive function. *Developmental Neuropsychology* **18**, 331–354.

Coppus, A., Evenhuis, H., Verrberne, G.J., Visser, F., van Gool, P., Eikelenboom, P.&van Duijin, C. (2006). Dementia and mortality in persons with Down's syndrome. *Journal of Intellectual Disability Research* **50**, 768–777.

Cornish, K., Sudhalter, V. & Turk, J. (2004). Attention and language in fragile X. *Mental Retardation and Developmental Disabilities Research Reviews* **10**, 11–16.

Cornish, K., Turk, J. & Hagerman, R. (2008). The Fragile X continuum: new advances and perspectives. *Journal of Intellectual Disability Research* **52**, 469–482.

Courtenay, K., Soni, S., Strydom, A. & Turk, J. (2009). Behavioral phenotypes and mental disorders. *Psychiatry* **8**, 391–397.

Deb, S., Hare, M. & Prior, L. (2007). Symptoms of dementia among adults with Down's syndrome: a qualitative study. *Journal of Intellectual Disability Research* **51**, 726–39.

Dover, C.J. & Couteur, A.L. (2008). How to diagnose autism. *Archives of Diseases in Childhood* **92**, 540–545.

Dunst, C.J. (1988). State transitioning in the sensorimotor development of Down's syndrome infants. *Journal of Mental Deficiency Research* **32**, 405–410.

Dykens, E.M. (2003). Anxiety, fears, and phobias in persons with Williams syndrome. *Developmental Neuropsychology* **23**, 291–316.

Dykens, E.M. (2007). Psychiatric and Behavioral Disorders in persons with Down syndrome. *Mental Retardation and Developmental Disabilities Research Reviews* **13**, 272–278.

Dykens, E.M. & Hodapp, R.M. (1997). Treatment issues in genetic mental retardation syndromes. *Professional Psychology: Research and Practice*, **28**, 263–270.

Dykens, E.M., Hodapp, R.M. & Evans, D.S. (1994). Profiles and development of adaptive behavior in children with Down syndrome. *American Journal of Mental Retardation* **98**, 580–587.

Dykens, E.M., Hodapp, R.M. & Finucane, B.M. (2000). *Genetics and mental retardation syndromes: A new look at behavior and interventions*. Paul H Brookes Publishing, Baltimore, MD.

Egeland, G.M., Katherin, P.H., Gessner, B.D., Ingle, D., Berner, J.E. & Middaugh, J.P. (1998). Fetal alcohol syndrome in Alaska, 1977 through 1992: An administrative prevalence derived from multiple data sources. *American Journal of Public Health* **88**, 17–24.

Elsabbagh, M. & Johnson, M.H. (2008). Infancy and autism: progress, prospects and challenges. *Progress in Brain Research* **164**, 355–382.

Esbensen, A.J., Seltzer, M.M. & Greenberg, J.S. (2007). Factors prediction mortality in midlife adults with and without Down syndrome living with family. *Journal of Intellectual Disability Research* **51**, 1039–1050.

Ewart, A.K., Morris, C.A., Atkinson, D., Jin, W., Sternes, K., Spallone, P., Stock, A.D., Leppert, M. & Keating, M.T. (1993). Hemizygosity at the elastin locus in a developmental disorder, Williams syndrome. *Nature Genetics* **5**, 11–16.

Fidler, D.J. (2005). The emerging down syndrome behavioral phenotype in early childhood: Implications for practice. *Infants & Young Children* **18**, 86–103.

Fidler, D.J., Hepburn, S. & Rogers, S. (2006). Early learning and adaptive behavior in toddlers with Down syndrome: Evidence for an emerging behavioral phenotype? *Down Syndrome Research and Practice* **9**, 37–44.

Fowler, A., Gelman, R. & Gleitman, L.R. (1994). The course of language learning in children with Down Syndrome. In: H. Tager-Flusberg (ed.), *Constraints on language acquisition: Studies of atypical children*, pp. 91–140. Lawrence Erlbaum Associates, Mahwah, NJ.

Garber, K.B., Visootsak, J. & Warren, S.T. (2008). Fragile X syndrome. *European Journal of Human Genetics* **16**, 666–672.

Geschwind, D.H. (2009). Advances of autism. *Annual Reviews* **60**, 367–380.

Goldstein, S. & Schweback, A.J. (2004). The comorbidity of pervasive developmental disorder and attention deficit hyperactivity disorder: results of a retrospective chart review. *Journal of Autism and Developmental Disorders* **34**, 329–339.

Gosch, A. & Pankau, R. (1997). Personality characteristics and behavior problems in individuals of different ages with Williams syndrome. *Developmental Medicine and Child Neurology* **39**, 527–533.

Hagerman, R.J. & Hagerman, P.J. (2008). Testing for Fragile X Gene Mutations Throughout the Life Span. *Journal of the American Medical Association* **300**, 2419–2421.

Hagerman, R.J., Berry-Kravis, E., Kaufmann, W.E., Ono, M.Y., Tartaglia, N., Lachiewicz, A., Kronk, R., Delahunty, C., Hessl, D., Visootsak, J., Picker, J., Gane, L. & Tranfaglia, M. (2009). Advances in treatment of Fragile X syndrome. *Pediatrics* **123**, 378–390.

Hayes, E.W. & Matalon, R. (2009). Fragile X syndrome. *Pediatrics* **124**, 790–792.

Hodpp, R.M., Evans, D. & Gray, F.L. (1999). Intellectual development in children with Down syndrome. In: Rondal, J.A., Perera, J.& Naedl, L. (eds.). *Down's syndrome: A review of current knowledge*, pp. 124–132. Whurr Publishers, London.

Johnson, C.P., Myers, S.M.& Council of Children with Disabilities (2007). Identification and evaluation of children with autism spectrum disorders. *Pediatrics* **120**, 1183–1215.

Jones, K.L. & Smith, D.S. (1973). Recognition of the fetal alcohol syndrome in early infancy. *The Lancet* **11**, 999–1001.

Kelly, S.J., Day, N. & Streissguth, A.P. (2000). Effect of prenatal alcohol exposure on social behavior in humans and other species. *Neurotoxicology and Teratology* **22**, 143–149.

Kodituwakku, P.W. (2007). Defining the behavioral phenotype in children with fetal alcohol spectrum disorders: A review. *Nuroscience and Biobehavioral Reviews* **31**, 192–201.

Kodituwakku, P.W., Handmaker, N.S., Cutler, S.K. Weathersby, E.K. & Handmaker, S.D. (1995). Specific impairments in self-regulation in children exposed to alcohol prenatally. *Alcoholism, Clinical and Experimental Research* **19**, 1558–1564.

Landa, R.L. (2008). Diagnosis of autism spectrum disorders in the first 3 years of life. *Nature Clinical Practice* **4**, 138–147.

Lee, K.T., Mattson, S.N. & Riley, E.P. (2004). Classifying children with heavy prenatal alcohol exposure using measures of attention. *Journal of the International Neruopsyhological Society* **10**, 271–277.

Leyfer, O.T., Woodruff-Borden, J., Klein-Tasman, B.P., Fricke, J.S. & Mervis, C.B. (2003). Prevalence of psychiatric disorders in 4–16-year-olds with williams syndrome. *American Journal of Medical Genetics Part B (Neuropsychiatric Genetics)* **141B**, 615–622.

Mantry, D., Cooper, S.A., Smiley, E., Morrison, J., Allan, L., Williamson, A., Finlayson, J. & Jackson, A. (2007). The prevalence and incidence of mental ill-health in adults with Down syndrome. *Journal of Intellectual Disability Research* **52**, 141–155.

Martin, J.A. (2010). Genetic Causes of Mental Retardation. In: Dryden-Edwards, R.C.& Combrinck-Graham, L. (eds.) *Developmental Disabilities from Childhood to Adulthood*, pp. 127–142. Johns Hopkins University Press, Baltimore, MD.

Martin, J.R. & Arici, A. (2008). Fragile X and reproduction. *Current Opinion in Obstetrics and Gynecology* **20**, 216–220.

Martinez-Pedraza, F. & Carter, A.S. (2009). Autism spectrum disorders in young children. *Child and Adolescent Psychiatric Clinics of North America* **18**(3), 645–663.

Mattson, S.N., Riley, E.P., Gramling, L., Delis, D.C. & Jones, K.L. (1997). Heavy prenatal alcohol exposure with or without physical features of fetal alcohol syndrome leads to IQ deficits. *Journal of Pediatrics* **131**, 718–721.

McCarthy, J. & Boyd, J. (2001). Psychopathology and young people with Down's syndrome: childhood predictors and adult outcome of disorder. *Journal of Intellectual Disability Research* **45**, 99–105.

McDougle, C.J. (2011). Psychopharmacological Treatment of Autism. In: Amaral, D., Dawson, G.& Geschwind, D. (eds.) *Autism Spectrum Disorders*. Oxford University Press, New York.

McDougle, C.J., Kresch, L.E., Goodman, W.K., Naylor, S.T., Volkmar, F.R., Cohen, D.J. & Price, L.H. (1995). A case-controlled study of repetitive thoughts and behavior in adults with autistic disorder and obsessive-compulsive disorder. *The American Journal of Psychiatry* **152**(5), 772–777.

McDougle, C.J., Kresch, L.E. & Posey, D.J. (2000). Repetitive thoughts and behavior in pervasive developmental disorders: treatment with serotonin reuptake inhibitors. *Journal of Developmental Disorders* **30**, 427–435.

Mendelsohn, N.J. & Schaefer, G.B. (2008). Genetic evaluation of autism. *Seminars in Pediatric Neurology* **15**, 27–31.

Merenstein, S.A., Sobesky, W.E., Taylor, A.K., Riddle, J.E., Tran, H.X. & Hagerman, R.J. (1996). Molecular-clinical correlations in males with an expanded FMR1 mutation. *American Journal of Medical Genetics* **64**, 388–394.

Mervis, C.B. & Morris, C.A. (2007). Williams Syndrome. In: Mazzoco, M.M.& Ross, J.L. (eds). *Neurogenetic Developmental Disorders*, pp. 199–262. MIT Press, Cambridge, MA.

Moldavsky, M., Lev, D. & Lerman-Sagie, T. (2001). Behavioral Phenotypes of Genetic Syndromes: A Reference Guide for Psychiatrists. *Journal of The American Academy Of Child and Adolescent Psychiatry* **40**, 749–761.

Myers, S.M., Johnson, C.P.& Council of Children with Disabilities (2007). Management of children with autism spectrum disorders. *Pediatrics* **120**, 1162–1182.

National Down Syndrome Society (NDSS) (2011). *What Causes Down Syndrome?* Accessed from www.ndss.org on 4–9–2011.

Newschaffer, C.J., Croen, L.A., Daniels, J. Giarelli, E., Grether, J.K., Levy, S.E., Mandell, D.S., Miller, L.A., Pinto-Martin, J., Reaven, J., Reynolds, A.M., Rice, C.E., Schendel, D. & Windham, G.C. (2007). The Epidemiology of autism spectrum disorders. *Annual Review of Public Health* **28**, 236–258.

O'Connor, M.J., Shaw, B., Whaley, S., Cronin, P., Gunderson, B. & Graham, J. (2002). Psychiatric illness in a clinical sample of children with prenatal alcohol exposure. *American Journal of Drug Alcohol Abuse* **28**, 743–754.

O'Malley, K.D. & Nanon, J. (2002). Clinical implications of a link between fetal alcohol spectrum disorder and attention-deficit hyperactivity disorder. *Canadian Journal of Psychiatry* **47**, 349–354.

O'Malley, K.D., Koplin, B. & Dohner, V.A. (2000). Psychostimulant response in fetal alcohol syndrome. *Canadian Journal of Psychiatry* **45**, 90–91.

Panagarikano, O., Mulle, J. & Warren, S. (2007). The pathophysiology of Fragile X syndrome. *Annual Review of Genomics and Human Genetics* **8**, 109–129.

Parmeggiani, A., Posar, A., Antolini, C., Scaduto, M.C., Santucci, M. & Giovanardi-Rossi, P. (2007). Epilepsy in patients with pervasive developmental disorder not otherwise specified. *Journal of Child Neurology* **22**, 1198–1203.

Pérez-García, D., Granero, R., Gallastegui, F., Pérez-Jurado, L.A. & Brun-Gasca, C. (2010). Behavioral features of Williams Beuren syndrome compared to Fragile X syndrome and subjects with intellectual disability without defined etiology. *Research in Developmental Disabilities* **32**, 643–652.

Pober, B.R. & Dykens, E.M. (1996). Williams syndrome: an overview of medical, cognitive and behavioral features. *Child and Adolescent Psychiatric Clinics of North America* **5**, 929–943.

Pueschel, S.M. & Scola, F.H. (1987). Atlantoaxial instability in individuals with Down syndrome: epidemiologic radiographic, and clinical studies. *Pediatrics* **80**, 555–60.

Raynham, H., Gibbons, R., Flint, J. & Higgs D. (1996). The genetic basis for mental retardation. *Quarterly Journal of Medicine* **89**, 169–75.

Reiss, A.L. & Hall, S.S. (2007). Fragile X syndrome: assessment and treatment implications. *Child Adolescent Psychiatric Clinics of North America* **16**, 663–675.

Roberts, J.E., Weisenfeld, L.A., Hatton, D.D., Heath, M. & Kaufmann, W.E. (2007). Social approach and autistic behavior in children with fragile X syndrome. *Journal of Autism and Developmental Disorders* **37**, 1748–1760.

Roberts, J.E., Mankowski, J.B., Sideris, J., Goldman, B.D., Hatton, D.D., Mirrett, P.L., Baranek, G.T., Reznick, J.S., Long, A.C. & Bailey, D.B. Jr., (2009). Trajectories and predictors of the development of very young boys with Fragile X syndrome. *Journal of Pediatric Psychology* **34**, 827–836.

Roebuck, T.M., Mattson, S.N. & Riley, E.P. (1999). Behavioral and psychosocial profiles of alcohol-exposed children. *Alcoholism, Clinical and Experimental Research* **23**, 1070–1076.

Rutter, M. (2006). Autism: its recognition, early diagnosis, and service implications. *Developmental and Behavioral Pediatrics* **27**, S54–S58.

Sampson, P.D., Streissguth, A.P., Bookstein, F.L., Little, R.E., Clarren, S.K., Dehaene, P., Hanson, J.W. & Graham, J.M. Jr., (1997). Incidence of fetal alcohol syndrome and prevalence of alcohol-related neurodevelopmental disorder. *Tetrology* **56**, 317–326.

Smith, D.S. (2001). Health Care Management of Adults with Down Syndrome. *American Family Physician* **61**, 1031–1038.

Spohr, H.L., Willms, J. & Steinhausen, H.C. (2007). Fetal alcohol spectrum disorders in young adulthood. *Journal of Pediatrics* **150**, 175–179.

Stigler, K.A. & McDougle, C.J. (2008). Pharmacotherapy of irritability in pervasive developmental disorders. *Child and Adolescent Psychiatric Clinics of North America* **17**, 739–752.

Stoler, J.M. & Holmes, L.B. (2004). Recognition of facial features of fetal alcohol syndrome in the newborn. *American Journal of Medical Genetics Part C* **127C**, 21–27.

Stratton, K.R., Howe, C.J. &Battaglia, F.C., Institute of Medicine (U.S.). Division of Biobehavioral Sciences and Mental Disorders. Committee to Study Fetal Alcohol Syndrome, National Institute on Alcohol Abuse and Alcoholism (U.S.) (1996). *Fetal alcohol syndrome: diagnosis, epidemiology, prevention, and treatment*. National Academy Press, Washington DC.

Streissguth, A.P., Aase, J.M., Clarren, S.K., Randels, S.P., LaDue, R.A. & Smith, D.F. (1991). Fetal alcohol syndrome in adolescents and adults. *JAMA* **265**, 1961–1967.

Streissguth, A.P., Bookstein, F.L., Barr, H.M., Sampson, P.D., O'Malley, K. & Young, J.K. (2004). Risk factors for adverse life outcomes in fetal alcohol syndrome and fetal alcohol effects. *Journal of Developmental and Behavioral Pediatrics* **25**, 228–238.

Switaj, D.M. (2000). *Identification and measurement of anxiety and obsessive compulsive tendencies in the Williams syndrome behavioral phenotype*. Temple University, Philadelphia, PA.

Terracciano, A., Chiurazzi, P. & Neri, G. (2005). Fragile X syndrome. *American Journal of Medical Genetics* **137C**, 32–37.

Thomas, S.E., Kelly, S.J., Mattson, S.N. & Riley, E.P. (1998). Comparison of social abilities of children with fetal alcohol syndrome to those of children with similar IQ scores and normal controls. *Alcoholism, Clinical and Experimental Research* **22**, 528–533.

Tsiouris, J.A. & Brown, W.T. (2004). Neuropsychiatric symptoms of fragile X syndrome. *CNS Drugs* **18**, 687–703.

Twedell, D. (2008). Autism: Part II. Genetics, diagnosis and treatment. *Journal of Continuing Education in Nursing* **39**, 102–103.

VanBorsel, J., Curfs, L.F.G. & Fryns, J.P. (1997). Hyperacusis in Williams syndrome: A sample survey. *Genetic Counseling* **8**, 121–126.

Volkmar, F., Chawarska, K. & Klin, A. (2005). Autism in infancy and early childhood. *Annual Review of Psychology* **56**, 315–336.

Wattendorf, D.J. & Muenke, M. (2005). Diagnosis and management of fragile X syndrome. *American Family Physician* **72**, 111–113.

Welt, C.K., Smith, P.C. & Taylor, A.E. (2004). Evidence of early ovarian aging in Fragile X permutation carriers. *Journal of Clinical Endocrinology and Metabolism* **89**, 4569–4574.

Winter, M., Pankau, R., Amm, M., Gosch, A. & Wessel, A. (1996). The spectrum of ocular features in Williams-Beuren syndrome. *Clinical Genetics* **49**, 28–31.

Yang, Q., Rasmussen, S.A. & Friedman, J.M. (2002). Mortality associated with Down's syndrome in the USA from 1983–1997: a population based study. *The Lancet* **359**(9311), 1019–1025.

Zafeiriou, D.I., Ververi, A. & Vargiami, E. (2007). Childhood autism and associated comorbidities. *Brain and Development* **29**, 257–272.

Zigman, W.B. & Lott, I.T. (2007). Alzheimer's Disease in Down Syndrome: Neurobiology and Risk. *Mental Retardation and Developmental Disabilities Research Reviews* **13**, 247–246.

Zigman, W.B., Schupf, N., Sersen, E., Silverman, W. (1993). Aging and Alzheimer's disease in Down syndrome. In: Bray, N.W. (ed.) *International Review of Research in Mental Retardation*, pp. 41–70. Academic Press, New York.

Zingerevich, C., Greiss-Hess, L., Lemons-Chitwood, K., Harris, S.W., Hessl, D., Cook, K. & Hagerman, R.J. (2009). Motor abilities of children diagnosed with fragile X syndrome with and without autism. *Journal of Intellectual Disability Research* **53**, 11–18.

Index

Aberrant Behavior Checklist (ABC)   18, 312
acetaminophen
   traumatic brain injury (TBI)   87
adenoma sebaceum   55
adrenoleukodystrophy   58
affect   19
affirmations   290
agenesis of corpus callosum   59
aggression   210–12
   assessment, emergency   223–4
      history taking   224–6
      management strategy   225
      organization   224
      summary   226
   assessment, multimodal model   223
   assessment, ongoing   226–7
   biopsychosocial model   220
      biological component   220–1
      psychological component   221–2
      social component   222
   clinical pearls
      patients with ID   244–5
      pharmacologic treatment   241
   cognitive processes   217–18
   comorbidities   216–17
      associated psychiatric and medical
         conditions   217
   comprehensive approach   241–4
   correlates in persons with ID   214–16
   differential diagnosis   228
   etiologies   228
   interpretations of behavior problems   242
   laboratory evaluation   221
   life transitions   219–20
   mood and anxiety disorders   218

   potential functions of problem behavior   224
   prevalence rates   212–13
   psychotic disorders   218
   risk factors   219
   syndromes associated with SIB   218–19
   treatment strategies   240
      electroconvulsive therapy (ECT)
         239–40
   treatment strategies, hormonal   239
   treatment strategies, non-
         pharmacological   227–9
      intervention levels   229
      psychotherapy   229–31
   treatment strategies, pharmacologic
      antidepressants   236–7
      antipsychotic medications   232–4
      benzodiazepines   237
      beta blockers   238
      mood stabilizers/anticonvulsants   235–6
      opioid antagonists   237
      overview   231–2
      psychostimulants   238–9
aging, premature   27
akathisia   33
alcohol-induced psychotic disorder   184
alcohol-related birth defects (ARBD)   346
alcohol-related neurodevelopmental disorders
      (ARND)   346
alopecia areata   27
altered consciousness (AOC)   77
Alzheimer's disease   27
amitriptyline   130
Angelman syndrome   52–3
anger facial expression   104
antecedent control   316

Psychiatry of Intellectual Disability: A Practical Manual, First Edition.
Edited by Julie P. Gentile and Paulette M. Gillig.
© 2012 John Wiley & Sons, Ltd. Published 2012 by John Wiley & Sons, Ltd.

Antecedent, Behavioral, Consequence (ABC) model 291, 309–12
anticonvulsants
aggression 236
ID 264–5
traumatic brain injury (TBI) 87
antidepressants
aggression 236–7
ID 266–9
antipsychotic medications 33, 64
antipsychotics 186
aggression 232–4
antisocial personality disorder (APD) 192, 201–3
distribution 193
anxiety disorders 146, 157–8
aggression 218
generalised anxiety disorder (GAD) 154–5
obsessive compulsive disorder (OCD) 150–2
panic disorder 149–50
post-traumatic stress disorder (PTSD) 152–4
presentation 148–9
prevalence 146–8
treatments 155
pharmacologic interventions 155–7
psychotherapeutic interventions 157
anxiolytics
ID 266–9
aripiprazole
Fragile X syndrome (FXS) 34–5
Asperger's syndrome
see also autism spectrum disorders (ASDs)
self-stimulation 169
assessment of patients see medical assessment;
psychiatric assessment
assistive devices 118
asylums 1, 3–4
ataxia 58
ataxia telangiectasia 56, 61
atomoxetine
aggression 239
atonia of corpus callosum 59
attention deficit hyperactivity disorder (ADHD)
attention span 112
fetal alcohol syndrome (FAS) 348
nonverbal behavior 103
attention span 112
inattention during evaluation 112–13
atypical antipsychotics 186
traumatic brain injury (TBI) 87
auditory hallucinations 171
Autism Speaks 4
autism spectrum disorders (ASDs) 59, 355
behavioral phenotype 357–8
cognitive functioning 357
genetics 356–7
medical issues 355–6

nonverbal behavior 103
psychopathology 358–9
self-stimulation 169
autoimmune disorders 27
automatic thoughts 290
avoidant personality disorder 192

Babinski reflex 62
Bachman–de Lang syndrome see Cornelia de Lange syndrome
baclofen 64
Bardet–Biedl syndrome 61
basal-ganglia-related disorders 59
baseline exaggeration 15, 17, 22–3, 95–7
Batten disease 61
behavior analysis
psychiatric assessment instruments 18
behavior support services
coordination 319–22
keys to success 322–3
plans 318–19
summary form 322
behavioral assessment 309–14
psychiatric problems 314–15
behavioral focus
aggression 230
behavioral intervention 315–16
benzodiazepines 33
aggression 232, 237
anxiety disorders 157
ID 267–8
psychotic disorders 186
bereavement 40
beta blockers
aggression 238
biopsychosocial model
aggression 220
biological component 220–1
psychological component 221–2
social component 222
psychotropic medications in ID 252
bipolar disorder (BD) 126
prevalence and predisposing factors 133–5
treatments 138–41
blink rates 151
blood vomiting 39
body manipulator nonverbal communications 104
body mass index (BMI) 37
borderline learning difficulties 9
borderline personality disorder (BPD) 192, 195–9
treatment 204
breast cancer 44
brief psychotic disorder 180
cultural issues 180–1
bupropion 130
bupropion-induced psychosis 185

buspirone
  anxiety disorders   156
  ID   268
  tardive conditions   65

café-au-lait spots   54
caffeine
  traumatic brain injury (TBI)   87
cancer   44–5
carbamazepine   139, 141
  aggression   235
  ID   264
  psychotic disorders   186
carbidopa   22
cardiovascular system   33–7
catatonic behavior   172
cerebellar disorders   59
cervical cancer   44
chain analysis   291
cherry red spots   61
Children's Depression Inventory (CDI)   18
citalopram   130
  anxiety disorders   156
clasped-knife finding   62
classification of ID (mental retardation)   5
clomipramine
  anxiety disorders   156
clonazepam
  anxiety disorders   156
clonidine
  tardive conditions   65
Closing The Gap   35
clozapine   34, 139
  aggression   233, 234
cognition   20
cognitive approaches
  aggression   230
cognitive behavioral therapy (CBT)   290–3
  mood disorders   129–30
cognitive disintegration   15, 95
cognitive processes   93
  concrete thinking   93–4
  egocentrism   94
  magical thinking   93
  pre-logical thinking   93
colon cancer   44
communication issues   283–5
  feeling states   285–6
communicative skill categories   92
competency to stand trial   334–6
compulsive behavior disorder   156
concrete operations   164
concrete speech   100
concrete thinking   93–4
confidentiality of patients   283
congenital hemiplasia   58

consciousness   290
consequences   316–18
constipation   39
Cornelia de Lange syndrome (Bachman–de Lang
      syndrome)   52, 60
  self-injurious behavior (SIB)   219
coronary heart disease   37
corpus callosum
  agenesis   59
  atonia   59
corticosteroid-induced psychosis   185
countertransference
  aggression   229–30
cranial nerve problems   60–2
cultural awareness and sensitivity   118–19
  beliefs about disability   119

dantrolene
  psychotic disorders   186
de Clerambault's Syndrome   179
delirium   171
delusional disorder   179
delusions   171–2
dementia   28
dementia praecox   170
dependent personality disorder   192
  distribution   193
Depo-Provera   42, 43
depression
  psychiatric assessment instruments   18
desipramine   130
development of discrepancy   289
Developmental Behaviour Checklist (DPC-P)   18
Developmental Behaviour Checklist for Adults
      (DBC-A)   18
diabetes mellitus   38
diagnosis of ID (mental retardation)
  see also medical assessment; psychiatric
      assessment
  assessment instruments, standardised   18
  criteria
    AAIDD definition   9
    DC-LC criteria for learning difficulties   9
    DSM-5 proposed criteria   10
    international classification   5–8
  differential diagnosis   21
  studies   20–1
diagnostic manual–intellectual disability (DM-
      ID)   170
diagnostic overshadowing   147
Diagnostic psychiatric assessment Schedule for
      Severely Handicapped-II (DASH-II)   18
dialectical behavior therapy (DBT)   204–7, 293–5
diazepam   39, 64
differential reinforcement of alternative behavior
      (DRA)   317

differential reinforcement of incompatible behavior (DRI) 317
differential reinforcement of low rates (DRL) 317
differential reinforcement of other behavior (DRO) 317
DiGeorge syndrome 53–4
dimenhydrinate
  traumatic brain injury (TBI) 87
disability benefits 331–2
disgust facial expression 104
divalproex sodium 141
dopaminergic drug-induced psychosis 185
doubling (psychodrama technique) 299
Down syndrome (DS) 27–8, 338–9
  behavioral phenotype 341
  cognitive functioning 340
  genetics 340
  interviewing techniques 105
  medical issues 339–40
  nutrition and activity education (NAE) 36
  psychopathology 341–3
doxepin 130
drooling 39
dynamic risk factors for aggression 219
dysarthria 58
dysmenorrhea 42

early menopause 27
echolalia 172
edema 29
egocentrism 94
electroconvulsive therapy (ECT)
  aggression 239–40
  mood disorders 131
emblem nonverbal communications 104
encephalotrigeminal angiomatosis 55–6
environmental setting conditions 223
epilepsy 67
estrogens 257
expressed emotion (EE) 118
expressing empathy 289
externalizing behavior symptom 212
extrapyramidal side effects (EPS) 33, 35
  quetiapine 34

facial expressions 103–4
fear facial expression 104
feeble-mindedness 6
fetal alcohol effects (FAE) 346
fetal alcohol spectrum disorder (FASD) 345–6
  behavioral deficits 349–51
  cognitive deficits 348
  diagnosis 346–7
  medical conditions 347–8
fetal alcohol syndrome 57–8
fluoxetine 130

aggression 237
anxiety disorders 156
fluoxetine-induced psychosis 185
folie à deux (shared psychotic disorder) 181–3
folie communiqué 181
fools 2
Fragile X syndrome (FXS) 28, 52, 60, 351
  behavioral phenotype 353
  clinical vignette 34–5
  cognitive functioning 352–3
  genetics 352
  interviewing techniques 105–8
  medical issues 351–2
  psychopathology 353–5
  stereotypies 58
Fragile X Tremor–Ataxia syndrome (FXTAS) 28
Functional Analysis Checklist (FAC) 18
Functional Analysis Interview Form (FAIF) 18
future projection (psychodrama technique) 299

gabapentin 139–40
gastric ulcers 40
gastroesophageal reflux disease (GERD) 29, 33, 39–40
gastrointestinal system 39–41
Gaucher disease 61, 62
gene silencing 52–3
general medical condition (GMC), psychosis due to 183–4
generalised anxiety disorder (GAD) 154
  clinical vignette 155
Glasgow Coma Scale (GCS) 77
Glasgow Depression Scale for people with a Learning Disability (GDSLD) 18
  Carer Supplement (GDS-CS) 18
grief and loss issues 298–302
group therapy 297–8
  aggression 231
guardianship 332–4
guided discovery 291

Haemophilus influenzae 39
hallucinations 171
haloperidol 139
  aggression 233
happiness facial expression 104
Healthy People 2010 35
hearing problems 46
heart failure 29
Helicobacter pylori 40
hemetesis 39
history of mental illness and intellectual disability
  pre-Enlightenment ideas 1–3
  reformers 3–4
history taking 16–18

histrionic personality disorder (HPD)   200–1
    distribution   193
hormonal treatment
    aggression   239
Huntington's disease (HD)   58, 61
hydrocephalus   61
5-hydroxyindoleacetic acid (5-HIAA)   232
hyperacusis   29
hypercholesterolemia   37
hyperlipidemia   34
hyperphagia   29
hyperprolactinemia   257
hypertension   34, 37
    white coat   47
hypogonadism   29
hypomania   17, 126
hypothyroidism   27, 29
hypotonia   27, 29

idiocy   3, 8
illustrator nonverbal communications   104
imbecility   7
imipramine   130
impulsive personality disorder
    distribution   193
incontinence   28
individual setting conditions   223
informed consent   327–30
    assessing capacity   328
    substitute decision-maker   328–9
intellectual disability (ID)
    behavioral presentations   30–1
    comorbid psychiatric and habit disorders
        256
    current treatment recommendations   4
    diagnostic criteria   5–8
    historical perspective   251
        biopsychosocial model   252
    historical perspective
        pre-Enlightenment ideas   1–3
        reformers   3–4
    interface with mental illness   11–12
    life expectancy   26–7
    nomenclature   8–10
    non-pharmacological interventions   252
    People First language   10–11
    pharmacological interventions   252–3
    prevalence and classification   4–5
    problem behaviors (PB)   253–6
    sexual aggression   256–8
intellectual distortion   15, 17, 94
interviewing techniques   15–16, 90–1, 121–2
    acquiescence   110–11
        management   111–12
    assistive devices   118
    attention span   112

inattention during evaluation   112–13
attitude of interviewer   119
baseline exaggeration   95–7
clinical pearls   122
cognitive disintegration   95
cognitive processes   93
    concrete thinking   93–4
    egocentrism   94
    magical thinking   93
    pre-logical thinking   93
cultural awareness and sensitivity   118–19
    beliefs about disability   119
expressed emotion (EE)   118
formal mental status examination   97
    summary   98–9
    guidelines   108–9
intellectual distortion   94
interpreting mental examination findings
    mild ID   97–101
    moderate ID   101
    severe/profound ID   102–4
language skills   91–2
    categories of communicative skills   92
level of ID   91
medical problems   116–17
memory   113–14
    interactions during treatment   114–15
    saliency   114
open-ended questions   115–16
perseveration   110
personality traits   105
psychological masking   95
psychotic disorders   163–5
responsiveness   115
sensory deficits   117
sensory hypersensitivity   117
serial order effects   113
setting the stage   92–3
social skills   115
specific disorders
    Down syndrome (DS)   105
    Fragile X syndrome (FXS)   105–8
    Williams syndrome (WS)   108
subvocalizations   110
suspects   120–1
victims   120–1
witnesses   120–1
intoxication
    nonverbal behavior   103
IQ
    AAIDD definition of mental retardation   9
    DC-LD criteria for learning disabilities   9
    international criteria for mental retardation
        6–8

journaling   291

Kayser–Fleisher rings   58, 61
Krabbe leukodystrophy   58

laboratory testing   32–3
Landau–Kleffner syndrome (LKS)   67
learning difficulties   9
learning issues   286
legal issues   325–6, 336–7
 evaluation of persons with ID   330–1
  competency to stand trial   334–6
  disability benefits   331–2
  petitions for guardianship   332–4
 treatment of persons with ID
  informed consent   327–30
  right to reasonable modifications   326–7
Lennox–Gastaut seizures   67
Lesch–Nyhan syndrome   219
levetiracetam-induced psychosis   185
levodopa   22
life expectancy of individuals with ID   26–7
Lisch nodules   54, 61
lithium   130, 141
 aggression   235–6
 ID   264
loss of consciousness (LOC)   77
Lowe's syndrome   61
luteinizing hormone releasing hormone (LHRH)
    agonists   257

macrocephaly
 mucopolysaccharidoses   56
 Proteus syndrome   57
 Sotos syndrome   56, 57
magical thinking   93
maintaining variables   223
major depressive disorder (MDD)
 differential diagnosis   128–9
 nonverbal behavior   103
 prevalence and predisposing factors   127–8
 traumatic brain injury (TBI)   81
 treatment   129–33
mania   17
Marfan's syndrome   61
matchbox sign   179
meclizine
 traumatic brain injury (TBI)   87
medical assessment   26–7, 46–7
 behavioral presentations   30–1
 clinical pearls   47
 interviewing techniques   116–17
 laboratory testing   32–3
 organ system review
  cancer   44–5
  diabetes mellitus   38
  gastrointestinal system   39–41
  menstrual-related issues   41–4

 metabolic changes and cardiovascular
    system   33–7
 osteoporosis   45
 pulmonary system   38–9
 sensory deficits   45–6
 prevalence of ID conditions   33
 primary care evaluation and preventive health
    planning   31–2
 side effects of medication   33
 syndrome-specific conditions
  autism spectrum disorders (ASDs)   355–6
  Down syndrome (DS)   27–8, 36, 339–40
  Fragile X syndrome (FXS)   28, 34–5
  Prader–Willi syndrome (PWS)   29, 36–7
  Williams syndrome (WS)   29–31, 344
medication side effects   33
medroxyprogesterone   257
memory issues   286
 evaluation   113–14
  interactions during treatment   114–15
  saliency   114
 memory aids   286–7
menopause, early   27
menstruation   41–4
 clinical vignette   43–4
mental defectives   1
mental examination   97
 interpreting findings
  mild ID   97–101
  moderate ID   101
  severe/profound ID   102–4
 summary   98–9
mental health (MH) care delivery systems   11
mental illness
 historical perspective
  pre-Enlightenment ideas   1–3
  reformers   3–4
 interface with intellectual disability (ID)   11–12
mental retardation see intellectual disability (ID)
mental weakness   170
metabolic changes   33–7
metabolic syndrome   38
metachromatic leukodystrophy   58
microcephaly
 fetal alcohol syndrome   57–8
 Rett syndrome   57
mild ID (mental retardation)   5
 clinical description   6
 diagnostic criteria   5
 diagnostic guidelines   6
 mental status examination findings   97–101
mild mental subnormality   6
mindfulness   294
mirror (psychodrama technique)   299
mirtazapine   22
mitral valve prolapse   28

modeling   291
moderate ID (mental retardation)   5
  clinical description   6–7
  diagnostic criteria   5
  diagnostic guidelines   7
  mental status examination findings   101
moderate mental subnormality   7
moderate oligophrenia   7
mood disorders   125–6, 141
  aggression   218
  bipolar disorder (BD) and ID
    prevalence and predisposing factors   133–5
    treatments   138–41
  MDD and ID
    differential diagnosis   128–9
    prevalence and predisposing factors   127–8
    treatment   129–33
mood stabilizers
  aggression   235–6
  ID   264–5
Mood, Interest, and Pleasure Questionnaire
      (MIPQ)   18, 19
Motivation Analysis Rating Scale (MARS)   18
Motivational Assessment Scale (MAS)   18, 312
motivational interviewing (MI)   287–90
mucopolysaccharidoses   56
myoclonus   59
myosis   28

nadolol
  aggression   238
naltrexone
  aggression   237
narcissistic personality disorder   192
neurocutaneous depigmented macules   55
neurofibromatosis   54–5
neuroleptic-induced movement disorders
  assessment and treatment   64–7
neuroleptic malignant syndrome   231
neurologic conditions   51, 68
  abnormal head circumference
    macrocephaly   56–7
    microcephaly   57–8
  dysmorphic features   51
    Angelman syndrome   52–3
    Cornelia de Lange syndrome (Bachman–de
      Lang syndrome)   52
    DiGeorge syndrome   53–4
    Fragile X syndrome (FXS)   52
    Prader–Willi syndrome   52
    velo-cardio-facial syndrome   53–4
    Williams syndrome (WS)   53
  examination of patients
    cranial nerves   60–2
    initial observation   60
    motor disorders   62

motor syndromes   58
  atonia/agenesis of corpus callosum   59
  Huntington's disease (HD)   58
  myoclonus   59
  Wilson's disease   58
neurocutaneous stigmata
  ataxia-telangiectasia   56
  encephalotrigeminal angiomatosis   55–6
  neurofibromatosis   54–5
  Struge–Weber syndrome   55–6
  tuberous sclerosis   55
neuroleptic-induced movement disorders, as-
      sessment and treatment   64–7
seizure disorders   67–8
soft signs   59
  autism   59
  basal-ganglia-related disorders   59
  cerebellar disorders   59
spasticity, management of   62–4
Niemann–Pick disease   61, 62
Nisonger Child Behavioral Rating Form
      (NCBRF)   18
nomenclature   8–10
non-steroidal anti-inflammatory drugs (NSAIDs)
  menstrual problems   43
nonverbal communication   15, 103
Noonan's syndrome   60
nortriptyline   130
nutrition and activity education (NAE)   36
nystagmus   61

obsessive compulsive disorder (OCD)   150–1
  clinical vignette   152
  research within ID population   151–2
oculogyric crisis   66
olanzapine   22–3, 34
  aggression   233, 234
  psychotic disorders   186
open-ended questions   115–16
opioid antagonists
  aggression   237
oppositional defiant disorder (ODD)   234
osteoporosis   45
Othello Syndrome   179
ovarian failure, premature (POF)   28

panic disorder   149–50
Papanicolaou tests   33
papilledema   61
paranoia   171
paranoid personality disorder   192
Parkinsonian syndrome   65
Parkinson's disease   22–3
paroxetine   139
  anxiety disorders   156
partial fetal alcohol syndrome (pFAS)   346

passive personality disorder 192
Pelizaeus–Merzbacher disease 61
People First 4
People First language 10–11
peptic ulcers 40
perphenazine
  aggression 233
personality disorders 21, 191–2, 207
  antisocial personality disorder (APD) 201–3
  assessment 193–4
    diagnostic criteria 194
    structured assessment of personality
      (SAP) 194
  borderline personality disorder (BPD) 195–9
  classification 192
  diagnosis in persons with ID 194–5
    DC-LD criteria 195
  histrionic personality disorder (HPD) 200–1
  prevalence 192–3
  treatment 203–7
    four-stage format 206
    invalidating environment 204, 205
personality traits
  influence on interview behavior 105
Pervasive Developmental Disorder Not Otherwise
    Specified
  self-stimulation 169
phakomas 61
phenobarbital 139
pneumonia 38
port-wine hemangiomas 55
Positive and Negative Syndrome Scale
    (PANSS) 18
post-traumatic amnesia (PTA) 77
post-traumatic stress disorder (PTSD) 152–4,
    303–4
  clinical vignette 153–4
  nonverbal behavior 103
  traumatic brain injury (TBI) 81–2
Prader–Willi syndrome (PWS) 29, 36–7, 52
  self-injurious behavior (SIB) 219
prazosin
  traumatic brain injury (TBI) 87
pre-logical thinking 93
premature aging 27
premature ovarian failure (POF) 28
prevalence of ID 4–5
preventive health planning 31–2
primary care evaluation for ID 31–2
profound ID (mental retardation) 5
  clinical description 7–8
  diagnostic criteria 5
  diagnostic guidelines 8
  mental status examination findings 102–3
    facial expressions 103–4
    nonverbal communication 103

profound mental subnormality 8
profound oligophrenia 8
progestins 257
propranolol
  aggression 238
prostate cancer 44–5
Proteus syndrome 57
psychiatric assessment 14–15, 23
psychiatric assessment
  see also diagnosis of ID (mental retardation);
    medical assessment
  challenges 15
  differential diagnosis 21
  history taking 16–18
  interview 15–16
    psychiatric assessment instruments,
      standardised 18
  mental status examination
    cognition 20
    diagnostic studies 20–1
    insight and judgment 20
    mood and affect 19
    observation 19
    orientation 19
    risk of harm 20
    thought disorder 19
  personality factors and disorders 21
  stressful life events 22–3
psychiatric assessment of Dual Diagnosis
    (ADD) 18
Psychiatric Assessment Schedule for Adults with
    Developmental Disabilities (PAS-
    ADD) 18
psychodrama techniques 299
psychological masking 95
Psychopathology Instrument for Mentally Retarded
    Adults (PIMRA) 18
  Informant (PIMRA-I) 18
  Self-report (PIMRA-SR) 18
psychosis
  psychiatric assessment instruments 18
psychosocial masking 15, 17
psychostimulants
  aggression 238–9
psychotherapy 278–9, 304–5
  barriers to treatment
    confidentiality 283
    lack of understanding of purpose 283
    multiple care provider involvement 282–3
    referral process 282
  communication issues 283–5
    feeling states 285–6
  issues related to ID
    impact on family 279–80
    impact on individual 280–1
  learning and memory issues 286

psychotherapy (*Continued*)
  collaboration with caregivers   287
  memory aids   286–7
  psychotherapy topics and ID
    grief and loss issues   298–302
    trauma   302–4
  treatment approaches   281–2
  types   287
    cognitive behavioral therapy (CBT)   290–3
    dialectical behavior therapy (DBT)   293–5
    group therapy   297–8
    motivational interviewing (MI)   287–90
    supportive psychotherapy (SP)   295–7
psychotic disorders   187
  aggression   218
  brief psychotic disorder   180
    cultural issues   180–1
  clinical pearls
    differential diagnosis   167, 169
  delusional disorder   179
  diagnosis   162
    caregiver interview   165–6
    diagnostic overshadowing   163
    patient interview   163–5
  diagnostic manual–intellectual disability (DM-
    ID)   170
  differential diagnosis
    clinical pearls   167, 169
    problem behaviors   167–9
    self-stimulation   169
  due to general medical condition (GMC)
    183–4
  exclusion from scientific literature   169–70
  historical perspective   161–2
  not otherwise specified (NOS)   185
  prevalence   162
  push for medication   166
  schizoaffective disorder   178–9
  schizophrenia
    clinical pearls   172
    current diagnosis   171
    delusions   171–2
    DSM-IV-TR and DM-ID diagnosis   173–6
    hallucinations   171
    historical perspective   170–1
    subtypes   177
    symptoms, disorganised   172
    symptoms, negative   172
  schizophreniform disorder   177–8
  shared psychotic disorder (folie à deux)   181–3
  substance-induced   184–5
  treatments
    medications   186
    psychotherapy   186
    safety   185
    treatment team involvement   186–7

Psychotic Symptom Rating Scales
  (PSYRATS)   18
psychotropic medications in ID   250–1
  anticonvulsants and mood stabilizers   264–5
    clinical effects and complications   264
  antidepressants and anxiolytics   266–9
  clinical pearls   271–2
  general principles   258–64
    circumstances for medication use   264
    relative receptor-binding affinities   262
  guidelines   270–2
  historical perspective   251
    biopsychosocial model   252
pulmonary system   38–9

Questions About Behavior Functions
  (QABF)   312
questions, open-ended   115–16
quetiapine   34, 141
  aggression   233, 234
  Fragile X syndrome (FXS)   34
  psychotic disorders   186
  traumatic brain injury (TBI)   87

reflective listening   290
Reiss Screen for Maladaptive Behavior
  (RSMB)   18
relaxation for anxiety disorders   157
responsiveness   115
Rett syndrome   57
  stereotypies   58
risk of harm   20
risperidone   22, 34, 139, 141
  aggression   233, 234
role reversal (psychodrama technique)   299
rolling with resistance   289
Rubenstein–Taybe syndrome   61

sadness facial expression   104
Sapir–Whorf hypothesis of language   10
schemas   290
schizoaffective disorder   178–9
schizoid personality disorder   192
  distribution   193
schizophrenia
  clinical pearls   172
  current diagnosis   171
  delusions   171–2
  DSM-IV-TR and DM-ID diagnosis   173–6
  hallucinations   171
  historical perspective   170–1
  subtypes   177
  symptoms
    disorganised   172
    negative   172
schizophrenic reaction   170

schizophreniform disorder   177–8
schizotypal personality disorder   192
scoliosis   29
selective serotonin reuptake inhibitors (SSRIs)
    aggression   232, 236
    ID   267
    premenstrual syndrome   43
    traumatic brain injury (TBI)   87
self-efficacy   289
self-injurious behavior (SIB)   212, 213
    associated syndromes   218–19
    persons with ID   214–16
    risk factors   219
Self-report Depression Questionnaire (SRDQ)   18
self-stimulation   169
sensory deficits   45–6, 117
sensory hypersensitivity   117
sertraline   130
    anxiety disorders   156
severe ID (mental retardation)   5
    clinical description   7
    diagnostic criteria   5
    diagnostic guidelines   7
    mental status examination findings   102–3
        facial expressions   103–4
        nonverbal communication   103
severe mental subnormality   7
severe oligophrenia   7
sexual aggression   256–8
shagreen patches   55
shared psychotic disorder (folie à deux)
        181–3
short stature   60
sialorrhea   39
side effects of medication   33
silencing of genes   52–3
skin picking   29
sleep apnea   27, 38
Smith–Magenis syndrome   219
smoking   37
social skills   115
    training for aggression   230
societal reaction to mental illness and intellectual
        disability   1–3
Socratic questioning   291
soliloquizing (psychodrama technique)   299
somatic delusional disorder   179
Sotos syndrome   56, 60
    clinical vignette   57
spasticity
    management   62–4
spinocerebellar degeneration   61
static risk factors for aggression   219
stereotypies   58
stimulants
    traumatic brain injury (TBI)   87

strength of recommendation taxonomy
        (SORT)   32
Stroptococcus pneumoniae   39
Struge–Weber syndrome   55–6
subacute sclerosing panencephalitis (SSPE)   59
substance-induced psychotic disorders   184–5
subvocalizations   110
summaries   290
supportive psychotherapy (SP)   295–7
surprise facial expression   104
sympathomimetic-induced psychosis   185
syndromes of ID   338, 359
    autism spectrum disorders (ASDs)   355
        behavioral phenotype   357–8
        cognitive functioning   357
        genetics   356–7
        medical issues   355–6
        psychopathology   358–9
    Down syndrome (DS)   338–9
        behavioral phenotype   341
        cognitive functioning   340
        genetics   340
        medical issues   339–40
        psychopathology   341–3
    fetal alcohol spectrum disorder (FASD)   345–6
        behavioral deficits   349–51
        cognitive deficits   348
        diagnosis   346–7
        medical conditions   347–8
    Fragile X syndrome (FXS)   351
        behavioral phenotype   353
        cognitive functioning   352–3
        genetics   352
        medical issues   351–2
        psychopathology   353–5
    Williams syndrome (WS)   343
        behavioral phenotype   344–5
        cognitive functioning   344
        medical issues   344
        psychopathology   345

tardive akathisia   65
tardive dyskinesia   64, 66
tardive dystonia   64
terminology   8–10
thorazine
    aggression   233
thought disorder   19
tics   58
topiramate   139
    ID   264
town idiot   3
trauma   302–4
traumatic brain injury (TBI)   75, 88
    assessment and treatment   84–7
    causes   78

traumatic brain injury (*Continued*)
  classification   78
  clinical pearls
    medications   86
    questions   85
    referrals   86
  clinical presentation   79
  compared with ID   76
  co-occurring mental illness   82–3
  definitions   76–7
  mental health presentation   79–82
  pharmacological management of symptoms   87
  symptoms   81
treatments   4
  aggression   240
    electroconvulsive therapy (ECT)   239–40
  aggression, hormonal   239
  aggression, non-pharmacological   227–9
    intervention levels   229
    psychotherapy   229–31
  aggression, pharmacologic
    antidepressants   236–7
    antipsychotic medications   232–4
    benzodiazepines   237
    beta blockers   238
    mood stabilizers/anticonvulsants   235–6
    opioid antagonists   237
    overview   231–2
    psychostimulants   238–9
  anxiety disorders   155
    pharmacologic interventions   155–7
    psychotherapeutic interventions   157
  bipolar disorder (BD)   138–41
    pharmacotherapy   139–41
  major depressive disorder (MDD)   129–33
    cognitive behavioral therapy (CBT)   129–30
    electroconvulsive therapy (ECT)   131
    pharmacotherapy   130–1
  memory   114–15
  personality disorders   203–7
    four-stage format   206
    invalidating environment   204, 205

  psychotherapy   281–2
psychotic disorders
  medications   186
  psychotherapy   186
  safety   185
  treatment team involvement   186–7
trepanation   2
tricyclic antidepressants   130
triptans
  traumatic brain injury (TBI)   87
tuberous sclerosis   55

ulcers   40
Usher syndrome   61

valproate/valproic acid   139
  aggression   235
  ID   264
  traumatic brain injury (TBI)   87
vanishing syndrome   223
velo-cardio-facial syndrome   53–4
venlafaxine   130, 141
Vineland Adaptive Behavior Scales   9
visual hallucinations   171
visual problems   45–6
vomiting blood   39

Williams syndrome (WS)   29–31,
      53, 343
  behavioral phenotype   344–5
  clinical vignette   53
  cognitive functioning   344
  interviewing techniques   108
  medical issues   344
  psychopathology   345
Williams–Beuren syndrome   59
Wilson's disease   58, 61

ziprasidone   34
  aggression   233, 234
zolpidem
  traumatic brain injury (TBI)   87

Printed and bound by CPI Group (UK) Ltd, Croydon, CR0 4YY

16/04/2025

14658460-0003